RAISING A VACCINE FREE CHILD

WENDY LYDALL

Published by Nangana Press.

ISBN 978-1-9793213-2-7

CONTENTS

FOREWORD

Wendy Lydall's book *Raising a Vaccine Free Child* exposes the myths of vaccination in no uncertain terms. It reveals many of the delusions and misconceptions that pervade this procedure in which my profession is involved. There is much in this fully referenced book that I previously did not know. The chapter on herd immunity contains valuable information that shatters the idea that parents who don't vaccinate are harming others.

Forty years ago I unquestioningly followed the "experts", and my daughters were routinely vaccinated. However, thanks to sleuths like Wendy Lydall and Hilary Butler in the New Zealand Immunisation Awareness Society, I became sufficiently enlightened to help my daughters make a genuine informed decision, and none of my 5 grandchildren (now aged 5-17) are vaccinated. Instead they sailed through those important childhood infectious diseases. They can participate in maintaining a vital cohort of healthy humans with intact immune systems to pass on to the next generation.

What a change there would be if Wendy Lydall's book was mandatory reading for every medical student. At the very least, they could rethink my profession's uncritical and seriously flawed reliance on the "magic bullet" of vaccination. Well done, Wendy, and thank you for making this information available to parents.

Mike Godfrey MBBS
Tauranga, New Zealand

"THE BENEFITS OF VACCINATION ARE WORTH THE RISKS"

Vaccine Myth Number One: Vaccination does sometimes cause adverse reactions, but these are much milder than the disease that the vaccine prevents.

When parents try to decide which if any vaccines to accept for their children, they are not given accurate information by the authorities. It is impossible for parents to weigh the risks of vaccination against the benefits when they are not told what the risks from a vaccine are, nor how much chance there is that the vaccine will actually prevent the target disease. In their zeal to persuade parents to vaccinate, the medical authorities misrepresent the threat from infectious diseases, and they and their lackeys in the media constantly repeat the myths of vaccination. These myths have been developed by the vaccine industry over two centuries, with great success at making a large proportion of the world's population believe that these myths are facts.

The first myth of vaccination is that the benefits outweigh the risks. Although more than two centuries have passed since vaccination was invented, neither the benefits nor the risks of any vaccine have been properly assessed, so there is no basis for making that claim. Scientists who attempt to research the long-term consequences of vaccination are actively hindered, and some are persecuted. Only a tiny proportion of severe reactions to vaccination are acknowledged by medical professionals, so the true incidence of adverse effects is not recorded.

When discussing the risks versus the benefits of vaccination, it is important to make a clear distinction between the two categories of infectious disease. These are *self-resolving infectious diseases* (often called the *childhood diseases*) and *infectious diseases that need intervention*. The issue of vaccination becomes muddled if the two categories of disease are lumped together. The self-resolving childhood diseases, like measles, mumps, rubella, and chicken pox, affect the immune system in a way that makes most people immune to the disease for the rest of their lives, while the diseases that need intervention, like TB and tetanus, do not do this. Vaccination is a partial copy of a natural infection, so when the germs of a self-resolving childhood disease are injected into the human blood stream, they create an artificial immunity that wears off and allows the person to catch the disease later on in life. There is a higher rate of complications with these diseases after the age of 15.[1]

The self-resolving childhood diseases do not need intervention, but they do need proper care while they run their course. They can develop complications if they are wrongly managed, and the complications can be as serious as pneumonia, encephalitis, or death. Parents need to know how to manage the self-resolving childhood diseases safely, and this book tells them how. Some people call the self-resolving childhood diseases "developmental diseases", because they bring about a jump in development.

When the germs of the diseases that need intervention are used for vaccination, they do create antibodies, but that is not the same thing as creating immunity. The vaccine industry describes a vaccine as "effective" if it is able to make antibodies. Further on I have described how the antibody threshold theory came to be the commercial backbone of the vaccine industry.

Parents have the right to be given accurate information about the effectiveness of vaccines, but whenever vaccines are dramatically seen to fail, the establishment throws its energy into making excuses, instead of acknowledging the real significance of the available data.

When my first baby was born I assumed that if I accepted a vaccine, it would mean that my child would not be able to catch the disease that the vaccine was supposed to prevent. After weighing up the risk of the polio vaccine against the risk of getting polio, I decided to let baby Chandra have the oral polio vaccine. I knew that homoeopaths can cure polio effectively and rapidly, but at that stage of our lives we spent a lot of time camping in the Drakensberg mountains of KwaZulu, where polio was endemic. If she had developed symptoms of polio it would have taken a long time for us to get from our camp site to a town with a homoeopath, so I felt that the risk of her possibly catching polio was greater than the risk of possible adverse effects from the vaccine. I believed that oral vaccines had fewer adverse effects than injected ones, and I knew that being breast-fed on demand reduced her chances of catching polio. What I did not know was that the vaccine would not make her immune to polio.

So in making the decision for Chandra, I had weighed up the risk of the vaccine against the risk of the disease, not realising that this was a faulty equation. As it happened, a polio epidemic did break out in South Africa while she was a baby, and I noticed some newspaper articles which said that the reason why vaccinated children were getting the disease must be because the vaccine had not been stored at a temperature that was low enough to prevent it from losing its virulence. At the time I paid little attention to the issue because it did not occur to me that anyone had a reason to lie.

The official literature that the health department had sent me said that three doses of oral polio vaccine would make my baby immune to polio. A few months after Chandra had had the third dose, a letter arrived from the city council informing me that it was time for her fourth dose. A while after I received the letter, the medical officer telephoned me to ask why I had not turned up for the fourth dose. She told me that Chandra was still in danger of catching polio because three doses were not enough to create immunity. That was my first inkling of the fact that the polio vaccine does not work. Since then, Chandra has never had any more doses of any type of vaccine.

The bullying was quite intensive in South Africa, so I decided that I needed to research vaccination more fully. As my research progressed I was surprised to learn that BCG, the vaccine for tuberculosis, does not prevent tuberculosis. I was even more surprised when I discovered that Edward Jenner's cowpox vaccine did not eliminate smallpox, and in fact I did not believe it at first. It was only when I read Jenner's own writings that I realised that cowpox inoculation does not create immunity to smallpox. It was a strange feeling when something that I had believed for all of my life got overturned in my mind.

My second baby was born at the beginning of the next polio epidemic in South Africa. By then we had moved to Cape Town, which is far away from the area where polio was endemic. My refusal to allow baby Kenny to swallow any doses of oral polio vaccine caused a flurry in the medical bureaucracy in Cape Town. They even sent a top ranking doctor from Groote Schuur Hospital to our house, and I have related the amusing details of that encounter further on in this book. By this time I had realised that vaccine enthusiasts are inclined to make statements that deviate from the truth, so I investigated the validity of the excuses given for the failure of the vaccine to prevent polio during that particular epidemic. The results of my investigation appear in Vaccine Myth Number Eight.

While Kenny was still a baby we moved to New Zealand, and then eight years later we moved to Australia, so I have had firsthand experience of the dishonest behaviour of the vaccine bureaucrats in three countries. I have also corresponded with medical authorities all over the world, trying to get them to answer awkward questions. They usually reply with an evasive answer, but sometimes their answers reveal that they know that there is no scientific evidence to support the claims that they are making. Dishonesty pervades the practice of vaccination in every country, and there are serious financial conflicts of interest in the higher ranks of the vaccine industry, and in the government agencies responsible for vaccine safety, vaccine licensing, and vaccination policies.

When trying to persuade parents to vaccinate, governments around the world tell outright lies about the safety of vaccines. An example of how extreme these lies can be appears in a booklet for parents printed by the Australian health department. It says, "serious reactions to Hib vaccines have not been reported."[2] At the time that the booklet was printed, the Therapeutic Goods Administration in Canberra had already received 1,161 official reports of serious adverse reactions to Hib vaccines in Australia, 16 of which were reports of death.[3] There are many other blatant lies told in this same booklet, and in other booklets and pamphlets produced by the Australian health department. Health departments in other countries indulge in the same deceptive behaviour.

Governments also exaggerate the danger from infectious diseases. This book provides information about how to bring children safely through the self-resolving childhood diseases, and discusses options for the prevention and treatment of the infectious diseases that need intervention. It also explains why doctors and nurses who have been trained in the pharmaceutical model fail to cure some diseases, and cause complications of the self-resolving childhood diseases.

Parents are not only told falsehoods about the safety and effectiveness of vaccines, they are also given false information about the law. In countries where vaccination is not compulsory, parents are routinely lied to and told that it is compulsory, or that it is compulsory for school attendance, or for obtaining welfare payments. The vaccine industry is pushing for vaccination to become compulsory in every country, and although they have not yet succeeded, medical tyranny is increasing in many countries.

Vaccination is a ritual that is held in awe by our modern society because the false history of vaccination is constantly repeated. Ever since writing was invented there have been people who have written down a false version of history in order to make people believe that events happened in a certain way, rather than in the way that they actually did happen. The Ancient Egyptian rulers did it, Stalin did it, the apartheid regime did it, and the vaccine industry does it. The false history of vaccination starts with the story that Edward Jenner proved that he could prevent smallpox by vaccinating a young boy with cowpox. The truth is that he vaccinated lots of people with all sorts of things, and did not prove that any of these things create immunity to smallpox. A boy named John Baker died from being vaccinated by Edward Jenner, but that is never mentioned in the glorified versions of vaccine history. In 2002 the British Medical Journal published an elaborate version of the false history of Edward Jenner, and as you will see further on in this book, they refused to correct the misinformation when I challenged them about it.

Following on from the false story of Edward Jenner there is the false story of Louis Pasteur, then the mythical story of typhoid vaccine, and the lies just keep on coming. The mainstream media, and most of the media that considers itself to be alternative, dutifully repeat the lies over and over again, while being reluctant to report any negative facts about vaccination. The excuses for vaccine failures are reported by the media as if they were scientific fact. When a vaccination policy is changed, a reason is given to justify the change, but then later a different reason is given for why the policy was changed, and the new reason is presented by the media as if it were the original reason. The dominant narrative is that vaccines are safe and effective, that they seldom fail, and that they only cause problems in one in a million people. However, all along, ever since vaccination started, there have been people saying, "Hey wait a minute, that's not true. Let's tell the story as it really happened!"

Millions of children are taught the false history of vaccination during their school years, and it is natural for people to assume that what they have been taught at school is true. Some of them grow into writers who repeat the myths in magazines, newspapers, pamphlets, and on Wikipedia. There is no point in trying to put the factual history of vaccination on Wikipedia because it will be removed within hours.

Repetition is the key to transforming a myth into a "fact". If people are told something often enough, they begin to believe that it is a fact, not an opinion or a falsehood. The principle of repetition, combined with the suppression of factual data, is what the vaccine industry relies on to keep millions of people around the world believing in the myths of vaccination.

Vaccination has religious status, and some people consider it a sacrilege to even question the claims made for vaccination. Many people hold the opinion that people who do not "believe" in vaccination are not only a danger to society, but that they are also crazy. Consumer advocates who try to educate the public face a problem that is similar to what medieval astronomers faced when they tried to make it known that the earth goes around the sun. The astronomers' claim sounded absurd at that time because, "Everyone can see that the sun goes round the earth." Nowadays the idea that vaccines are beneficial is regarded by believers as a universal truth. It is considered quite "obvious", because everyone can see that smallpox and diphtheria are no longer with us, and the adverse effects of vaccination are not at all obvious because they are labelled with different names.

"SIDE EFFECTS ARE RARE"

Vaccine Myth Number Two: Sometimes vaccination does have side effects like a rash, a fever, or a swelling at the site of injection. Serious adverse effects are extremely rare. Only one in a million has a severe reaction.

The medical establishment has an effective way of ensuring that the official figures for vaccine reactions remain small. When confronted with a case of vaccine damage, they simply deny that there is a relationship between the vaccine and the symptoms. They even resort to denial when a large number of people suffer the same severe reaction to the same vaccine at the same time.

There are five ways that adverse reactions to vaccines develop;

* Mild symptoms appear soon after vaccination, and then clear up after a few days. The child suffers no permanent effects.

* Serious symptoms appear soon after vaccination, and they do not clear up after a few days. The child either dies or remains permanently damaged in some way.

* Symptoms are mild at first, but slowly get worse, so that the full extent of the damage only shows up long after the date of vaccination. This is often how it happens when vaccination causes epilepsy or intellectual brain damage. A toddler has staring episodes the day after the injection, stops using language the next day, becomes "clumsy" a week later, and has the first grand mal seizure five weeks after the injection. Intellectual disability is confirmed much, much later. The medical establishment gives the excuse that the epilepsy only started five weeks after vaccination, so therefore there is no connection between the vaccine, the epilepsy, and the brain damage. When a tiny baby has this slowly developing type of reaction it is difficult to pinpoint the moment when the halt in development occurred, because it was not yet doing things

like talking and walking at the time of vaccination.

* No symptoms appear at first, but a deep-rooted problem, which takes a long time to surface, is set in motion by the vaccine. Autoimmune diseases are an example of this.

* A child is "not the same" after vaccination, with mild symptoms that persist for years, affecting the child's health, and lowering the child's quality of life.

Vaccinators are happy to acknowledge the adverse effects that are not serious and go away after a while, like fever and swelling at the site of injection, but they are not keen to acknowledge adverse effects that alter a person's ability to enjoy life. I used to assume that the incidence of adverse effects was researched before a vaccine was used on the public, but now I know that vaccines are approved for marketing without proper studies having been conducted on their adverse effects. This situation has prevailed from the days of Edward Jenner up until the present. Furthermore, once a vaccine is in use, the real incidence of serious adverse effects is not recorded.

There is a simple way to find out whether or not there is a relationship between vaccines and chronic diseases. You take a few thousand people who have had the vaccine, and a few thousand people from the same geographical area who have not had the vaccine, and you count what percentage of each group suffers from, or has died from, the disease you are investigating. So questions like, "Does hepatitis B vaccine cause diabetes?" "Does Hib vaccine cause brain damage?" "Does MMR vaccine cause leukemia?" "Does the new whooping cough vaccine cause sudden infant death syndrome?" could be answered, if the medical establishment wanted to know the answers. It is remarkable that vaccination has been practiced on billions of people for more than two hundred years without these basic studies ever having been done.

The pharmaceutical industry and governments are the groups that have the money that is needed to fund research. Governments have a moral responsibility to ensure that vaccines are properly tested for adverse effects before they foist them on the public, but all governments fail dismally in this duty. They prefer to take the easy option of just believing what the manufacturers say about their products. The way that the pharmaceutical industry conducts its "research" is discussed in Vaccine Myth Number Eleven, and the way that governments fail to monitor vaccines is discussed in Vaccine Myth Number Twelve. Governments should fund scientifically sound research into the relationship between vaccination and all chronic diseases, instead of just adding more and more vaccines to their schedules.

Most of the evidence of the damage done by vaccines lies in parents' accounts of what happened to their children after they were vaccinated. The vaccine establishment scorns such testimonies, dismissing them as "anecdotal evidence". They claim that parents or doctors who report serious adverse effects are mistaken. They say that the symptoms that appear after vaccination are "just a coincidence", and that parents who think that there is a connection between the vaccine and the symptoms are ignorant. Only a tiny proportion of doctors actually report the vaccine reactions that they see to government agencies like VAERS in the USA, the HPFB in Canada, the MHRA in Britain, and the TGA in Australia. These reports are also dismissed as being anecdotal evidence, and are not taken seriosly by the medical establishment. The vaccine establishment would have the right to disregard anecdotal evidence if they had done studies which show that the anecdotal evidence is wrong.

Before the advent of the internet, the parents of vaccine-damaged children were isolated from one another. Radio, TV, newspapers, and glossy magazines rarely allow stories about vaccine-damaged children to be broadcast or printed, so it was usually impossible for the parents of vaccine-damaged children to find out about other parents whose children had suffered the same reaction to the same vaccine, and who were also being told by their doctor that the timing was "just a coincidence." This situation has changed with the advent of the internet. Parents of vaccine-damaged children can now tell their story online, and can make contact with other parents of vaccine-damaged children. The vaccine industry is worried by the fact that it has lost control of the flow of information, and it is taking a variety of steps to counteract the resultant loss of profits.

I grew up knowing about the existence of vaccine damage because of victims within my family, but I thought that vaccine damage was rare and that we were just a susceptible family. It was only in 1991 that I became aware of just how common severe reactions to vaccination are. I was living in New Zealand, and my phone number was published in a health magazine at the end of an article about vaccination. In the following weeks I received scores of phone calls from people whose children had reacted badly to a vaccine, and had gone on to suffer permanent damage. These parents had been rejected and shunned by the medical establishment, and they were relieved to be able to tell their story to someone who did not disparage them. The families of vaccine-damaged children need emotional support as much as they need financial help. None of them had received any type of support from the official channels that are supposed to take responsibility. This flood of phone calls jolted me into the realisation that vaccine damage is shockingly common.

Now when I give talks or publish articles I am no longer surprised by the number of terrible stories that I hear. Old people have stories to tell of what they saw the smallpox vaccine do, whereas younger people relate events concerning the modern vaccines. In between talks and articles I receive a steady stream of phone calls and messages from parents who are faced with someone trying to jab another vaccine into their already damaged child, or into another child in the family. When a baby or child has died from vaccination, I find that it is never the mother who contacts me. It is someone further removed from the victim, like an aunt or a grandmother.

The fact that parents of vaccine-damaged children can now tell their story on the internet serves as a warning to other parents, but so far it has not made the people who make and market vaccines accountable, nor has it made governments improve their method of collecting data about vaccine damage. Most doctors and nurses still brush aside the cases of vaccine damage that they personally encounter, and do not report them. There is a definite pattern of reactions from each vaccine, or combination of vaccines, but the most consistent thing that parents report to me is that doctors deny that the vaccine was responsible for the reaction. When parents move on to other doctors in the hope of getting help, they usually meet more denials that the vaccine could have been the cause. Sometimes doctors do admit it, but although they might say it verbally, they are not keen to put it in writing. They have good reason to fear the consequences if they speak out publicly about vaccine damage, but they know that they will not be punished for merely submitting a passive report. Doctors cannot be expected to report the adverse effects of vaccination that appear long after the vaccine has been administered, but if there were honest reporting of adverse effects that show up during the first few weeks, a whole new picture would emerge.

Many governments rely on the American Food and Drug Administration (FDA) to ensure that the medical products that they buy are safe. The FDA is supposed to protect the American consumer from dangerous substances, but as I will show further on, it fails to perform this function. The FDA should encourage research into the long-term effects of vaccination, but instead it actively discourages long-term research. For instance, Dr. Anthony Morris, a virologist and bacteriologist who was employed by the FDA, began some research into the long-term effects of vaccination. His research displeased the FDA, and in 1976 he was fired for going to the press and warning the public not to accept the dangerous swine flu vaccine that had been manufactured for use that year. The FDA took the opportunity to physically destroy his long-term research in his laboratories.[4]

Another example of obstruction of research by the medical establishment occurred when a professor at Otago University in New Zealand applied for permission to study changes in the blood after vaccination. The research required a heel-prick to take a blood sample from each baby soon after birth, and then another heel-prick sample to be taken months later. Permission was denied on the grounds that it would be "too invasive". Heel-prick samples are taken from babies for all sorts of frivolous reasons, but it is not permitted when there is the possibility that the results may show that vaccination alters the immune system in an undesirable way. If the vaccine industry felt confident that vaccination seldom causes detrimental effects, they would not feel the need to suppress research. They are afraid of the consequences of subjecting vaccination to proper scrutiny.

Back in the 1980s when the whole cell whooping cough vaccine was still in use in Western countries, two professors at Florida University in the USA examined the blood of seven children who had been brain damaged by the vaccine, and found that six of the seven children had a particular tissue typing antigen. This made them think that some children might be genetically predisposed to reacting to this vaccine, so they applied for funding to research the matter. Funding was refused with the flimsy excuse that there is "no evidence" that the vaccine causes brain damage.[5] In the 1980s there was already heaps of evidence that the vaccine caused brain damage, and curiously, now that the whole cell vaccine has been replaced with a less dangerous vaccine in affluent countries, the vaccinators are willing to admit that the whole cell vaccine was dangerous.

Despite this type of obstruction, some research does get through. A study that compared the rate of chronic disease of the intestines in the vaccinated and the unvaccinated was published in 1995.[6] With the help of a statistician, three doctors at the Royal Free Hospital School of Medicine in London compared the rate of Crohn's disease in people who had received measles vaccine with the rate in people who had not received it. The doctors had become suspicious that measles vaccine causes Crohn's disease because measles virus persists in the tissue of the intestines of some people with Crohn's disease,[7,8] and because there had been a three-fold rise in Crohn's disease in Scotland in the fifteen years after mass vaccination against measles was introduced in Britain.[9] Crohn's disease is a mysterious and horrible affliction of the intestines, which bears no resemblance to measles. The British Medical Research Council had done a trial run of measles vaccine (not MMR) in 1964,[10] and thirty years later 3545 of these children could still be traced. The parents of the trial children had been questioned about adverse effects in the third week after vaccination, but after that they were only questioned about whether the child got measles. Thirty years after the trial the doctors in London compared the rate of Crohn's disease in the 3545 children who had been injected with single measles vaccine with the rate of Crohn's disease in 2541 people of the same age who had not been vaccinated against measles.[6] They also compared the rates of ulcerative colitis, coeliac disease, and stomach ulcers in the two groups.

When I first read the study, I thought that the researchers were silly to include peptic ulcers and coeliac disease, because *obviously* measles vaccine could not cause those. Then I realised that I had the wrong attitude. The researchers were right to investigate those two diseases as well as Crohn's disease and ulcerative colitis, because you cannot *know* whether a medical intervention causes a long-term chronic disease unless you study it. The study revealed that measles vaccine makes a person 3 times more likely to get Crohn's disease, and 2.5 times more likely to get ulcerative colitis, but does not increase the risk of coeliac disease nor stomach ulcers. So that means that two out of every three of those people with Crohn's disease, which drastically reduces a person's quality of life, would not be suffering from it if they had not been injected with measles vaccine in 1964. There is a possibility that natural measles also causes Crohn's disease in some people, but even if it does, the results of this study show that the vaccine increases the risk far more than natural measles could. Eighty nine percent of the unvaccinated people in the study had had measles before the age of eleven, yet they had a very low rate of Crohn's disease.

Health conscious parents can be grateful to this group of doctors for stepping out of line and doing this research, but the vaccine establishment was far from grateful. The study annoyed the vaccine zealots, and they tried to discredit the method used,[11,12,13,14,15,16,17] but their endeavors flopped.[18]

Dr. Andrew Wakefield was one of the doctors who took part in the study. Later on he and twelve other doctors conducted a study of some children with autism, the results of which suggested that there may be a connection between MMR vaccine and autism. The writers of the study expressly stated that their study does not prove that MMR vaccine can cause autism, but they did call for studies that investigate a possible connection to be done. This infuriated the vaccine industry, and the authors of the study were told to recant. Ten of the authors capitulated to protect their careers, but three stood their ground, and have been persecuted by the vaccine establishment and vilified by the mainstream media.

In 2012 four Polish doctors published a review of the medical literature in which they looked at case reports of vaccine damage, types of adverse reactions, toxicity of ingredients, and trends in chronic disease in relation to vaccination.[19] They came to the conclusion that the harmful effects of vaccination "are disproportionate to the benefits of vaccination in the elimination of dangerous diseases in childhood".[19] If these doctors had been based in Britain or the USA they would have been punished for publishing this information in a medical journal.

While measles vaccine was still used on its own, some of the deaths that it caused were acknowledged,[20] but the actual number of deaths it caused will never be known because vaccine-related deaths are deliberately concealed. Nowadays measles vaccine is given at the same time as other vaccines, and deaths are always brushed off as "coincidence". Of course deaths from other causes can occur coincidentally after vaccination, but deaths that are part of an obvious reaction to vaccination are not coincidental.

In some countries parents who want compensation for permanent disability caused by vaccination have to sue the drug company that manufactured the vaccine. The onus is on the parents to prove that the vaccine caused the symptoms, while the drug company does not have to prove that it supplied a safe vaccine. In other countries the law provides for compensation to be paid at taxpayer expense, but in these countries the system is designed to prevent victims from obtaining the compensation to which they are legally entitled. New Zealand is an example of a country in which victims of vaccine damage are supposed to be paid compensation by the taxpayer. According to the law, compensation should automatically be paid whenever a child suffers permanent damage from vaccination. In theory all that has to happen is that the parents have to fill in form M46, and get it signed by any medical doctor. They then have to hand the form in to the Accident Compensation Corporation (ACC), which gets a panel of experts to investigate the case and decide whether or not compensation should be paid.

The ACC has a lot of money at its disposal. It does not hesitate to pay for reconstructive surgery if someone breaks a knee while playing a recreational game of rugby. It awarded a large amount of compensation to someone who suffered stress because a bank refused him a loan to start a business. It even paid a prisoner $10,000 compensation because he broke his legs when he jumped from the prison wall in an attempt to escape. However, when someone applies for compensation for vaccine damage, the behaviour of the ACC changes completely.

Before the parents of a vaccine-damaged child get to the point of applying to the ACC, they have to cross the hurdle of getting form M46 signed by a doctor. The catch for parents is that even doctors who do not get angry at the suggestion that vaccination is not perfect are usually unwilling to sign the form, because they are afraid of the effect that signing the form might have on their career. Parents have no chance of getting compensation to help them cope with the financial costs of their child's disability when all the doctors they approach for help refuse to formally acknowledge the cause of the disability.

To demonstrate the resistance that doctors have to acknowledging what are patently obvious adverse effects of vaccination, I will describe four of the cases with which I was associated during my years as a campaigner in New Zealand. I am choosing these stories from New Zealand because they show how doctors go into denial to protect the reputation of vaccination even when neither they nor a drug company can be sued.

In 1991 I interviewed the father of a girl who was perfectly normal until a combination of DPT and hepatitis B vaccines made her unable to sit up, unable to hold up her head, and unable to control her limbs. The only thing she could do was to make crying type noises when she was hungry. I could not tell whether or not her intellect had been damaged. Perhaps her mind was working normally and only the motor part of her brain had been destroyed. I saw an expression in her eyes that made me feel she was experiencing an emotional reaction to the conversation around her. She could not speak, nor control the direction in which her eyes looked. My interview with her father was filmed by a TV cameraman, but never shown on TV.

Auckland is the biggest city in New Zealand, and this family lived on an island close to the city. One day their doctor set off for the mainland saying that he was going to find out how they could obtain financial compensation. He returned to the island a frightened man, saying that the vaccine could not have been the cause.

When the family applied for compensation, the public health nurse said that she would support their claim. Then she was told that her job would be in jeopardy if she did that, because, "your action would make it appear that you are not supportive of immunisation policy." When I interviewed the father in front of the television camera, he related how the specialists who were supposed to be helping him submit his claim for compensation had treated him with suspicion, disrespect, and dishonesty. The thing that amazed me about this interview was that despite all his experiences with the medical conspiracy, the father still believed that it was quite rare for a child to be affected in the way that his child had been. When I told him afterwards about the other cases we know about from the area, he was surprised to learn that his child was not "one in a million". If TV stations would allow that sort of footage to be aired, the public would become more aware of the extent of vaccine damage.

In another case, a 15 month old girl had the measles, mumps, and rubella vaccine (MMR) injected into her hip. The hip and leg became swollen and painful, a lump of pus developed in the hip joint, and the cartilage disappeared from the joint. She also suffered a systemic reaction which put her in hospital for three weeks. Before the injection she had been toddling with free movements, but afterwards she could not put weight on that side.

The rubella component of MMR has a predilection for attacking the cartilage in joints,[21,22,23] but the lump of pus that was surgically removed seven days after the injection implied that the needle had hit the bone. (Babies have very small hips and syringe needles are long). The surgeon who carried out the operation to remove the lump of pus met the girl's father and granny in the hospital corridor after the operation. He said to them, "That needle went in too far."

According to New Zealand law, the child is eligible for compensation for pain and suffering, for the travel costs to have her treated, for a plastic hip joint, for physiotherapy, and for whatever else she needs to cope with the consequences of the injection. The parents filled in form M46, but the doctor who administered the vaccine would not sign it, even though under New Zealand law he is immune from litigation if the finding is that he did put the needle in too far. No other general practitioner in the town in which they lived would sign the form. The surgeon who said after removing the lump of pus that the needle had gone in too far would not sign the form, and no other doctor in the hospital would sign the form. The parents lived in a small town on the South Island of New Zealand, where all the medical people know each other. The parents could not afford to travel to another town to try to find an honest doctor, so they contacted the consumer group of which I was a member for help. We were able to put them in touch with one of the three doctors in New Zealand who have enough backbone to sign form M46.

Even when parents have managed to get a doctor to sign the application form, they then have to face the problem that the Accident Compensation Corporation does not want to pay for vaccine damage. The ACC places the burden of proof on the victim, and then rejects whatever material the victim comes up with as being "insufficient evidence". The average young couple does not have the time nor the money to research the history of a vaccine and compile a scientific case proving that the vaccine was the cause of that specific set of symptoms. When they try, their effort is just brushed aside anyway.

A tiny proportion of vaccine-damaged children do get financial compensation because of intervention by consumer activists. One of those was a child who was born 12 weeks prematurely. He spent six weeks in intensive care, where he had to be vigorously stimulated more than a hundred times because he had stopped breathing. After he was moved into the regular prem unit the parents were told that he was thriving, so he could go home in a few days. They were also told that he must be vaccinated because he was very susceptible to disease. Although it was still six weeks before he should have been born, the parents naively gave permission for him to be injected with DPT vaccine.

After the jab in the morning he would not wake up for feeds. That night he was blue, but the doctors told his mother not to worry. At 3 am a nurse walked past his cot and noticed that he was very blue. He was rushed back to intensive care and put on a respirator. At the time the doctors mentioned the vaccine as a possible cause of the relapse. He spent two weeks in intensive care, and then went home to a life of "spastic quadriplegia" and "cerebral palsy".

It took a whole year for the parents to get form M46 signed so that they could apply for accident compensation. The doctors were not keen to admit on paper that DPT vaccine was the cause of the child's condition, but they were in a quandary. The doctors who had assessed the baby before he was vaccinated had all put it in writing that the baby's prognosis was very good. When the baby's future turned to disaster, they were made to look stupid for giving such a good prognosis. So they wanted it known that their prognoses had been made before the baby had been injected with DPT. It seems that doctors are willing to tell the truth about DPT to protect their own reputations, but not when it is merely to help the victim get financial help in meeting the costs of the disability. The doctors' signatures made it possible for the family to apply to the ACC.

The parents had two other things in their favour. One was that the reaction had occurred in hospital, under the eyes of lots of medical people. The other was that Hilary Butler, who is a voluntary worker with a huge knowledge base, spent eighty hours of her time combing the medical literature, and writing an argument that the timing was not "just a coincidence", and that it was in fact the vaccine that had caused the condition.

The bigwigs at the ACC were convinced by Hilary's evidence, and they ruled that compensation should be paid. However, a person lower down in the ACC hierarchy did not like the ruling, and sent a letter to the parents saying that compensation had been denied. It was only by chance that one of the bigwigs of the ACC found out about this letter, and the lump sum compensation was paid three days later. None of the doctors who had agreed to admit that the vaccine was the cause of the little boy's disabilities reported the reaction to the Adverse Reactions Committee.

Another distressing case involved the death of a 32-year-old woman. She had developed an enlarged heart and an enlarged liver after giving birth in Auckland hospital. Many tests were done during the eight months of her illness, but her family did not receive an explanation for her condition. She was moved to Greenlane Hospital to have an operation in which they were planning to replace some swollen heart tissue with plastic. Before she was due to have the operation, she was injected with a vaccine that contains the outer shells of 23 strains of germ that can cause pneumonia. She went into a coma, and her body swelled up and turned red.

The doctors apologised profusely to the family for giving her the vaccine, because the official line on that vaccine is that it should not be given to anyone who is sick. But nothing was put on paper. Not only did the doctors fail to document the fact that she had reacted to the vaccine, they also failed to document that she had ever been given the vaccine. All they did was to write "operation cancelled" on the patient card, and send her back to Auckland Hospital.

When she came out of the coma her skin was very painful to the touch, and it developed the appearance of a snow burn. The skin condition began to subside, but it flared up again when she had the heart operation. It was still there when she died of cardiac arrest 25 days after the vaccination. This had been a very severe and painful rash; a sign that there was a serious disturbance within the body. The family believes that she would have survived the heart condition, had it not been for the vaccine. They are powerless against the medical establishment. What was a vaccine that is not supposed to be given to sick people doing in a fridge in intensive care? There is no accountability for what goes on in the name of "immunisation".

THE CRUCIAL DIFFERENCE BETWEEN THE SELF-RESOLVING INFECTIOUS DISEASES AND THOSE THAT NEED INTERVENTION

Discussion about the effectiveness of vaccination becomes muddled unless a clear distinction is made between the two categories of infectious disease. Infectious diseases are usually classified according to the type of germ that causes them, so it is said that there are bacterial diseases, viral diseases, rickettsial diseases, protozoal diseases, and so on. However, that method of classification does not help us understand the effects that infectious diseases have on humans. From the point of view of prevention, treatment, and immunity, it is more useful to divide infectious diseases into two groups based on how they interact with the human immune system, rather than on what type of germ causes them. In the first group are the *self-resolving childhood diseases* that you expect a child to get before the teenage years, like measles, mumps, and chicken pox. There are eight of them. In the other group are the *diseases that need intervention*, like polio, diphtheria, and TB. Some medical people mistakenly refer to polio and diphtheria as childhood diseases. Polio does occur in children more often than it does in adults, but that is not the case with diphtheria. Polio, diphtheria, and TB are not self-resolving diseases; they need interventions to make them come to an end as quickly as possible.

When the self-resolving childhood diseases are handled correctly, they have a beneficial effect on the child's long-term health. When wrongly treated, they can develop complications that can harm or even kill the patient. They do not need any action to be taken to make them come to an end. They automatically come to an end by themselves. They cannot be prevented by good nutrition, but the level of nutrition affects the way that the child copes with the disease. One dose of the disease creates life-long immunity. The vaccines that are intended to prevent these diseases have a different effect on the immune system to the natural infection. They create a flawed kind of immunity that wears off in time, so that vaccinated people are vulnerable to getting the diseases when they are teenagers or adults.

Self-resolving Infectious Diseases	Infectious Diseases that need intervention
Infantum roseola	Polio
Rubella	TB (tuberculosis)
Mumps (parotitis)	Diphtheria
Measles (rubeola)	Tetanus
Chicken pox (varicella)	Cholera
Whooping cough (pertussis)	Typhoid
Slapped cheek roseola	Meningitis
	Typhus
	Hepatitis A
	Hepatitis B
	Hepatitis C
	Rabies
	Haemophilus
	Smallpox
	Yellow fever

The infectious diseases that need intervention are the ones that we do not calmly "expect" our children to get. They are diseases that cause a panic, and rightfully so. Tetanus, tuberculosis (TB), polio, diphtheria, cholera, rabies, bubonic plague, typhoid, typhus, and yellow fever are diseases that give absolutely no benefit to a person who gets them. Some of these diseases can be prevented by hygiene, but the germs of the airborne diseases cannot be avoided during an outbreak. However, airborne germs will only be able to cause disease in a person who is susceptible, and good nutrition is an important protective factor.

A significant feature of this category of infectious disease is that catching one of them, and surviving, does not mean that the person cannot catch it again at a later date. The medicinenet website revealed more than they night have intended when they said this about tetanus, "After recovery, patients still require active immunization because having the tetanus disease does not provide natural immunization against a repeat episode." The Australian medicrats put it more simply, with, "Having tetanus does not make you immune, so you should be immunised."

When my son Kenny was three he got measles. He did not like the spots because they spoiled his appearance. The sight of himself in the mirror made him upset. I consoled him by telling him that when it was all over he would never get measles again. A few months later he got gastric flu, and he felt terrible. With a sad look he said, "At least it means I'll never get it again." I had to tell him the bad news that gastric flu does not cause immunity to itself, and the germs that cause it often come into the air, so he could get it again.

One can only get a disease when the germs for that particular disease are in the environment. The vaccine industry would like us to believe that if it were not for the protection of vaccination, people would be accosted by deadly germs wherever they go. However, the germs that cause infectious diseases are not always present in the environment, and when they are present, their virulence increases and decreases.

Self-resolving Infectious Diseases	**Infectious Diseases that need intervention**
Are self-resolving diseases that need proper care to prevent complications, but no intervention.	Are not self-resolving diseases and without intervention death is a possible outcome.
Cannot be prevented by good nutrition.	Good nutrition helps with prevention.
Cannot be prevented by hygiene.	Some can be prevented by hygiene.
Can be prevented by total quarantine.	Can be prevented by total quarantine.
Create life-long immunity to themselves.	Do not create immunity to themselves.
Vaccines create temporary artificial immunity.	Vaccines are either ineffective or have no proven efficacy.

The germs that cause the infectious diseases that are not self-resolving come from three different sources; some live in water, some float in the air, and some can only be caught from another person's blood. In some countries it is safer to assume that cholera and typhoid are always in the environment. Typhoid and cholera lurk in water that is contaminated with sewage, and the only sure way to avoid getting sick is to ensure that all the water you consume is not contaminated. Being fit and well-nourished is no guarantee that the germs of cholera and typhoid will not be able to overcome your immune system.

The germs that cause self-resolving childhood diseases float in the air, and there is a concentration of them in the air space around a person who is incubating the disease or who has the disease. The germs infect everybody, but not everyone gets the disease. Some people have already had it and are immune, while others are never going to get it, or are going to get it at a later date. Some children are repeatedly exposed to the germs by parents who are keen for their children to get the self-resolving childhood diseases behind them, but their bodies obstinately refuse to catch the disease.

A child's nutritional status has no bearing on whether or not he or she catches a self-resolving childhood disease, but it does make a difference to how he or she handles the disease. It annoys me when anti-vaxxers tell parents that a child who was breast-fed and given only wholesome food will not get measles. That is not true.

Well-meaning people might advise you to "cure" the self-resolving childhood diseases with homoeopathy or high doses of vitamins. Further on I will explain why that is bad advice.

Health-conscious communities have "measles parties" to give as many children as possible the opportunity of catching measles. This has to be done in a way that is sensitive to the needs of the sick child. Sometimes children who do not even like each other have to play together. Despite all this effort, there will be some children who just do not get it. This is very vexing, because if a person gets a self-resolving childhood disease in adulthood, the risk of complications is much higher.[1] An exception to this is whooping cough. A young baby is vulnerable to the complications of whooping cough if the disease is not handled wisely, whereas complications seldom occur in older people, even with the worst medical treatments.

My mother-in-law had three brothers who all had mumps when they were children, but she did not get it. All seven of her children had mumps at one time or another, and she cared for them closely, but did not catch it. It would have been difficult for her if she had got it during her child-caring years. Then, much to her amusement, she got it from one of her grandchildren when she was 62. She knew exactly what to do. She took herself off to bed and read books and caught up on her knitting until it was safe to get up again. She lived with a daughter who kept her well supplied with nourishing soup. People of any age with mumps need to be well cared for, but an adult with mumps who does not stay in bed is especially vulnerable to complications.

We have been conditioned to fear the self-resolving childhood diseases, instead of being taught how to treat them. Parents who fear the self-resolving childhood diseases wonder what the *risk* is of their child catching one of them. Once liberated from the fear that has been cultivated by the vaccine industry, they change their thinking and wonder what the *likelihood* is of their child catching a childhood disease. Once we know how to treat them safely, we do not need to fear them. However, we do need to have a healthy, well informed respect for the infectious diseases that do not resolve themselves and need to be dealt with swiftly if they put in an appearance.

FEVER IS A FRIEND

These days parents are taught to fear fever as if it were a disease, and to make it go away when it appears in a child. However, suppressing fever, either by the use of drugs or by chilling the patient, is a dangerous practice, which sometimes causes the patient to die. This is because raising a fever is one of the ways that the body protects itself when it is invaded by a germ or by a toxin. If fever is suppressed during the course of an infectious disease, the patient becomes more vulnerable to the germ that is causing the disease. Infected humans who experience fever have a better survival rate than infected humans who do not experience fever.[27,28,29,30,31,32] Suppressing fever also increases the risk of pneumonia developing as a complication of an infectious disease.[33]

Many parents believe that if they do not bring down a fever, their child will have a convulsion and suffer brain damage. This belief is promoted even though scientific research has shown that it does not happen. When a patient has a fever, the fever rises, stays at a high point for a while, and then goes down again. There is no danger from the increased temperature because it will stop rising when it reaches the right level to achieve what it needs to achieve.[34,35] Hyperthermia, on the other hand, can be dangerous. Hyperthermia is where the body becomes too hot because of too much exercise, or because the air temperature is too hot, like when someone is locked in a car on a hot day. This is different to fever, which is when the body deliberately makes itself hotter than normal as a reaction to invasion by a germ or a toxin. A person who is too hot from overheating, like from doing excessive exercise in hot weather, should be cooled down, but a person should not be chilled when the body is deliberately creating a fever.

The immune system is still not fully understood, but some of the mechanisms by which fever helps to protect the body during germ invasion are known. Leukocytes are an assortment of cells in the immune system that fight unfriendly germs. They also fight the toxins that unfriendly bacteria make. Leukocytes move faster when the temperature goes up,[36,37] and they can eat invader germs at a faster rate.[38] When foreign germs invade the body, some leukocytes manufacture a protein called endogenous pyrogen.[39,40] There is disagreement about exactly how this protein stimulates fever, but the fact that it is what provokes the fever is not disputed. Once the fever starts, the level of iron in the blood becomes reduced so that foreign bacteria cannot feed on it.[41,42,43] The movement of iron out of the blood is not caused directly by the rise in temperature; it is a separate defence mechanism that works co-operatively with the fever to defeat germs.[44] The body also starts producing interferons,[45] which are substances that kill viruses and bacteria, and make leukocytes more active.[45,46] Interferons work faster at a higher temperature,[47] and are three times more effective at 40°C than at 39°C.[47] Antibiotics are also more effective in the presence of fever.[48] Vitamin C helps leukocytes kill germs, and when the temperature is higher, the effect of vitamin C is greater.[49]

Leukocytes also respond faster and more effectively when the temperature goes up to 40°C,[50] and they move to where they are needed faster and stay at the site where they are needed when the temperature is elevated.[45,51] T cells are an important type of leukocyte which are manufactured in the thymus gland. When fever is present the thymus produces more T cells.[52,53,54] Bacteria get weaker and are easier to kill at a higher temperature.[55,56]

Reptiles do not generate much body heat, so they need warmth from the sun or another source to warm themselves up. When reptiles are infected with harmful germs, they move to a warm spot. If they are prevented from moving to a warm place, they die.[57] This shows that they need a raised body temperature to successfully fight the infection. Very young mammals, like human babies or puppies, are similar to reptiles in that their own bodies cannot produce enough warmth. They are instinctively kept warm by their mothers, but if they become infected with harmful germs, and are not kept warm, they die.[34,38,58] Debilitated humans of any age who cannot produce a fever, die from infection.[48]

Drugs that reduce fever place both reptiles and mammals at a disadvantage. A study was done in which twelve iguanas were infected with a bad germ and kept in a warm environment, but they were also given aspirin. In five of these the aspirin did not work, and their temperatures went up, and they survived. In the other seven, the aspirin succeeded in preventing a rise in body temperature, and they all died.[59] Giving drugs to rabbits to reduce fever increases the death rate from infection.[60]

At a hospital in Miami twelve doctors decided to, "evaluate the impact of antipyretic therapy strategies on the outcomes of critically ill patients", because, "despite the large body of evidence suggesting a beneficial role of fever in the host response, antipyretic therapy is commonly employed for febrile critically ill patients."[61] "Antipyretic therapy" means giving drugs to suppress fever. They commenced a study in which one group of patients was allowed to have a fever of 40 degrees, but no higher, while the other group of patients had their fever aggressively suppressed. The experiment had to be halted on ethical grounds after only 82 patients had been studied because the death rate was 6 times higher in those who had had their fever aggressively suppressed. The results of this study were published in a medical journal in 2005, but hospitals continue to kill people by suppressing fever.

The medical establishment will not change its ways for two reasons. One is that they are relentlessly brain washed by the drug industry into believing that fever must be suppressed; the other is that they have an aversion to admitting that what they have been doing all along is harmful. Dr. Panagiotis Kiekkas is a Greek doctor who has tried to educate the medical profession about the benefits of fever. He reports how nurses at his hospital were more interested in suppressing fever than in managing pain, providing nutrition, or practicing hygiene, and when he tried to get them to base their actions on science rather than on tradition, he met with huge resistance.[62]

A 2011 study of critically ill patients in hospitals in Britain, New Zealand, and Australia provides yet more evidence that fever helps with the survival of people who have an infection. The higher the temperature was in the critically ill patients who had an infection, the less likely they were to die.[63] The opposite happened with critically ill patients who did not have an infection. The higher their temperature was, the *more* likely they were to die.[63] There are some serious non-infectious conditions, including brain injury, for which the patient needs to have their temperature kept below 39°C.

There was a time when every culture on earth supported fever as part of their care of a sick person, but now there are only a few traditional forms of medicine that still support fever to help a sick person recover. The idea that fever is harmful was set in motion when aspirin began to be commercially produced. Aspirin started its life as a pain killer, but it was soon discovered that it had the side effect of reducing fever, so the manufacturers of aspirin promoted the idea that bringing down fever is the right thing to do. The use of aspirin for fever suppression is now discouraged, and the fashion is to prescribe paracetamol or ibuprofen instead. Paracetamol is called acetaminophen in the US, Canada, Japan, and Iran, but it is most commonly called by one of its two hundred trade names. Some trade names are Tylenol, Calpol, Panadol, Panado, Pamol, and Tempra. In this book I will refer to the drug as paracetamol/tylenol.

In 1980 an American paediatrician conducted a survey in which he found that many parents believed that fever could cause brain damage and other forms of serious permanent damage, including death. Many of the surveyed parents also believed that the fever would just continue to rise if there was no intervention.[64] The paediatrician says, "Health education to counteract 'fever phobia' should be a part of routine pediatric care". In another article he says, "Parents clearly need to be educated about fevers."[65] He is right, but the problem is that the drug companies are the ones that are doing the "educating". Drug companies make billions from selling fever-suppressing drugs, so they use magazines, TV, and radio to "educate" parents that fever should be suppressed. They also control what doctors and nurses are taught during their training, so medical personnel come out of the mill believing that fever should be suppressed. The doctors who want to introduce science into the belief system (and there are many) are up against serious opposition. It is not surprising that in 2001 another survey of parental beliefs about fever found that many parents still believed that fever is a disease that can cause brain damage and death, and that the temperature would keep on rising in left untreated.[66] The authors of the 2001 study conclude, "Fever phobia persists."

There is a myth that having a fever makes a person feel uncomfortable, and cooling them down with water or cold air will make them feel more comfortable. That is the opposite of the truth. It is the onlookers who feel uncomfortable about the fever, not the person who is experiencing the fever. Mere observation is enough to know that people with a fever feel more comfortable when they are warm, but to my great joy someone has actually done a scientific study that proves it.[67] The people with fever in the study, and they all reported that they felt more comfortable when they were warmed up, and less comfortable when they were cooled down. The study found that cooling a person who has a fever not only causes discomfort, it also increases oxygen intake, it activates the autonomic nervous system, it increases blood pressure, and it makes stress indicators appear in the blood. The study authors call this a "substantial metabolic cost".[67]

A child in a high fever with measles is not uncomfortable. The child's behaviour is different to normal, mainly because he or she just lies there doing nothing. But the child feels okay. If pain or discomfort is present with measles, it means that something is wrong. When something is wrong it is not the fever that needs to be dealt with. Reducing the fever will only make the child more vulnerable to whatever is wrong. Suppressing the fever in someone who has measles increases the risk of complications developing. Giving paracetamol/tylenol to a child with chicken pox makes the spots more itchy, and makes the illness last longer,[68] yet parents are routinely advised to give paracetamol/tylenol to a child with chicken pox. It becomes downright dangerous when hospital staff give a cancer patient who catches chicken pox a drug to suppress fever. Suppressing the fever of someone who has meningococcal meningitis is also extremely dangerous, yet this is what doctors do when someone turns up at hospital with the disease. Paracetamol/tylenol makes a cold worse,[69] yet many people are programmed to take paracetamol/tylenol when they have a cold. Paracetamol/tylenol cripples neutrophils, basophils, and eosinophils, which are white blood cells that play a crucial role in fighting bacterial, viral, and parasitic infections.[70] In fact all drugs that suppress fever have a detrimental effect on the immune system.[71,72,73,74] All of this means that when a person with an infectious disease is given a drug to suppress fever, they are being harmed in two ways. They are being deprived of the benefit of fever, and at the same time their immune system is being disabled by a drug.

By mindlessly reducing fever in patients with infections, the medical profession is sabotaging the body's attempt to defend itself. The result for well-fed, affluent children is that they become immunocompromised for a few hours, and consequently become more vulnerable to harm from the infecting germ. While the child's body is dealing with the lack of fever, he or she is in a similar situation to what impoverished, under-fed children are in all the time. The immune system of a child who is severely malnourished cannot raise a fever to fight invader germs. The inability to raise a fever causes many children in impoverished countries to die from infectious diseases. Most children in affluent countries do not eat a wholesome diet of organically grown, unrefined, unprocessed food, but they do get *enough* food to make their immune systems work. As a result of eating the artificially fertilised, refined, and highly processed foods, affluent children grow up to get the diseases that are now considered "normal" in people over 50, like type 2 diabetes, cancer, heart disease, and arthritis. But at least they can fight off germs long enough to grow up and get the diseases of modern civilisation. Children who have kwashiorkor (severe malnutrition) cannot make pyrogen, and consequently they do not raise a fever when they get infected with germs.[75,76] "Infections in these circumstances are frequently fatal."[75] Dr. G. J. Ebrahim has worked extensively with these children, and he says,

> The child with malnutrition is very susceptible to infection. The body's defences are unable to mount an adequate response to microbial challenge so that the mildest infection tends to spread and become life-threatening. In severe cases the clinical response to infection, like fever and phagocytosis, may be absent and the first sign of widespread infection may be sudden deterioration in the general condition, refusal to take food and hypothermia.[77]

Hypothermia means getting colder. So instead of getting a fever when something like measles starts, the body of a malnourished child gets colder. Measles without fever is a dangerous situation. Most well fed children survive having the fever artificially reduced, but they do not all survive.

A child who is in a fever because of a self-resolving childhood disease needs quiet surroundings, and needs to know that a parent or primary caregiver is nearby. A baby might want a parent present all the time while awake. A person with a fever needs to be given frequent drinks, and to be lying down, and be covered with warm bedding. The patient instinctively pulls the bedding up to the chin as the fever rises, and pushes it back when the fever recedes. Babies cannot adjust their covers, so they need adult help to ensure that they do not get too cold or too hot. Shivering is a sign that the fever is building up and warmth is needed. Sweating is a sign that the fever is over and the body is cooling itself down. Don't force a sweating child to stay under the covers, but also don't do anything that would make him or her cool down any faster than nature intends. The body will do it at the correct rate. When fever is achieved, the pyrogen shuts off its own production.[78] Then when fever is needed again, the pyrogen stimulates the production of fever. That is why the fever comes and goes during the illness, instead of remaining constant.

By recognising the role of fever in infectious diseases, we are better equipped to help the patient recover. In Europe there was a long-standing tradition that, in certain circumstances, a disease could be cured by stimulating a fever. The Zulus also treated illness that was accompanied by fever by warming people up. Dr. Henry Francis Fynn described his experience of Zulu medicine in 1823.

> I discovered that their chief, Shaka, resided at too great a distance from there for me to reach him. Apart from this I became considerably indisposed, hence went back to where our vessel was, upon which I was immediately laid up with a severe attack of fever. During my absence, Maynard had sent for the schooner, hence I found myself left with only the sailor who had been with me the whole time. I obtained possession of a hut like those at Delagoa and there I lay for several days. I must have become delerious, for the first thing I remember was being taken from the hut by a native doctor and several women. On coming to an open space, they lifted me up and placed me in a pit they had dug and in which they had been making a large fire; grass and weeds had been placed therein to prevent my feet from being burnt. They put me in a standing position, then filled the pit with earth up to my neck. The women held a mat round my head. In this position they

> might have kept me for about half an hour. They then carried me back to the hut and gave me native medicine. I felt I was recovering. On the third day, I was able to communicate with the vessel.[79]

Two hundred years ago a group of Bunurong first nation Australians used a similar method to help a sick European man whom they found wandering around in the wilderness.

> On seeing Buckley ill, they scooped out a depression in the ground, lit a fire all along it, later swept the fire out and laid Buckley in it, covering him with the warm soil. This method proved successful and he recovered fully.[80]

There is also an account of Native Americans restoring a European to health by warming him up when he had a fever.[81]

In the 1940s Dr. Benjamin Spock wrote a book on childcare which revolutionised the way Western children were brought up. In this book he devotes four and a half pages to telling parents how to take a child's temperature, then says, "on the other hand a dangerous illness may never have a temperature higher than 101°F. So don't be influenced too much, one way or the other, by the height of the fever." Then he goes on to advise giving aspirin and chilling the child with water, and then says, "remember the fever is not the disease. The fever is one of the methods the body uses to help overcome the infection."[82] Bring on the psychologists.

Measuring the temperature when a child has a fever does not provide information that helps with making decisions about care. The child's condition is what matters. It is normal for a child with fever to lie down, have glazed eyes, and not be talkative. Those symptoms are not a sign of danger. The symptoms that go with a self-resolving infectious disease are also not signs of danger. But pain, stiffness, seizures, vomiting, confusion, unresponsiveness, or a rash of tiny reddish purple dots are signs of danger, and the cause needs to be investigated and treated. If a drug is given to suppress fever it will work against the helpful treatments.

Fever often gets higher at night during a self-resolving childhood disease. Sleeping near the child means that you will be woken if he or she needs a drink. At night a baby with roseola will want to drink more than usual. If the baby is breast-fed there is no need to "supplement" with water. In the 2001 survey, 85% of parents said that they wake their sleeping child to give a fever-suppressing drug.[66] The child should be left to sleep and the fever should be left to do its job. If the fever is caused by a dangerous underlying condition, then emergency treatment is needed. It is not the fever that needs treating, it is the underlying condition that needs treating.

When a child has frequent low-grade fevers it could mean that there is something seriously wrong, like lupus or cancer. Giving drugs to suppress the fevers does not fix the problem. When recurrent fevers are treated homoeopathically, the objective should be to remove the underlying problem, not just to stop the fevers. This can only be done by choosing a remedy that matches all of the symptoms that are present. Mindlessly giving potentised *aconite* or potentised *belladonna* for every fever is almost as bad as giving aspirin or paracetamol/tylenol. *Aconite* and *belladonna* are brilliant remedies when they are used correctly, but they should not be used for the sole purpose of suppressing fever.

Malaria is a disease that is characterised by recurring fevers. It is easy to cure homoeopathically by giving homoeopathically potentised quinine (*china officinalis 30*). This makes the body kill the parasite that causes malaria. Non-homoeopathic quinine, or one of its derivatives, makes the fever temporarily subside, but it does not cure the underlying disease. It can also cause serious adverse effects, including psychotic violence, whereas homoeopathic quinine has no side effects. There are also herbs that boost the immune system, like *olive leaf, garlic,* and *echinacea.* Herbs can be used to help support a person with repeated low-grade fevers, but should not be used to abort acute fevers.

HYPERTHERMIA

Hyperthermia is different to fever in that the body heats up because of an outside influence, and it can get hotter and hotter until cell damage or death occurs. When the body feels itself becoming too hot it instinctively tries to reduce its temperature, by, for example, sweating, or moving into the shade, or drinking cold liquid. Young babies are unable to rectify the situation if they are too warmly wrapped up, and overheating is associated with sudden infant death syndrome.[83,84,85] Leaving a child in a car can cause brain damage or death from overheating, and adults can experience hyperthermia from doing too much exercise. When a person is suffering from heat stroke everyone around should help to reduce that person's body temperature, even if it involves pouring cold water over the person. Drugs like cocaine and heroin can make the body produce a fever in an attempt to defend itself, but those drugs disable the hypothalamus so the temperature gets hotter and hotter. The high temperature contributes to the damage done by the drugs, and the patient, who is usually unable to stand, should be cooled down, along with the other treatments that are needed.

FEBRILE CONVULSIONS

There is a popular myth that if a child has a fever it is necessary to get rid of the fever or else the fever could cause a febrile convulsion that would result in permanent brain damage. (Febrile means "from fever".) Febrile convulsions and febrile seizures are the same thing. A large-scale study, in which 54,000 children from a variety of backgrounds were studied from birth to the age of seven years, was published in 1978.[86] The study found that 4% of the children experienced febrile seizures before the age of seven, and none of the seizures resulted in death, brain damage, nor epilepsy. One third of the children who had a febrile seizure had at least one more febrile seizure before the age of seven.

The authors of the study offer a suggestion as to how the myth that febrile convulsions cause brain damage has arisen. They suggest that it may have arisen because the only data that was in existence before their study was done, involved children who had neurological problems. Some of these children had had a febrile convulsion in their past, and this led to the wrong assumption that the convulsion had caused the neurological problems.

Twenty years later another large-scale study confirmed that children who have febrile convulsions do just as well academically, intellectually, and behaviourally as other children.[87]

People who have a low seizure threshold are more likely to have a convulsion during fever than people with the usual threshold.[88,89] Febrile convulsions do not cause epilepsy,[90,91] but they are alarming to observe. Parents suffer shock and stress from seeing their child have a febrile convulsion.

Some people believe that convulsions are sparked off not by the height of the fever, but by a rapid rise or a rapid fall in temperature. Some nurses and some paramedics believe that giving drugs for fever increases the likelihood of a convulsion, because when the drug takes effect it makes the fever drop very sharply, and when it wears off it makes the fever rise suddenly. The makers of fever-suppressing drugs have not yet funded a study on the issue. The paramedics that I know never feel that their time has been wasted when they are called out because a child has had a convulsion, because they know how frightening it is for parents.

The pharmaceutical industry over-emphasises the danger from convulsions caused by natural fevers, while trivialising convulsions caused by vaccination. Many children are put on anti-epileptic drugs for years after just one febrile convulsion, even though the drugs make no difference to the child's long-term neurological condition.[92] In 1997 it was officially confirmed in the USA that febrile seizures are harmless, and that fever-suppressing drugs do not prevent them.[93] The information has not been passed on to doctors, nurses, and parents, because drugs are big money spinners.

DANGEROUS FEBRILE DISEASES

If a dangerous disease is brewing, suppressing the fever is not going to help the patient. The disease itself must be treated, not the symptom of fever. Some life-threatening, fast-acting diseases produce a fever if the person's immune system is working properly. For example, polio and meningococcal meningitis are diseases that usually produce a fever, and if a person who is suffering from one of these diseases takes paracetamol/tylenol, the drug helps the germ attack the body. On the other hand, lack of fever does not mean that there is no cause for alarm. Polio, meningococcal meningitis, typhoid, hepatitis A, and many other life-threatening diseases can progress quite far before the fever puts in an appearance. It is dangerous to think there is no problem when there is no fever.

There are many strains of virus and bacteria that can cause meningitis. The ones caused by bacteria can be successfully treated with antibiotics. Haemophilus, pneumonia, legionnaires' disease, and some types of streptococcal infection can also be treated with antibiotics, but if the doctors give fever-suppressing drugs at the same time, they are undermining their own treatment. As well as directly protecting the patient from the germs, fever helps antibiotics to be more effective.[48,55]

If a rash that looks like little reddish purple dots or like mottled bruising appears, it could be a symptom of meningococcal meningitis, which can kill a person in a matter of hours if it is not treated. Unfortunately meningococcal meningitis does not always produce a rash. There are many tragic stories of people with meningococcal meningitis going to hospital because they feel terrible and are almost collapsing, and being told by the overworked staff to go home, which they do, only to die a few hours later.

Meningitis occurs when there is infection and inflammation of the meninges. The meninges are the three layers of membrane that are around the brain and spinal cord. Encephalitis, on the other hand, is inflammation of the whole brain and spinal cord. Encephalitis usually starts suddenly, and the first symptoms are the same as meningitis. Symptoms of meningitis are a stiff neck and headache, the neck going rigid, pain all over which gets worse and worse, drowsiness, vomiting, fever, confusion, and sensitivity to light.

Convulsions are usually not present with meningitis, but some people do get them. Sometimes the head goes backwards and the back begins to arch. That is a very bad sign. Some germs bring on meningitis really quickly, while others make it creep up slowly and insidiously. Bringing down the fever only makes it more difficult for the body to fight the germs.

Babies can be under attack from meningitis germs without showing any signs other than high fever, so a prolonged high fever in a baby with no obvious cause should be medically investigated, or treated by an experienced, properly qualified homoeopath. People who tell you to use homoeopathic belladonna for every fever do not know what they are doing. If a baby's fontanel is not yet closed over, watch it for signs of trouble. If it sinks in, it is a sign of serious dehydration. If it bulges out, it could be meningitis.

CHILLING

Bringing down the fever with drugs knocks down the body's defences, and prevents the body from dealing with the underlying problem. Bringing down the fever by chilling the patient carries many more risks, the most obvious being pneumonia. However, this is not obvious to people brainwashed in the ways of modern medicine. Advice from them is to remove clothing and place the child in a draught. This advice is taken seriously by followers of modern medicine. I once heard a couple debating which was the draughtiest position in their house, so that they could sit their baby who had roseola in it. Bronchitis and ear infections are the most common consequences of the medical obsession with chilling, but pneumonia can develop very quickly. The modern delusion is that the germs that cause bronchitis, ear infections, and pneumonia act independently of their environment.

My husband's cousin's baby was admitted to the Red Cross Children's Hospital in Cape Town with croup, and was given a wild assortment of drugs, which provoked a fever. He was then stripped to his nappy, and placed in front of an open window. Cape Town is notorious for wind, so at any window you can be sure of a good draught. The baby promptly developed pneumonia, and one of the nurses said to his mother, "Don't worry. It's normal for a baby in hospital to have pneumonia."

CATCHING A CHILL

The way that catching a chill can make a person succumb to germs is still a mysterious process, and the idea that a chill can adversely affect the immune system is vehemently denied by some people. The denialists tend to be people who feel that their identity is tied up with "science". Their "logic" is that colds, flu, and lung infections have been proven to be caused by germs, so therefore no other factors can play a part. That is not logical, but it is currently politically incorrect to even talk about catching a chill. There is a difference between getting chilled and "catching a chill". When someone "catches a chill" there is an on-going effect after the feeling of being cold has gone away. Some people are so hardy that they never catch a chill, no matter what they do. Others are extremely susceptible to catching a chill, and will even get sick from short exposure to a draft from badly designed air conditioning. People also have different levels of susceptibility to chills at different times, and having a fever is one situation that increases susceptibility. The mechanism involved in catching a chill is not a popular topic for research, but a start was made when some scientists from Yale University infected some human lung cells with the viruses that cause colds, and they found that when the lung cells were warm, the immune response was better able to fight off the viruses.[94]

A study in Wales compared the rate of colds in people who had their feet severely chilled for twenty minutes with the rate of colds in people who did not have their feet chilled. The participants were not deliberately infected with the viruses that cause colds, they just had normal exposure to whatever germs were floating around in the community at the time. Overall very few of them developed colds, but the rate of colds in the group who had their feet chilled was much higher than the rate in the group whose feet were not chilled. The study authors concluded that, "Acute chilling of the feet causes the onset of common cold symptoms in around 10% of subjects who are chilled."[95] They go on to say, "Further studies are needed to determine the relationship of symptom generation to any respiratory infection." Flu, bronchitis, and pneumonia can be triggered by catching a chill, but we might have to wait a hundred years for any studies to actually investigate what proportion of people are susceptible to being catapulted into these conditions by catching a chill. In the meantime sensible people will protect themselves and their children from sore throats and "ear infections" by wearing scarfs and beanies when they are out in cold weather. Animals can also get sick from catching a chill, and sensible horse owners are careful to not let their horses catch a chill after a hot run. When a chill has been caught the homoeopathic remedy *aconite 30* can nip any consequences in the bud, if it is given early enough. It works with horses too.

I suspect that more than 10% of adults are susceptible to getting a chest infection or earache from a cold wind. Babies and young children are more susceptible to catching a chill than adults, but a trial that subjects babies to cold drafts would be unethical because it is known that cold drafts can make a baby sick. Even people who deny that the phenomenon of catching a chill exists are aware that it would be unethical to subject babies to cold drafts for research purposes. Some people believe that bacterial cystitis can be triggered by chilling, and the matter has been partially investigated[96] but not yet properly studied.[97]

Measles, mumps, rubella, infantum roseola, chicken pox, whooping cough, and slapped cheek roseola cannot be triggered by catching a chill as these diseases do not need the immune system to be suppressed before they take hold of a person. However, catching a chill while you have one of them is a serious matter, and, as I have elaborated elsewhere, can cause complications like bronchitis, pneumonia, and death.

Feelings of nausea are worsened by getting cold, but that is not the same as having the immune system depressed by catching a chill. As a teenager I went on a cruise over the cold, cold sea, and a fellow passenger who had just qualified as a doctor told me that I should wear slacks on deck when it was rough, because having cold legs would make my seasickness worse. He had been taught that at medical school, which surprises me as it is very politically incorrect. I was grateful for the advice because it worked.

"FEED A COLD AND STARVE A FEVER"

This wise old adage is dismissed by pharmaphiles, but in the real world it can be observed that a fever causes loss of appetite, while a person with a cold feels ravenously hungry. While experiencing a fever, children do not want solid food, they want, and need, liquid. During the fever they must take in enough liquid, or else they will dehydrate and can die. At the height of the fever a child might be too floppy to ask for liquid, so offer a drink frequently. One of the consequences of too little liquid intake can be that the body fails to maintain the fever, so the invading germs can take over.

After the fever subsides in a self-resolving childhood disease, the child begins to feel hungry. The more intense the fever has been, the more ravenous the hunger will be. This is the time to feed your child with loads of good wholesome food, not with ice cream and white bread.

THE THEORY THAT THE SELF-RESOLVING CHILDHOOD DISEASES ARE BENEFICIAL

Children take a jump in development during the course of one of these diseases, which is why some people call them the developmental diseases. Sometimes these diseases make a chronic condition suddenly clear up, and reports of this happening have even been published in medical journals. There is an age old theory that a natural dose of one of the self-resolving childhood diseases makes a person less likely to get cancer and other degenerative diseases later in life, and now there is enough research on the matter to state with confidence that the theory is correct.

Numerous German studies have shown that febrile infectious childhood diseases protect against cancer.[98,99,100,101,102] A Swiss study found that each of measles, mumps, rubella, whooping cough, scarlet-fever, and chicken pox were protective against carcinomas, except for breast cancer.[103] An Italian study found that measles, mumps, rubella, chicken pox, whooping cough, and scarlet fever reduced the risk of Hodgkin lymphoma, and that measles also reduced the risk of non-Hodgkin lymphoma.[104] A review of published studies found that measles, mumps, rubella, and chicken pox reduced the risk of cancer in later life, while chronic infections without fever increased the risk of cancer.[105] This review also found that the level of protection against cancer increased with the frequency of acute infections.[105]

Interest in the idea that mumps may protect against ovarian cancer was sparked by a study published in 1966 which found that women with ovarian cancer were significantly less likely to have had mumps, compared to women with benign ovarian cysts.[106] A number of small studies followed, including one that found a significant protective effect from measles and rubella, as well as from mumps.[107] A 2010 review of all available studies on mumps and ovarian cancer found a 19% decrease in the risk of ovarian cancer associated with a history of mumps.[108]

Studies show that natural chicken pox significantly reduces the risk of developing the most common type of malignant brain tumour.[109,110,111,112]

The studies have focused on cancer because of the age old theory about the relationship between childhood diseases and cancer, but now there is evidence that these diseases also protect against heart disease. A study done at a Swedish university hospital found that enterovirus, herpes simplex, and chlamydia pneumonia increased the risk of heart disease in later life,[113] while measles, mumps, rubella, scarlet fever, chicken pox, and glandular fever (infectious mononucleosis) protected against heart disease in later life.[113] The study also found that the greater the number of the self-resolving childhood diseases a person has had, the more they were protected. Two self-resolving childhood diseases reduced the risk by 40%, four by 60%, and six by 90%.[113] So the "bad" diseases increased the risk of heart disease, and the "good" diseases reduced the risk. A Japanese study of 103,000 people found that measles and mumps reduced the risk of heart disease, and having both measles and mumps reduced the risk even more.[114]

A study of fity thousand men found that measles reduced the risk of Parkinson's disease.[115] Apart from cancer, heart disease and Parkinson's, there may be other life-spoiling conditions for which the risk is reduced by having measles or one of the other self-resolving childhood diseases.

Less serious conditions that have also attracted research are allergies, asthma, and eczema. People with a history of chicken pox are less likely to have eczema, asthma, and hayfever,[116,117] but are not less likely to have food allergies.[116] The chicken pox vaccine, however, does not reduce the risk of eczema, asthma, and hayfever.[117] A British study found that children who had a history of measles had a reduced risk of asthma, and it found that for those who had been vaccinated against measles before getting measles, the reduction in the risk was not as great as it was for those who had not been vaccinated before getting measles.[118] This study also found that whooping cough, mumps, and croup increased the risk of allergies.[118] Studies in Turkey, Northwestern Europe, and Guinea-Bissau found that a natural dose of measles reduces the risk of developing allergies,[119,120,121] but a study in Finland found more asthma and eczema in people who had had measles.[122] Clearly further studies on the long-term effects of febrile infectious diseases need to be done in which data about the drugs given to the patients are collected. This would make it possible to differentiate the effects of the drugs on the outcome of the diseases from the actual effects of the diseases. Drugs that suppress fever during the self-resolving childhood diseases are only one type of drug that might sabotage the long-term benefits of the diseases.

A big study in Tasmania that was started in 1964 and followed participants into middle age found that rubella, mumps, and chicken pox protected against asthma for decades, but measles and whooping cough protected against asthma only during childhood.[123] This study found that childhood pneumonia increased the risk of asthma, but when the effects of pneumonia were lumped in with the effects of the other diseases, there was an overall benefit.[123]

The positive results of all of these studies suggest that similar outcomes might be found if the relationship between the self-resolving diseases and other chronic conditions were to be studied.

The other side of the coin is that these diseases can cause pre-existing chronic diseases to clear up. The effect of a self-resolving childhood disease is quite striking when it clears up a chronic condition that already exists. I know a little boy who suffered from eczema from birth, but it cleared up completely, never to return, when he got chicken pox. It was an intense case of chicken pox, with his whole body covered in pustules. When the chicken pox pustules went away, the eczema had gone too, and it never came back. The doctor had prescribed Zovirax for the chicken pox to make it "a lighter case", but his mother had not given it to him because she had looked up Zovirax on a medical site, and found that it should only be given to the elderly, or to people with compromised immune systems, and should not be given otherwise. No wonder BigPharma hates the internet.

Reports of measles making psoriasis clear up have been published in medical journals.[124,125,126,127,128]

There is a published report of chicken pox curing rheumatoid arthritis in a 65-year-old man,[129] and one of it curing a seven-year-old girl who had juvenile rheumatoid arthritis.[130]

People who have cancer are sometimes cured or put into temporary remission by catching measles,[131,132] and the same has happened with rubella.[131] It has also been observed that paediatric nephrotic syndrome can be cured or sent into remission by deliberately infecting children with measles,[133,134] as well as by a natural dose of measles[135] and by natural chicken pox.[136]

Measles sometimes cures Hodgkin lymphoma (a type of cancer), and sometimes makes it go into lengthy remission.[137,138,139,140] Burkitt's lymphoma is another type of cancer that has gone away because of measles.[141,142]

If you can access the Lancet of 1971, you can take a look at photos of a little boy who was rapidly cured of cancer when he caught measles in hospital. The first photo shows him with a tumour over and around his right eye. In the second photo he is spotty with measles rash and the tumour is already smaller. In the third photo the measles is over and the tumour is gone. Four months later when the article was written the boy was still "in complete remission", having had no cancer treatment.[142]

Some types of cancer are more amenable to being cured by measles than others. Not all people who have cancer react in the same way when they catch measles;

* Some survive the measles, although they may die later from the cancer.

* Others die right away because the cancer, or the cancer treatment, makes them unable to cope with measles.

* Others are cured of cancer by having measles.

Some people believe that measles is a process of elimination. At present there is no research on the matter, so the idea has neither been supported nor refuted. A child with measles begins to smell absolutely terrible when the rash appears. The putrid smell is strong enough to be noticeable from an adjacent room. Some people speculate that the smell is caused by something unwanted being eliminated from the child's body.

After the measles virus enters the body through the mucous membranes, it travels around and multiplies in the lymph system.[143] When it moves from one cell to another it does so by breaking through the cell walls and temporarily making two cells into a big cell.[143] This phase lasts 10 to 14 days, and although it is not obvious that the child has measles, an observant parent will notice that the child's behaviour is different. Some of the measles viruses get broken up while others remain intact.[143] At the end of the incubation phase, the viruses move into the blood, Koplik spots appear in the mouth, and other types of spots also appear on the mucous membranes.[143] After 1 or 2 more days the typical measles rash appears on the skin.[143] Antibodies begin to appear in the blood at this time if they are going to appear at all,[143] and the measles viruses move from the blood to the skin, where they can be found in large numbers during the first 4 days of the rash.[144] The number of viruses in the skin decreases, and then they disappear completely before the rash fades.[144]

None of this explains the horrible smell that comes out of the skin. So the issue of whether the process of measles actually benefits the cells of the human body remains unresolved, until more research is conducted into what the virus is doing as it passes through the different types of cells.

Unless the patient was severely malnourished before the measles started, the measles virus is gone from the body 12 days after the rash first appeared.[145] In some well-nourished individuals the measles virus is not eliminated from the body, and it goes on to cause chronic diseases like SSPE or Crohn's. When the measles virus is injected directly into the blood stream, as in the case of measles vaccination, it does not undergo that first 10 to 14 days of being processed by the immune system in the lymph glands. SSPE and related disintegrative disorders are more common after measles vaccine than after measles,[146] and Crohn's is hugely more common after the vaccine than after the disease.[6] The mode of entry of the virus is a possible reason.

When the acute phase of measles is over, the child becomes ravenously hungry, with a particular need for protein. Lots of good wholesome food is needed to fuel the growth spurt that follows measles.

Children undergo a jump in maturation during the course of a self-resolving childhood disease. The fact that these diseases cannot be prevented by good nutrition strongly implies that nature considers the self-resolving childhood diseases to be beneficial.

Despite the lack of research, the idea that measles strengthens the immune system of an already healthy person is a widely held belief. The Pharmacy Guild of New Zealand said on a promotional flyer in 1989,

> "...common infections like measles and chicken pox are still around. These childhood diseases help build up immunity to fight off infections in later life."[147]

I was startled to see this opinion emanating from such a source, so I wrote to them and asked them how they knew. They backed off and said they had not meant it.

Here are some comments made by parents about their subjective observations of the effects of measles, rubella, or chicken pox, "He seemed to become more solid in himself," "Might be age-related, but it seems there was a spurt in development," "There was something more tangible about his personality," "She seems to have come on so quickly, understanding what I say more, being independent, and standing up herself," "When he came out of the fever he had lots more words and better sentences. How did that happen?" "It makes me wonder, when you consider that these diseases cause a jump in development, and that vaccines made from these germs sometimes cause developmental regression, whether the regression is actually the vaccine doing the opposite of what a natural dose does, and not simply a result of neurological insult."

My daughter Chandra had measles when she was three years old. She baked with an intensive fever for two and a half days, but her temperature did not remain constant. It peaked and dipped, sometimes being very high, sometimes being low. I did not measure the level it reached at any stage, because I knew that the actual temperature was irrelevant to her well-being. However, out of curiosity, I now wish that I had measured how high it went when it peaked. When she emerged from the fever on day three she was markedly different. Her sense of humour had changed. It was still childish, but different. She no longer wanted to sleep in our bed, which was a great relief because she had been an awfully wriggly bedfellow. The sound of her cry had changed too, and it took me a while to become familiar with the new sound. Two weeks after the acute phase, while she was still recuperating, four mothers and their youngsters came round for morning tea. The children were playing in her room, and each time someone started crying, I would have to get up to see if it was Chandra. It is very strange for a mother not to recognise the sound of her own child's cry, but it took me a while to become familiar with the new sound. She also ate voraciously, and she blossomed in many ways that are not easy to measure.

She had caught measles from her three-year-old friend Reuben. One day he asked his mother, "Was it Chandi's birthday?"

"No," said his mother.

"Then why did I give her measles?" he asked.

In a way, it really was a gift.

"BUT CHILDREN DIE OF MEASLES"

Before measles vaccine was introduced in Britain the death rate from measles was one in 5000,[1] but in some affluent countries the death rate from measles goes as high as 1 in 2000. The latter statistic is used to promote vaccination, but the public are not told the full facts. A child only dies of measles if he or she;

* had a serious underlying condition before catching measles, or
* suffers from severe calorie/protein deficiency, or
* is accidentally or deliberately chilled while having measles, or
* is given drugs to suppress the fever.

Doctors and nurses are taught during their training that a child with measles should be chilled and given drugs to suppress the fever. Parents of children with measles are advised to chill their children and administer fever-suppressing drugs. Both the chilling and the drugs are harmful for a child with measles. Chilling carries the risk of causing pneumonia, while fever-suppressing drugs inhibit the work of the immune system.[70,148,149,150,151,152,153] Pneumonia is a complication of measles, not a symptom of measles, but if a child dies of this complication, it is said that he or she died of measles, not of pneumonia.

Fever-suppressing drugs have a direct effect on the cells of the immune system, paralysing them so that they cannot do what they are designed to do.[70,148,149,150,151,152,153] A patient with a fever who is given one of these drugs is harmed in two ways. The patient suffers because the drug inhibits the immune system, and then on top of that, the patient suffers because of the lack of fever. I have explained above how fever is part of the body's defence mechanism, and how a patient without fever is more likely to die from an infectious disease. Modern medicine kills countless people who are struggling against infectious diseases by sabotaging the body's natural defence mechanisms. It is not only people with measles who get killed by not being kept warm enough and by being given inappropriate drugs.

In impoverished communities the death rate from measles is higher than 1 in 2000. In severely malnourished children the symptoms of measles are different to the symptoms of classical measles, and the risk of death is higher. Vaccine defenders often say that people whose ancestors are not European are particularly susceptible to dying from measles, but this is not true. High susceptibility to death from measles is not genetically determined;[154] it is determined by poverty.[154]

In 1984 the measles virus became virulent in New Zealand, and two children died during the ensuing epidemic. This was used to terrify parents in both New Zealand and Australia. The scaremongers did not mention that both the children had terminal illnesses before they caught measles, and one of them was "fully immunized".[155]

The next measles epidemic in New Zealand, which occurred in 1992, had been in progress for three months before a child died. As soon as the death happened, the propaganda machine swung into action. After the death toll reached 3, there was a correction, and the official number of deaths went back to 2. Then it rose again to 4. On the day that death number 3 was revoked, I spoke to a chiropractor who lived in the town where the death had occurred. He said that the child had been vaccinated against measles, and when the medics discovered this, they decided to change the cause of death. I was on the committee of a consumer group called the Immunisation Awareness Society (IAS), and we monitored the situation as closely as we could. Although the health department's pre-planned propaganda campaign only lasted a week, for the next few months the media kept repeating that "four babies" had died of measles because not enough children had been vaccinated.

While the epidemic was still in progress, a health magazine published an article[156] that I wrote about measles, in which I predicted that the authorities would never let the full facts about these measles deaths be published. It was a safe prediction. The only thing that the official report let slip was that one of the "babies" that died was 12 years old. A member of IAS wrote to the 12-year-old's general practitioner and asked about the circumstances of the death. He replied, "My case was a very rare complication of measles and unlikely to happen again." He did not say whether or not the child had been vaccinated. A nurse who worked in the Wellington hospital where one of the babies died told us that the baby had been hospitalised for pneumonia, and had caught measles in hospital. So that is two out of the four that we managed to confirm as not having just upped and died of measles. I am sure that if our spy network had been good enough, we would have learned similar facts about the other two.

IAS wrote to the Ministry of Health and asked;

* whether the children who died of measles were old enough to have

been vaccinated,

* whether they had any underlying health problems prior to contracting measles,

* and what their vaccination status was.

They refused to supply the information, although it was illegal for them to withhold it.

In November 2012, a measles outbreak started in Britain. Five months into the outbreak a 25-year-old man who had measles died from pneumonia. The unfortunate man had all the risk factors for dying while he had measles; he was an adult, not a child, he had two serious chronic diseases before he caught measles, he was severely malnourished (which is unusual in Britain), and he had the complication of pneumonia. On top of all this he had been advised to take paracetamol/tylenol. The day before he died his mother had taken him to a medical centre because he had a measles rash, a high fever, an infected chest, and he found it difficult to stand up. Even though there was hysteria in the community about measles, it did not occur to the three GPs who examined him that he might have measles and that his chest infection might be pneumonia. They told his mother to take him home and give him paracetamol/tylenol, which she did, and he died during the night. Because he was an unhealthy person he might have died from the pneumonia without the extra burden of paracetamol/tylenol, but it did not help that the paracetamol/tylenol crippled his immune system, and made him less able to fight the pneumonia. If he had been put in a hospital bed with an electrolyte drip, been given an antibiotic for the pneumonia, and been given vitamin A because he was severely malnourished, he would have had a good chance of survival, even though they would have given him paracetamol/tylenol as well. The official cause of death was given as pneumonia. Medicrats used the poor man's death to create fear about measles and to promote MMR vaccine. They failed to mention the factors that led to his death, and that the official cause of death was pneumonia. Naturally the doctors whose negligence resulted in the man's death were not made accountable.

In New Zealand I sometimes had the opportunity to speak about vaccination to groups of Public Health nurses. When Chandra was ten years old I took her with me to one of these lectures, because she had the flu and was off school. The flu was well under control because she had already been in bed for a few days, and she had been having organic lemon and honey drinks, and lots of vitamin C. I knew that taking her with me to the lecture would not cause a relapse, because she would go from a warm house to a warm car to a warm lecture theatre. She had caught the flu by playing netball in the rain, then walking home in a cold wind, at a time when a nasty flu virus was felling people. If there had been a polio virus in the air, I would have been more conscientious and forbidden her to play netball that day, despite the negative social consequences that such an action would have provoked.

When we got to the lecture theatre I settled her down at a desk in the front corner with her art gear. She got busy producing works of art, but her ears were listening to the goings-on in the room. One of the nurses said that she was not sick and she should be at school. Others nodded. They are clueless about how to prevent an infection from turning into a serious illness. There were quite a few aggressive ladies in this group and they were angered by almost everything I said. When I said that TB is caused by wrong nutrition and damp housing, they all started barking that TB is caused by immigrants. This was in line with a campaign that was being waged against immigrants in the newspaper at the time.

When I said that suburban children do not die of measles unless there is something else wrong with them, one of the ladies tried to refute it by telling the story of a child she had nursed who had died of measles. "He was a perfectly healthy child. There was nothing wrong with him. And I so clearly remember, I was feeding him jelly and ice cream just before my shift ended. He had to be fed because he was on a ventilator because he had bronchitis. The next morning I heard on the radio that he had died."

A loud whisper came from the art factory in the corner, "Mommy, Mommy. Jelly and ice cream, jelly and ice cream." Chandra was concerned that I may not have noticed that the nurse had said that she had been force-feeding the child with substances that worsen bronchitis. Not only do the ingredients in jelly and ice cream increase the amount of mucus in the lungs, but they also suppress the immune system.[157] (Jelly is known as jello in North America.)

I told the nurses why Chandra was pointing out the mention of jelly and ice cream, and a hubbub ensued. One nurse called out scathingly, "So are you saying that (name) caused the child's death by giving him jelly and ice cream?"

"Yes," I replied, "It certainly contributed to the death, and probably caused it." The hubbub turned into a near riot.

This gathering was Chandra's first experience of that type of mass hostility, and all the irrationality that goes with it. On the way home in the car she talked energetically about the nurses, and one of the questions she fired at me was, "Why do they think that someone with bronchitis is perfectly healthy?" I have to leave it to the psychologists to answer that one, but I am grateful to the nurse for speaking up, because she proved my point beautifully.

SICK CHILDREN NEED PROPER CARE

A child who is sick needs to get enough rest and needs to be cared for by an adult until he or she has fully recovered. This might seem like an obvious statement, but many modern parents have been groomed to believe that if a sick child is given the right drug, the child can carry on with his or her usual routine. It can be difficult for a parent to stay at home and look after a sick child if there is a risk of getting fired or losing crucial income, but in those circumstances it would be ideal if a trusted caregiver could be at the home of the child during work hours.

Health departments distribute pro-pharmaceutical propaganda to parents, instead of teaching them how to bring their children safely through colds, flu, and the self-resolving childhood diseases. The people who work for health departments are unable to give the right advice because they have been trained in the pharmaceutical model, and they do not know how to treat the self-resolving childhood diseases safely.

A child who has a fever because of flu or a self-resolving childhood disease needs to be lying down, and needs to be kept warm. If the fever is caused by a dangerous infectious disease, medical or homoeopathic intervention is needed, and the child must not catch a chill or become exhausted in the process of acquiring that intervention. Most importantly, the child must not be given a drug to suppress the fever, nor be cooled down with water or a draught.

The way that modern medicine treats the self-resolving childhood diseases increases the risk of complications and death. Drugs that cripple the immune system are given to bring down the fever, and chilling is recommended when the child actually needs to be wrapped up warmly. The need for bed rest and a quiet environment is not emphasised, and food is forced on a child during the acute phase of the illness, instead of waiting until the hungry phase of convalescence. The need for a period of convalescence is not even recognised. In short, they have got it all wrong. Some doctors have enough common sense not to do these things, but they are few and far between.

Suppressing fever is one of the most dangerous things that orthodox medicine does, which is why I have explained the function of fever in such detail in the section called "Fever is a Friend." If a child with measles is not kept warm and in bed it can result in the development of bronchitis, pneumonia, ear infections, or encephalitis. The last two can end up as deafness or brain damage. Mumps can also result in brain damage and deafness if the child is allowed to run around, and it can damage the pancreas and cause sterility in a person past puberty. Scarlet fever can damage the kidneys and the heart, and chicken pox can end in brain damage if the patient is not kept quiet during the few days of acute disease.

If the patient with a self-resolving childhood disease is a teenager or an adult, the danger of complications is greater. It can be very difficult to make a teenager or adult who feels driven by responsibility stay in bed during the acute phase, and to take it easy during convalescence. School and sporting commitments can put as much pressure on a teenager as earning a living or caring for children puts on an adult. Like adults, teenagers are at risk of wanting to get up and carry on with their usual routine, instead of resting while they are sick. During the winter months the radio and TV broadcast adverts for drugs that partially suppress the symptoms of colds and flu. The adverts advise people to take these drugs so that they can carry on with their family obligations and business affairs. When people die from following that advice, their families cannot sue the drug manufacturers, because there is no accountability.

Sick children should not be bombarded with stimulation. If they are lolling about it does not mean that they are bored, it means that they need to rest. Teenagers who are normally addicted to pop music do not want it on when they have measles. When they start wanting the beat again, it shows that they are returning to normal. A child should not be sent back to school as soon as he or she is "well enough to cope". The concept of convalescence has almost disappeared from modern society. Getting a child "right" in as short a time as possible is perceived as a great achievement, but it is not good for the child.

One day when I was helping at the afternoon session of a kindergarten there was a little boy flopping about instead of playing. The teacher telephoned his mother and told her to collect him. When the mother arrived she told us that the boy had had a fever in the morning, and she had given him paracetamol/tylenol at lunch time so that he could come to kindergarten. After she had left another mother expressed her anger to me, saying that the woman did not care about her child, and had sent him to kindergarten just to get rid of him for a few hours. I happen to know that that mother cares very much for her child, and it is just ignorance that made her do that. Fortunately the fever was not the beginning of anything serious, or the child would have been in trouble.

Ignorance about fever caused some friends of mine to take their son who had measles out to see fireworks on a very cold night. He had a convulsion at 9 pm, supposedly from the coldness of the water he had been given to drink down his next dose of paracetamol/tylenol. It flabbergasts me to think that parents will take a feverish child out into the open on a cold night, but I have to remember that if circumstances had not led me to research vaccination, I might have done the same.

A child with a fever does not interact with parents or caregivers in the usual way, but is nevertheless aware of the caregiver's presence. As well as providing a sense of security for the child, it is good to have someone keeping a close eye on a patient with a self-resolving childhood disease, so that if any symptoms that are not a normal part of the disease show up, quick action can be taken to prevent them from developing into serious complications like pneumonia or encephalitis. A fever should also be watched in case it is the beginning of something serious. Diseases like polio, diphtheria, and meningococcal meningitis can start off looking quite innocuous at first, and if they are allowed to progress too far before intervention begins, the outcome can be grim.

Self-resolving childhood diseases do not need intervention, they just need to be endured. However, they do need to be endured in the right way, or else they can develop complications. Complications need intervention, but the diseases themselves do not. Some people use homoeopathic remedies to shorten the self-resolving childhood diseases. This is not wise. People who have measles, but do not have it in full, are more likely to suffer chronic disease in later life.[158] It is appropriate to use homoeopathy to treat any complications that develop, but it is not right to use homoeopathy nor any other means to stop the natural process of the self-resolving childhood disease. Homoeopathy is also appropriate when a self-resolving childhood disease does not finish off properly, for example when a child is chesty every winter after whooping cough, or when chicken pox re-emerges as shingles.

If someone is in danger of dying from an infectious disease, the first intervention should be injections of vitamin C.[159,160,161] Dr. Archie Kalokerinos has intervened with vitamin C injections to save the lives of children in Australia.[159,160,161] He has tried to educate the medical establishment, but they do not want to know. He has met with vilification and even persecution. One night I mentioned Archie's work to a group of nurses in Auckland, and one of them turned on me with a vicious character assassination of Archie. Why does a nurse in New Zealand feel so threatened by a doctor who is saving children's lives in the Australian outback? Archie published *Every Second Child* in 1974. Hundreds of thousands of babies and children have died unnecessarily since then because the medical establishment is too arrogant to use his discovery.

CARING FOR A CHILD WITH:

INFANTUM ROSEOLA

This disease only happens during the first three years of life, and usually during the first year, if it happens at all. The symptoms are fever and a rash that looks like the measles rash.[162] Some people call it "baby measles," and some doctors misdiagnose it as measles, which makes the parents think the child is getting measles for a second time when he or she actually does get measles. Some doctors are unaware that infantum roseola exists. The virus that causes roseola is called HHV-6. When a vaccine containing this virus has been manufactured we will start hearing that infantum roseola is a dangerous disease that needs to be prevented.

Some babies develop a high fever when they have roseola, while others experience a fever so low that the roseola is only noticed once the rash appears. The fever starts before the rash, and usually the rash only appears when the fever is ending. Sometimes there is a gap of a whole day between the fever and the rash. The baby needs to be kept warm and quiet until the symptoms have gone. If you have to go out, wrap the baby very warmly for the excursion and protect the face from the wind. Frequent breast-feeds or another source of liquid is all that is needed for nourishment during the fever stage. If the baby has already started on solids, give no solids while the fever is present.

This illness should be allowed to run its course and resolve itself with no medical, herbal, homoeopathic, or vitamin interventions. Using any means to suppress fever is not helpful, as explained in the section on fever. The disease will end by itself, but care must be taken for the child to not catch a chill and not get overtired.

MEASLES

Measles is a disease that must be treated with respect. Complications like bronchitis, pneumonia, encephalitis, ear infections, blindness, and death can occur when a child with measles does not receive proper care. The child must be kept exceptionally warm during the middle stage of measles, and must not be expected to follow his or her normal routine during any stage. While it is wrong to try to prevent measles either by vaccination or by homoeopathic means, it is important to prevent complications. No medication is necessary for the prevention of complications; proper care is enough. Suppressing fever with drugs increases the risk of complications, and deliberately chilling the child is extremely dangerous. The use of an inappropriate homoeopathic remedy can also cause problems.

It is important for parents to know the difference between the symptoms of measles and the symptoms of the complications of measles. Classical measles in an unvaccinated person has the symptoms of fever, a putrid smell, red puffy eyes, a skin rash that starts as separate dots and then becomes mottled, a shallow cough, eye sensitivity, and extreme tiredness. Too often parents who do not know what to expect from measles get a shock when this happens to their child, and they rush off to hospital, where the staff sometimes cause complications by chilling the child and giving drugs that suppress fever.

Classical measles has three stages. First there is the incubation period when the disease is brewing. Then there is the acute phase when the child has a fever and needs to be tucked up in bed. After that there is the convalescent phase when the child can get out of bed to play but still needs a lot of rest. Getting it right during the convalescent phase is just as important as getting it right during the acute phase. When a person who has been vaccinated against measles gets measles, the symptoms are not the same as classical measles, and they are certainly not "milder". Measles in a vaccinated person is called "atypical measles", and it manifests in a variety of ways which I will discuss further on. Individuals who are severely malnourished when they get measles also experience symptoms that are different to classical measles. This is called "severe measles", although the term "severe measles" is also used by some medical people when referring to measles with complications.

The first indication that a child is infected with the measles virus is that he or she starts to grizzle and becomes clingy. While the child is still grumpy there will be a faint smell of putrefaction, which can go unnoticed. Then the nose becomes runny, there is a shallow but persistent cough, a red rim develops around the eyes, and the child is generally "watery." Most children are still miserable towards the end of this phase, but some become cheerful. They begin to lose their appetite during this phase, and they have almost no appetite during the next phase, which is the acute phase.

Fever and rash are the main features of the acute phase. Usually the fevers start before the rash appears, but sometimes the two start together. As soon as there is the first fever the child will need to lie down and be covered with warm bedding. At first the rash consists of small red dots on

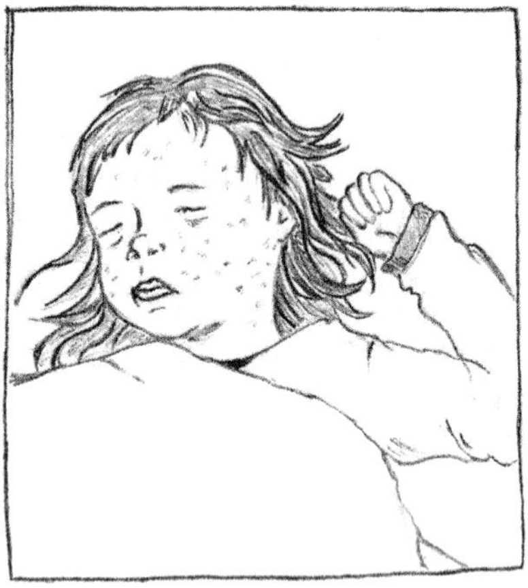

Chandra with measles.

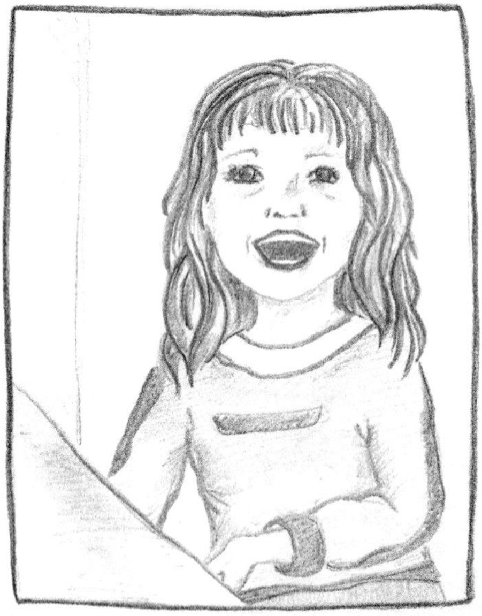

Chandra one month after measles.

the face and then the tummy. The whites of the eyes become reddish, the face becomes puffy, the eyelids swell, and the putrid smell becomes stronger. The eyes become sensitive to light, but in babies the sensitivity is usually milder than in children. White flecks called Koplik spots make a brief appearance inside the mouth.[163] The Koplik spots help to differentiate measles from rubella. The trouble with Koplik spots is that they are difficult to see if the child is not co-operative, and they vanish quickly. Their presence confirms measles, but their absence does not exclude it. With rubella, glands behind the ears and at the back of the neck swell up, which does not happen with measles. The rash of measles is darker than that of rubella. Measles rash spreads from the face downwards, and changes from small red spots to big mottled blotches. The spots on the feet are the last to fade. In atypical measles the rash might start on the hands and feet and move inwards and upwards, and it might be slightly raised, and it can even haemorrhage. Haemorrhaging of the rash often occurs in severely malnourished children.

The only demands that a child with a high fever will make will be for water, juice, and fruit, or for breast-milk if he or she is still suckling. Don't try to force the child to eat normal food. Keep offering liquid. Non-acidic tropical fruits are good if they are ripe, otherwise try tomatoes or cucumber, or just stick to water. Many children like to drink warm water with a teaspoon of honey dissolved in it. It is preferable to use honey from an organic source, which has not been filtered or heated before bottling. The child will instinctively know how much food to eat, so don't try to persuade him or her to eat more than he or she wants. Do keep offering a drink though, because often the child is too tired to ask for one. Get a good supply of protein and whole foods ready for the convalescent phase, because once the fever phase is over the child will have a voracious appetite.

During measles the fever can become very high, and it comes and goes over a period of about three days, sometimes longer. It is crucial that the child be kept exceptionally warm during the fever stage. Warm does not mean hot. Great care must be taken to ensure that he or she does not catch a chill. A cold draught that lasts for three minutes can start the patient down the slippery slope of bronchitis, ear infections, and pneumonia. It is often difficult for caregivers to focus attention on preventing draughts because an adult who feels fit and well does not notice the movement of air. Even just walking barefoot over a cold floor to the bathroom can make a child with measles catch a chill, which enables the germs that cause bronchitis and pneumonia to take advantage of the vulnerability of the child.

Once the fever sets in, the horrid smell of measles becomes strong, and parents feel tempted to wash the child. They often convince themselves that the child would be more comfortable if he or she were washed, when it is really the parents' hang up about the anti-social smell that motivates the bath. Some people consider it a social disgrace to skip bathing for three days, but there is no need to bath the child. The neighbours won't know, so don't run the risk of complications. The smell will go away of its own accord. When Chandra had measles I took photos of her spotty face, and I wanted to take a photo of her tummy because it looked so funny with the rash, but I refrained. With those old non-digital cameras it took about a minute to organise a photo in a dark room, and having her tummy uncovered for that length of time would have run the risk of her catching a chill.

Medical doctors and nurses are taught to scorn the concept of catching a chill. Chills lead to pneumonia, and pneumonia is the most common cause of death with measles.[164,163]

The conventional medical treatment of measles is antibiotics and drugs that suppress fever. The antibiotics reduce the risk of bronchitis and pneumonia, while the drugs that suppress fever reduce the effectiveness of the antibiotics. In some hospitals the staff try to force-feed children who have measles, and they strip them and blow cold air at them. Most doctors and nurses do not understand the difference between the symptoms of measles and the symptoms of the complications of measles. Newspaper articles that scaremonger about measles sometimes mention IV drips and multiple injections for children who are in hospital with measles.

Well meaning people who want to "cure" measles will proudly tell you that if you give high doses of vitamin C, the eyes will stop being red and watery, the shallow cough will disappear, the bouts of fever will stop, and the rash will not develop. This intervention leaves the patient vulnerable to measles during adulthood,[143] and increases the risk of chronic diseases like cancer in later life.[103,104,105,158]

The intensity of light must be drastically reduced to protect the eyes of a child with measles. If the curtains are thin, pin a blanket or dark cloth onto them so that more light is excluded. You can also stick brown paper over the windowpanes as well as closing the curtains. When Kenny had measles he was in our room, and we left the brown paper on the small side windows for a long time afterwards because it gave the room a nice hue.

Once the fever phase is over the child becomes extremely hungry. This is because measles is always followed by a period of rapid growth. The child will instinctively want to eat lots of protein. Measles causes a sudden halt in growth, which is followed by rapid catch up growth.[166] Children who do not get enough protein and calories during the convalescent phase never grow to the full size of their genetic potential.[167] In impoverished communities the children who survive measles, but do not have sufficient food available during the convalescent phase, never grow to their correct height.[167] Many children in impoverished countries die during the convalescent phase of measles because of insufficient food during this time of increased need.

When the fever subsides the child wants to get up and play. Convalescence is a difficult phase to manage because it is necessary to strike a balance between the child's desire for activity and need for rest. The immune system is suppressed for quite a few weeks after measles, so parents must be vigilant that the child does not catch a chill while playing out of bed. He or she wants entertainment and food, but gets tired easily, and needs a quiet lifestyle for at least two weeks. Warm clothing is essential during this phase, and the child must not play outside unless the air is warm and still. Medical folklore still promotes the idea that "fresh air" is good for measles. Even if you live in the tropics, "fresh air" can be exactly the thing that starts bronchitis or pneumonia. Also, a slight wind can bring on earache, which is very painful. Followers of pharmaceutical medicine believe that germs are the sole cause of earache, so they see no reason why a child with a suppressed immune system should not play outside on a cold, windy day. Armed with the knowledge about the danger from chills, use your discretion in regards to playing outside.

For centuries it was observed that measles makes children susceptible to secondary infections, and the first attempt at trying to find out why was published in 1908.[168] Despite much research it is still not known exactly what the immune system is doing during measles.[169] It is known that during the three weeks after the rash appears, NK lymphocytes become greatly reduced in the blood, and the few that remain become less active.[170] Other aspects of the immune system are also depressed for several weeks after infection.[169] The observable changes in the immune system have been shown to be clinically significant.[164,163] Pharmaceutical medicine fails to acknowledge that when this lowered immunity is combined with a deficiency of warmth, the person becomes even more vulnerable to germs.

The eyes usually remain sensitive to light for a week after the fever subsides, but sensitivity can last for up to five weeks. When Chandra had moved out of the fever stage my uncle showed her how to make a doily. That started an epidemic of doily making. We closed all the curtains so that she could move about the house, and in every room there grew a pyramid of doilies that had been cut from discarded print-out paper. She did not want us to throw away a single precious piece, not even the bits that had been cut out to make the patterns. Whenever I think of measles, I think of a pyramid of paper in every room. It was an ideal activity to keep her busy indoors. Her little brother is not so keen on art and crafts, so we had to entertain him during his convalescence from measles.

The modern tendency is to send children back to kindergarten or school as soon as they can no longer infect other children. That is very unwise because the child is not given an opportunity to recuperate. Children remain sensitive to noise for about two weeks, and they suffer pain from sounds that are a normal part of a kindergarten or classroom. Remember that the immune system is suppressed for at least three weeks after the rash appears.[169,170] For hundreds of years nothing was known about what the immune system was doing during measles, but it was known that it was foolhardy to force children back into their usual routine before they had finished recuperating from measles.

It is unwise to use a homoeopathic remedy to try to "cure" measles. People who want you to get rid of measles as soon as it appears might tell you to use potentised *pulsatilla*, because *pulsatilla* fits the symptoms of redness of the eyes, clinginess, lethargy, and melancholy in a person who is normally cheerful. This advice comes from people who do not understand that these are normal symptoms of measles, and are part of a process that should be left alone to resolve itself. The famous Cape Town homoeopath, Dr. Jimmy Jones, told me that giving *morbillinum*, which is the potentised measles virus, to a child with measles, can cause seizures. Don't do it.

If you know the remedies well, or if you have someone who can prescribe for you, it is alright to use a remedy to prevent complications. For instance, in a child who tends to be chesty, *drosera 30* could prevent bronchitis, without aborting the measles. If the rash takes too long to appear, or does not develop into a proper measles rash, *bryonia 30* can help it blossom and get it over with. If chest, eye, or ear complications develop, call in a homoeopath to rectify the situation. The homoeopath should visit the child at home. A homoeopath who expects a child with measles to be taken out of bed has little experience of measles. The same cannot be said for a pharmaceutical doctor who expects a child with measles to be taken to a clinic. Doctors have lots of experience of children with measles, but they consider it "normal" for a child with measles to have complications.

These days it is fashionable in some circles to say that children with measles should be given vitamin A, but think carefully before you follow that advice. Vitamin A supplementation is a life saver when children who are severely malnourished get measles. Vitamin A deficiency is common in impoverished communities where the people do not have fats and nutritious vegetables in their diet. The water supply in these communities is often contaminated with diarrhoea-causing bacteria. When children in these communities get measles, many of them die from the complications of pneumonia or diarrhoea. Studies have been done which show that it is beneficial to give vitamin A supplements to severely malnourished children when they have measles, especially if they are less than two years old.[171,172,173] The World Health Organisation recommends that two doses of 200,000 IU of vitamin A should be given to every severely malnourished child with measles, and when this recommendation is followed, it does reduce the death rate.[174,175,176] This does not automatically mean that a child who is *not* severely malnourished should be given vitamin A when he or she has measles. Under normal circumstances vitamin A only becomes toxic in huge doses, but a child who has measles can get sick from a dose that is much lower than the toxic dose.[177,178] A little too much vitamin A can cause headache, nausea, and vomiting,[177,178] which causes unnecessary stress for a child with measles. Any kind of vitamin A or fish oil will cause insomnia in a person with or without measles if too much is given, even if it is only slightly too much. Also the correct dose can cause insomnia if it is given after midmorning. Children need to be able to sleep when they have measles. If you think that your child has a deficiency of vitamin A, don't wait until measles comes along before you do something about it.

Measles is inconvenient for parents because the child needs a lot of attention during the acute phase, and needs surveillance for about two weeks afterwards. The glib solution is to vaccinate to prevent measles. However, vaccination is no guarantee that measles will not occur during childhood, and it makes measles more likely to happen after childhood. The adverse effects of measles vaccine can also result in a child needing special care for the rest of his or her life. That is far more inconvenient than having a child out of school for two or three weeks. Teenagers and adults with measles need the same intensity of care as a child with measles.

Measles is not a disease to be feared if it is properly managed. Watch how your child takes a jump in physical and emotional development after measles. Remember that the fever is part of the immune system's response to help fight the germs. Don't give any drug, homoeopathic remedy, or herbal remedy to reduce the fever. Don't wipe the child down with cold water. Keep the child warm and cosy.

MUMPS

Do not underestimate the potential of mumps to cause long-term damage. A child with mumps must stay indoors and get a lot of rest to avoid complications. An adult with mumps is even more vulnerable to complications. Mumps affects the salivary glands so that the jowls swell up and the person looks hilarious. The virus can also cause inflammation in the pancreas, the ovaries, the testicles, the brain, and the ears. Consequently, diabetes, sterility, brain damage, or deafness can result from improper care of a person with mumps.

By affecting the pancreas, the virus can cause diabetes. This was first documented in 1899.[179] The ovaries and testicles cannot be damaged in a person who has not yet reached puberty, which is one good reason for getting mumps over with in childhood. An adult male is the most vulnerable to mumps, which is a problem because some men find it difficult to rest in bed for a few days. While trying to persuade me that vaccinating my children against mumps would be a good idea, a neighbour told me about a famous New Zealand athlete who developed encephalitis from mumps, and was left partially paralysed. When I pressed him for details, it emerged that the athlete had run a race while the mumps was acute. Once upon a time people knew that they must not run a race when they have mumps. An old-fashioned medical book states,

> The testicles are swollen, painful and very tender. When the inflammation subsides, it may be found that the patient has been made sterile. This is especially liable to happen if he has not taken proper care of himself during the acute stage of the inflammation.[180]

Vaccination increases the risk of sterility, because it makes people get mumps when they are older.

Much of the scaremongering about mumps focuses on the fact that mumps can cause deafness. It would be helpful if proper records were kept so that we could find out whether the use of fever-suppressing drugs increases the risk of deafness. The vaccine promoters also say that there is a high incidence of encephalitis with mumps, without mentioning that this can be avoided with proper care. When MMR vaccine replaced measles vaccine in New Zealand, a medical bigwig said on the TV that mumps needed to be prevented because it causes encephalitis in one in seven cases. We wrote to him repeatedly asking for the reference, and eventually he admitted that what he had said was not true. The person who told this lie on New Zealand TV is now a high ranking vaccine promoter with the World Health Organisation.

The swelling of the jowls can be very painful, but the pain can be reduced by applying heat or cold to the swollen area. Trial and error will show whether a particular child is helped by cooling or warming of the jowls. The tinctures or oils of *arnica*, *calendula,* and *hypericum* (*St John's Wort*) reduce the pain of swollen jowls. These are extracted from European plants, and conveniently bottled for worldwide distribution, but nature has provided every continent with plants that can be used for the purpose. It is just a matter of knowing which they are. The tinctures and oils are for external application, not for swallowing. Any medication must be applied gently, as too much pressure will cause pain.

Children with mumps should be fed according to their appetite, not according to how much they usually eat. The fever is not as intense as it is with measles, but they will have no appetite while fever is present. All food should be liquidized because chewing is painful.

Although children with mumps do not look very sick once the fever phase is over, be careful. Keep them inside, keep them warm, and keep them quiet. They need to recuperate.

RUBELLA

Rubella is usually less intense than measles or mumps. The fevers are usually not very high and do not last very long, but while fevers are coming and going, the child must be kept warm and in bed. After the fevers stop coming, the child needs to lead a quiet life for a few days. He or she can safely get out of bed for some of the day, and can even play at another child's house if the mother is not pregnant. Avoid sudden changes in temperature, like going from a warm car into a place that is air-conditioned. Going to the supermarket is a bad idea for the sake of the child as well as the sake of the public. Pregnant women can get rubella no matter what their vaccination status is. From the child's point of view there is too much stimulation at a supermarket, and the air is cold. The risk of complications is lower than with measles or mumps, but complications can happen, with sufficient provocation. Chills are less dangerous to a child with rubella than to a child with measles. A mild chill would just cause a cold or flu, making the child feel sick and miserable, but it is not likely to cause bronchitis or death like it can during measles.

Playing quietly does not include activities like jumping on a trampoline. Chandra's little friend Sarah felt so well with rubella that she forgot she had it. After a few minutes of jumping she developed a bad headache which lasted the rest of the day. Too much activity can bring on convulsions and vomiting. The symptom of sore joints often accompanies rubella, and this can progress to arthritis if the patient does not take care.

The rash looks like the measles rash but it is fainter. It also moves from the face downwards, but it moves and disappears more quickly. The way to differentiate rubella from measles is by the swollen glands at the back of the neck or behind the ears. Rubella often goes undiagnosed in children with dark skin because the rash can be too faint to show up. The parents of a dark skinned child notice that the child is tired and listless, and a bit feverish, but unless they see the swollen lymph glands at the back of the neck, they might not realise it is rubella.

Because rubella is such a mild disease, the vaccine was introduced with the excuse that it was needed to prevent congenital rubella syndrome. Congenital rubella syndrome is the name given to a variety of problems that a baby can be born with if the mother gets rubella during the first three months of pregnancy. The virus that causes rubella can damage the heart, ears, eyes, and brain during the first three months of prenatal development. Having a high level of antibodies to rubella before becoming pregnant does not mean that a woman will not give birth to a baby who is deformed by congenital rubella syndrome.[181,182,183,184,185,186] It is best for a girl to have rubella when she is a child, so that she can develop natural immunity to the disease, and will be far less likely to get it when she is pregnant. Mass vaccination of pre-adolescent girls did not eliminate congenital rubella syndrome, and mass vaccination of infant boys and girls, followed by revaccination of boys and girls during childhood, has also failed to prevent congenital rubella syndrome. The vaccinators want all adult women to be revaccinated.[187]

Rubella vaccine causes acute and chronic arthritis in some adults.[23,188,189] The call for revaccination of women does not include a call for women to be informed of possible adverse effects, nor for women to be informed that the vaccine is made from aborted baby. Rubella vaccine was one of the first to be made with lung cells taken from the body of an aborted baby.[190,191]

WHOOPING COUGH

The incidence of whooping cough has been decreasing for more than a hundred years, which means that very few children get it nowadays. However, every parent needs to know how to keep a child with whooping cough comfortable and safe, in case their child is the one who gets it. Whooping cough in a baby presents different problems to whooping cough in a child, so I will start with caring for a child with whooping cough.

The first two weeks of whooping cough seem like a bad cold with mild fever, and occasional fits of coughing. Suddenly the cough becomes more intense, and the child starts waking at night with spasms of coughing. When you hear that first "whoop" you know that whooping cough has arrived, and it cannot be ignored. It is time to batten down the hatches and get ready for broken nights and long days. If you try to "cure" it with herbs, homoeopathy, drugs, or vitamins, you could interfere with the development of life-long immunity. Supporting the child through the illness with non-drug interventions is not the same thing as trying to terminate the disease prematurely.

Two things make whooping cough more bearable; a firm resolve and a plastic bowl. The first few whoops are alarming to observe, but you soon get used to them. If you panic you make the child tighten up and gasp all the more. Whooping cough is far worse for the parents than for the child. The sooner you settle in to a happy routine of throwing up and cleaning up, the easier it will be for the family. (The child does the throwing up, you do the cleaning up.) The coughing spasms are not glamorous affairs. The eyes bulge and the breath is pulled in through a constricted throat, causing that awful whoop sound. At the end of each spasm the child vomits up thick mucus, and sometimes food. Between spasms he or she sleeps soundly, or is cheerful and chirpy. Whooping cough does not cause the grumpiness that measles and mumps cause. The whoop sound is not always present in babies under six months of age, but the tongue will protrude and the eyes will bulge, and the cough will bring up mucus and food. There are some bad coughs that are not whooping cough, and in babies they are commonly misdiagnosed as whooping cough. This leads the parents to believe that the child has acquired immunity to whooping cough.

The two worst problems when dealing with a child with whooping cough are that the parents become exhausted because they are woken frequently at night, and that the child can become malnourished because of repeatedly throwing up. The solution to the latter problem is to feed the child immediately after he or she throws up. Don't wait ten minutes, do it immediately, and then the food will stay down. Avoid foods with crumbs, because they irritate the throat and cause vomiting. Things like nuts which get bitty after chewing also cause vomiting. Just a little food after each spasm will keep up the child's calorie intake, and prevent too much loss of weight. Observe which type of food suits the child most. Some prefer fatty foods, some starchy. At night give a sip of water after each spasm.

Make sure the child sits up every time the coughing starts so that he or she cannot choke on vomitus. The father of a child who was severely brain damaged by whooping cough vaccine told me that the brain damage made it really difficult to convince the child to stay sitting up during each whoop, although she was four years old when she got whooping cough. Sleeping near the child makes things easier, and means you get the child upright quickly when coughing starts. Keep a plastic bowl at hand so that bedding does not get soiled. When Chandra had whooping cough I did not wash the plastic bowl at night. I just put it on the floor after every whoop, and went back to sleep as soon as she was settled. Then in the morning I would hurl the contents under a bush and wash the bowl.

At the beginning the spasms occur every half-hour, then they become less frequent. They can go on for 6 weeks or 6 months, but usually it is all over in 10 weeks. A family in Australia had three of their four children come down with whooping cough at the same time. All four children had been fully immunised before getting whooping cough. Granny and an aunt flew in from New Zealand to do night shifts, so that the parents could function properly during the day. If all families could be that supportive, whooping cough would have a less detrimental effect on parents' health.

Excitement or physical exertion will bring on a coughing spasm. Visitors are usually greeted by the sight of a red-faced child gasping for breath with bulging eyes, and then retching up large globs of revolting mucus. The parents smilingly explain that this is all happening because the child is pleased to see them.

Don't let anyone pollute the air with tobacco smoke near a child with whooping cough. That would increase the number of spasms. Some parents give their children an electrolyte solution to drink to prevent dehydration. It is a good idea, although not essential. Electrolyte solution can be bought from the chemist, and it tastes nice.

Antibiotics shorten the length of time that coughing lasts if they are given at the beginning, but they make no difference if given once the cough has set in,[192,193,194] and as is always the case with antibiotics, the germ is becoming resistant to them.[195] Sometimes antibiotics are given to try to prevent pneumonia, or to try to prevent the spread of the whooping cough bacteria. There is no evidence that giving antibiotics to patients prevents the spread to close contacts.[194] Antibiotics kill the good bacteria in the intestines that help digestion. Killing these bacteria does not strike me as a sensible idea when there is a need for optimum uptake of nutrients from a limited amount of food.

There is no need for the child to stay in bed all day after the first week of whooping. Lack of warmth is not as dangerous with whooping cough as it is with measles, but a child with whooping cough is far more vulnerable to getting bronchitis, ear infections, and pneumonia from a chill, than a child who does not have whooping cough. Some doctors think it is normal for a baby with whooping cough to have the symptoms of a cold, because they are accustomed to seeing babies that have not been kept warm enough. Pneumonia will not set in from the mild type of chill that results from a minute's distraction, but consistently being cold makes a baby or child vulnerable to pneumonia. Sometimes parents do not realise that their child is not dressed warmly enough. Ninety percent of deaths from whooping cough are actually caused by pneumonia.[196]

Vaccinated children with whooping cough are sometimes officially diagnosed with "croup" to hide the failure of the vaccine, but the symptoms of croup are quite different to those of whooping cough. Croup is a serious condition that can be caused by a variety of bacteria and viruses. Susceptibility lies within the individual. The throat swells so that air cannot get through. Homoeopathy can cure the acute condition, and it can convert a child who is prone to getting croup to one who does not experience this horrible and life-threatening condition. Medical doctors can treat the acute condition by inserting a tube into the throat to allow air to pass through, but all they can do about the susceptibility is to wait for the child to outgrow the tendency. Croup is quite different to whooping cough. The throat closure in whooping cough comes in a spasm and then it opens up again. In croup the lips can turn blue and death can result from lack of oxygen. As far back as 1860 the difference between whooping cough and croup was clearly understood, but now the difference is being fudged to obscure vaccine failures.

A child with whooping cough does not enjoy going out until the disease is almost over. He or she is especially bothered by moving air. What feels like a mild breeze to an adult feels like a gale to a child with whooping cough. Even a child who is normally discontented and bored without social contact will play happily at home when he or she has whooping cough. People will tell you that your child needs "fresh air" after being cooped up inside for a couple of weeks, but your child does not need "fresh air".

If the complication of pneumonia arises, antibiotic treatment should be started without delay. The homoeopathic remedy *drosera 30* helps the antibiotic do its work against pneumonia, but the idea of using *drosera 30* to "cure" whooping cough is a different matter. *Drosera 30* is a homoeopathic remedy that is sometimes recommended for whooping cough because the symptoms of whooping cough are similar to the symptoms caused by eating the drosera (sundew) plant. Eating the sundew plant (which no one in their right mind who is not part of an experiment would do), causes a deep cough, so homoeopathically potentised drosera is an excellent remedy for deep coughs.

If the child is older than one year, it is not a good idea to try to make the whooping cough go away, for two reasons. It could prevent the development of immunity, and it could also mean that when the person gets full blown natural whooping cough later on, they still cannot develop immunity.

When a person who has been vaccinated against whooping cough gets natural whooping cough, they cannot develop life-long immunity to whooping cough, because the vaccine has primed their immune system wrongly.[197,198] Both the whole cell and the acellular whooping cough vaccine do not create natural immunity, and on top of that they prevent the immune system from creating natural immunity in the future.[197,198] So even when a vaccinated person gets full blown natural whooping cough, that person's immune system cannot create natural immunity, and the person remains susceptible to getting whooping cough again and again. Aborting whooping cough with massive doses of vitamin C or a homoeopathic remedy may have a similar effect, because full natural immunity takes two weeks or longer to develop during the natural disease. However, giving oral vitamin C to a baby with whooping cough to avoid complications is preferable to allowing the baby to develop life-long immunity, even though the baby may later get whooping cough a number of times throughout life.

When a young baby gets whooping cough it is very stressful for the parents. The baby has to be held upright so that he or she can cough out the mucuc successfully. When my elderly neighbour heard Chandra whooping, I expected her to lean over the fence and give me a blast for not having her "immunised". But instead she told me about how she had suffered when her son Johnathan got whooping cough at the age of three weeks. "We had just moved to Joh'burg. I was feeling weak from the birth, Ted had to go away on business, and I had to hold Johnathan upright on my shoulder all through the night. Sometimes I sat in a chair and dozed between whoops, and sometimes I walked up and down patting his back. It was terrible. I'll never forget it." I was amazed to hear this, because at that stage of my life I thought that young babies were supposed to die from whooping cough. The baby she was describing was by then a man whom I often saw visiting his parents with his wife and children.

I have since learned that in previous generations parents used to know that they must hold a baby with whooping cough upright at night, and that they must keep him or her warm. Millions of children have enjoyed the books about Noddy, The Famous Five, and The Secret Seven, which were all written by Enid Blyton. Enid Blyton got whooping cough when she was three months old, and her father stayed up at night to keep her upright and warm during the acute phase of the disease.[199] He believed that she would have died if he had not.[199] By holding her he was also giving her the benefit of his body warmth, which was important in an unheated house in London in winter.

The germ that causes whooping cough produces a toxin that can be dangerous for a baby. The toxin can set in motion processes that, among other things, adversely affect the heart, the lungs, and the brain. There is much discussion in the medical literature about which drugs and treatments to use when a patient who is suffering from the effects of this toxin is admitted to hospital, but the benefits of vitamin C are ignored. In 1936 it was first demonstrated that vitamin C detoxifies the toxin, reduces the virulence of the whooping cough germ, and improves the condition of patients with whooping cough.[200] There followed a string of articles in which doctors who used small amounts of vitamin C reported small improvements in their patients. It did not seem to occur to them that larger amounts would have caused larger improvements. The fact that small doses of vitamin C caused greater improvements in babies than in bigger children is one of the things that should have made the researchers think of using larger doses.

Dr. Suzanne Humphries has successfully used high doses of vitamin C for whooping cough in babies, and now she travels the world trying to educate doctors and parents. She recommends oral, not injected, vitamin C for whooping cough. She says that one of the benefits of using oral doses is that it is easier to monitor whether you are giving too much, and to know when the next dose is needed. Too much would cause diarrhoea, which would cause dehydration, which is not good with whooping cough.[201] Oral vitamin C also detoxes the bowel and the liver more effectively than injected vitamin C.[201] She is in favour of using injected vitamin C for other infectious diseases, but, "Whooping cough on the other hand requires steady high (not mega like IV) doses all day and night and continuous dumping of endotoxin out in stool".[201] This regime prevents toxic shock. In a crisis situation, like when a baby with whooping cough is already experiencing toxic shock, both oral and injected vitamin C should be used, but once the crisis is over, careful use of oral vitamin C will keep the toxin under control.

The suggestion that vitamin C should be used for whooping cough causes fury among the trolls on social media, but most doctors do not react because they consider anything that they were not taught at medical school to be beneath their contempt. In 2008 an article in the British Medical Journal described the treatments of two babies who died from whooping cough in hospital.[202] About one baby they say, "Within 24 hours of admission to paediatric intensive care, the infant died despite maximum treatment." About the other baby they say, "She died within 30 hours despite being given maximum treatment, including inhaled nitric oxide and inotropes." Those babies were not given maximum treatment, because they were not given vitamin C. I wrote to one of the authors of the article:

> Please will you inform me whether you would consider investigating the usefulness of vitamin C as an intervention for infants with whooping cough. Vitamin C is able to dismantle toxins, and it might be particularly helpful for infants who are suffering from, or in danger of suffering from, the effects of pertussis toxin.

> During the 1930s doctors reported moderate success with

small doses of vitamin C for pertussis, and now there is unpublished anecdotal evidence of great success when large enough doses are used. A proper trial needs to be conducted. The aim of vitamin C for pertussis is not to terminate the illness, but to ensure survival without sequelae.

Please will you inform me whether you would be willing to study the effects of large enough doses of vitamin C for infants with pertussis at your hospital.

As expected, he did not reply.

The typical behaviour of doctors regarding vitamin C is reflected in the story of Allan Smith whose life was saved by the fact that he had three assertive sons.[203] Allan had swine flu that was complicated by pneumonia, and the doctors told the family that nothing could be done and that they should agree to switch off his life support. The doctors refused to treat him with vitamin C, so Allan's sons contacted a lawyer who forced them to treat their dad with vitamin C. Some doctors give the impression that they would rather have their patient die than face up to the fact that there is something important that they were not taught at medical school. Allan recovered "miraculously".

Not content to let it be, the Pharma shills are still carping that Allan was turned onto his tummy at the same time as the vitamin C treatment started, so it could have been the change in position that made the viral pneumonia suddenly go away. If turning someone over is such a great cure for viral pneumonia, it is odd that the doctors did not think of turning him over before they campaigned to have his life support switched off.

One of the problems with hospitals is that they do not keep a baby with whooping cough warm enough. This causes the complication of pneumonia, and pneumonia is the biggest cause of death with whooping cough.[196] In 1992 the New Zealand Immunisation Awareness Society held its first international symposium on vaccination. While we were organising it, committee member Judy Gilbert telephoned a paediatrician at Auckland hospital and told him it was his duty to attend the symposium. He shouted into the phone, "I'll come to your symposium if you'll come to my hospital and see all the children with whooping cough." We were very keen to go to the hospital to see the children with whooping cough. We wanted to know what drugs they were being given, whether they were being held upright during whoops, why the parents had sent them to hospital, how many doses of vaccine each child had had prior to getting whooping cough, and, most importantly, whether they were being kept warm enough to prevent pneumonia. But the visit never materialised because there were no children in the hospital with whooping cough. He still refused to come to our symposium.

Medical textbooks recommend some treatments that are harmful and useless, like immune serum globulin, and some treatments that are helpful, like a constant warm room temperature. Some deaths from whooping cough in the early days of modern medicine were caused by the dreadful treatments that were used, like injections of ether. Nowadays chilling is the biggest cause of death.[196]

The vaccine industry tries to frighten parents into believing that whooping cough carries a high risk of death. In many countries vaccine promoting pamphlets say that one out of 200 babies under six months of age with whooping cough will die. This sounds very frightening, as it is designed to do. Some parents are told that the risk of brain damage from vaccinating is one in a million, while the risk of death from not vaccinating is one in 200. When doctors and nurses say this, they are being very deceitful.

That figure of "one in 200" is used consistently in many countries, so I thought it must be based on something, not just made up, like some official figures are. I found it difficult to track down the source, because most people who were using it were just repeating it from other unreferenced sources. Eventually I found that it came from information on whooping cough gathered in the USA during the years 1986 to 1988.[204] During these years one out of every two hundred babies that were less than six months old, and who were reported as having whooping cough, ended up dying. The published report says that the rate of complications like pneumonia and encephalopathy was higher in this age group than in any other group, but it does not say what the rate of complications was. Not surprisingly the report does not tell the reader how many of the babies that died during those years had been vaccinated. It does tell us that 85% of cases in all age groups were given an antibiotic, but it does not tell us whether those who died were given antibiotics, nor does it mention the use of fever-suppressing drugs and chilling. The report admits that 90% of cases of whooping cough in the USA are not reported.

It is deceptive to say that every baby has a one in 200 chance of dying if it is not vaccinated. It is also dishonest to say that every baby who gets whooping cough has a one in 200 chance of dying. The risk of death is affected by the type of care provided, and by other factors. In Sweden there were 19,000 cases of whooping cough in an epidemic that ran from 1977 to 1979, with no deaths.[205] If I were to use this statistic to print a pamphlet saying that young babies with whooping cough have no chance of dying, I would be behaving as dishonestly as the vaccinators behave.

Most of the children who died in the 1974 and 1977 outbreaks of whooping cough in England were already chronically ill when they developed whooping cough.[206] People trying to encourage vaccination often repeat the claim that when the vaccination rate fell in Britain in 1976, it caused a big epidemic of whooping cough and lots of deaths. This is a lie that I have dealt with in the section on herd immunity.

Droplets of saliva are infectious for six weeks from the time the mucousy symptoms start. A child or adult with whooping cough should be kept away from babies and severely malnourished children, regardless of whether the babies or severely malnourished children have been vaccinated.

When Chandra was no longer infectious, and had recovered enough to want to go out, I always took the plastic bowl with me. She kept it on the seat beside her in the car, and once she had thrown up we knew we had time to do some shopping before the next spasm. One day she threw up during her violin lesson, and the teacher shouted at me for not having her "immunised". Thanks to the plastic bowl, no harm was done to the teacher's carpet.

After 11 weeks we travelled from Cape Town to Johannesburg by car. We drove at night so that she could sleep while travelling and would not moan about boredom. We stopped for petrol in a desolate Karroo town, and she woke up when the motion of the car stopped. She then whooped, and the petrol attendant got a terrible fright. He probably thought she was choking to death. He did not understand English, so we could not explain that it was only the tail end of whooping cough. He was disturbed by our casual attitude, and looked very worried as we drove off into the night.

Her very last whoop was 13 weeks after the first. While we were in Johannesburg we visited the minitown that is a replica of the city, and as we arrived the minitrain was about to set off. We ran to catch it, and the excitement and exertion brought on a whoop. There was no plastic bowl as she had not needed it for ages, so I cupped my hands and she threw up into them. She then forgot all about me and enjoyed the thrill of rattling along in a minitrain through a minitown, while I sat there wondering what to do with this handful of mucus. As we crossed a minicreek I dumped it, and then I used my one and only paper handkerchief to clean my hands. These are the tribulations of parenthood that I would far rather endure than coping with a brain damaged child, or grieving for a life cut short by the vaccine.

CHICKEN POX

Chicken pox varies in intensity. A child who has it mildly can play with a playmate between fevers, but a child who feels tired and has high peaks of fever needs continual bed rest and warmth. Chicken pox can develop serious complications if it is not properly managed. The risk of complications is higher in adults than in children, and very much higher in adults who smoke. It is essential for an adult with chicken pox to stay in bed for three days, otherwise complications can develop. With uncomplicated chicken pox, adults usually suffer emotionally from the itchiness and the bouts of dizziness, but when it is over they feel wonderful. They can describe the feeling of being cleansed and renewed, whereas children do not stop to tell you.

Doctors, nurses, chemists, glossy magazines, and neighbours tell parents to give paracetamol/tylenol to children with chicken pox. Like many medical practices, this treatment became dogma without being tested. In April 1984 a year-long study was commenced to investigate whether paracetamol/tylenol affects the duration or severity of chicken pox.[68] This was the first time that the use of paracetamol/tylenol during chicken pox had been studied. The study found that the drug made the itching a little bit worse, it made the illness last one day longer, and it made absolutely no difference to vomiting, insomnia, headaches, abdominal pain, or fussiness. The results were published in 1989, and this would have been a good time for the medical establishment to inform everyone that it is not helpful to give paracetamol/tylenol to a child with chicken pox.

The study was done at John's Hopkins, which is a prestigious medical outfit in the USA. The Johns Hopkins website advises parents to give paracetamol/tylenol to a child with chicken pox, which shows how little they care for science. Their own science shows that giving paracetamol/tylenol to a child with chicken pox is a bad idea, yet they recommend just exactly that.

The spots that chicken pox causes are quite different to those caused by measles, roseola, or rubella. Each spot starts off looking like a little pimple, then it forms a yellow, watery blister on top. This top changes to a crust that eventually comes off cleanly. Care needs to be taken to refrain from knocking off the crusts before they are ready to come off. The spots are itchy, unlike the spots of measles, rubella, and roseola, and the patient feels tempted to scratch them. If the spots become infected from scratching they will form scars. Uninfected spots generally do not leave scars, but a few rogue spots end up leaving little scars. On some children the spots get very big and leave scars when they burst, but this is rare. When the skin has healed over, you can apply vitamin E oil or hydrogenated lanolin to help the scar tissue convert to normal tissue.

Another way that the spots differ from those of measles, roseola, and rubella is that new batches of them appear when the older spots are already quite mature. If the spots are too itchy for the child to bear it is a good idea to dab on something like calamine lotion, rhus tox ointment or rhus tox tincture, paste made from oatmeal, or gentian violet (which stains the sheets) to stop the itch. Whatever you use will only have a temporary effect, and it has to be dabbed onto each spot over and over again. Sometimes it has to be repeated after only half an hour. There are liquids and ointments that stop the itching that is caused by things like urticaria or flea bites, but do not stop the itch of chicken pox. If a substance you are using does not stop the itch, don't persevere with it - try something else.

Chicken pox does not need to be "cured". People who recommend the use of homoeopathy or vitamin C to shorten or "cure" chicken pox are misunderstanding the role of the self-resolving childhood diseases. Sometimes the chicken pox does not finish off properly and the virus lingers on in the body. Later it can reactivate and cause a painful skin condition called shingles. Homoeopathy can cure shingles.

In the era before vaccination most cases of chicken pox occurred in children under the age of fifteen.[207] The death rate from chicken pox in the USA was 1 per 25,000 of the population.[207] The death rate was 25 times higher among adults than among pre-schoolers,[208] and it was 4 times higher among babies than among pre-schoolers.[208] The majority of the deaths occurred in people who did not have a pre-existing immunocompromising disease, and the main causes of death were pneumonia, central nervous system complications (including encephalitis), secondary infection, and hemorrhagic conditions.[208] The medics thought that Reye's Syndrome was a natural complication of chicken pox[207] until they realised that it was being caused by aspirin. The majority of complications of chicken pox that were recorded as encephalitis may actually have been Reye's Syndrome.[208] Paracetamol/tylenol and ibuprofen do not cause Reyes Syndrome with chicken pox, but they do suppress the immune system, and they increase the risk of complications.

The chicken pox vaccine is manufactured on tissue from aborted babies.[209,210,211] It causes horrendous, life-spoiling adverse effects,[212,213] the extent of which is not acknowledged by post-marketing surveillance exercises nor by passive reporting.[212,213] As is the case with all vaccines, the majority of severe reactions to chicken pox vaccine are simply ignored by the vaccine industry. Using their false data they conclude that the risk of damage from natural chicken pox is greater than the risk from the vaccine. They arrive at this conclusion by ignoring three important factors; many complications from natural chicken pox are caused by orthodox medical treatment, no one knows the actual risk from the vaccine, and properly managed chicken pox reduces the risk of cancer and heart disease in later life.[109,110,111,112,113] Under proper care most complications of chicken pox can be prevented, whereas it is extremely difficult to prevent long-term damage in a child who is experiencing an acute severe reaction to the vaccine.

Vaccination of children shifts chicken pox to adolescents and young adults,[214] so there has been the inevitable introduction of more doses.[215,216,217] The reduction of chicken pox among children has caused an increase in shingles in older people.[218] The vaccine industry has responded by introducing a vaccine for shingles. It contains human protein, pig protein, and calf serum. Studies that want to "prove" that there has been no increase in shingles do not include cases of shingles from GP records, they only look at hospital admissions. People are five times more likely to die from shingles than from chicken pox.[219]

In some countries that have introduced the chicken pox vaccine the disease is presented as a "killer disease", while in other countries the authorities are being more coy, and are saying that the vaccine is necessary because it is bad for the economy when caregivers take time off work to look after a child with chicken pox.

Britain is one of the countries that has announced that it is not going to introduce the chicken pox vaccine. A British mum called Katy told me this story,

> I was at my doctors last week asking for the packet inserts of the vaccinations and the nurse started to tell me how dangerous childhood illnesses were. I told her I had had measles, chicken pox and rubella as a child as all my friends had, so I think that not every case will be as dangerous as she described. I also mentioned that in the US they vaccinate against chicken pox and they are now scaring people into thinking chicken pox is dangerous. The nurse and doctor both said there was absolutely nothing to worry about with chicken pox, it is one of the mildest childhood illnesses, it is good to get it as a child and it is ridiculous to vaccinate against it. (They missed my point - I wasn't worried about it, I wanted to illustrate how two countries with different underlying motives have totally different views and therefore how can I take what you are saying about anything else seriously!? But their answers illustrated my point perfectly anyway.) It made me reflect that if we do introduce the vaccine here in the UK I'll bet both of those medical people will tell me how dangerous chicken pox is as they will get financial rewards for their surgery for doing so.

SLAPPED CHEEK ROSEOLA

This disease is caused by a virus called parvovirus B19. It is also called erythema infectiosum. It comes in epidemics, and when it spreads through schools and pre-school centres, it causes comment because it gives children a comical appearance. However, it does not make them feel very sick. The most striking feature is that the cheeks and side of the jaw become bright red. They do not really look as if they have been slapped, because the redness is too solid and extensive. Kenny was little when he had it, and he called it "slap-cheek-roll-me-over."

A rash that is mottled and lacy appears on the body, and a peculiarity of this disease is that the rash comes and goes. The rash itches some of the time, and having a shower makes it itch more. However, it does not get nearly as itchy as chicken pox. The fever does not become as high as it does with measles, and the tiredness is not as extreme as it is with measles. Nevertheless children should not be given paracetamol/tylenol and expected to meet their usual commitments; they should be allowed to rest. Some children even cope with going to school while they have it, but sporting activities should definitely be avoided.

Adults who get the disease sometimes suffer from sore joints. The pain can be quite severe, and in rare cases can last for a long time before it goes away.

"WHEN VACCINATED CHILDREN GET THE DISEASE THAT THE VACCINE WAS SUPPOSED TO PREVENT, THEY GET IT LESS BADLY"

~~~~~~

Vaccine Myth Number Three: Vaccinated children sometimes get the disease that the vaccine was supposed to prevent, but when they do, the severity of the disease is greatly diminished.

~~~~~~

Whenever I hear an apologist for vaccine failure say the above, I am tempted to ask if death from measles is less severe in the vaccinated than in the unvaccinated. A vaccinated child with measles does not experience the typical symptoms of classical measles, but gets what is called "atypical measles". Unvaccinated children with measles have a more comfortable time than those who experience atypical measles.

The rash in a vaccinated child is often paler than a normal measles rash, which is not a reason for celebration. A Danish researcher has found that a lack of rash in people with measles antibodies is associated with cancer and degenerative diseases later on in life.[158] The subjects in his study averaged 38 years of age, and none of them had been vaccinated. Those who had not had measles, but had antibodies to measles, either from being infected with the wild virus without developing symptoms, or from being injected with immune serum globulin, had a much higher rate of a wide range of degenerative diseases than those who had had measles with a proper rash.

The first measles vaccine contained a killed measles virus instead of a live measles virus. When people who were injected with the killed virus vaccine catch measles, the symptoms can be so different to ordinary measles that it is often difficult to diagnose what is wrong. The rash does not look like a measles rash, and it does not start on the face and move downwards. It starts on the hands and feet and moves inwards. It can look like a severe allergic reaction, or like chicken pox, and it itches and stings. It is sometimes mistaken for meningitis, scarlet fever, Rocky Mountain spotted fever, an allergic reaction to drugs, pleurisy, or lung cancer. The greatest danger from having atypical measles after the killed virus vaccine is that doctors might do harmful invasive tests to try to find out what is wrong. If left alone, the sickness will heal itself spontaneously, although it can persist for months before it suddenly clears up.

I am intrigued by the fact that a person who has been injected with a dead virus gets a worse form of atypical measles than a person who has been injected with a live virus. There is speculation in the medical literature about why this happens.

Figures from Zambia showed that the death rate from measles during an epidemic was higher among the vaccinated than among the unvaccinated.[220]

In the USA the vaccine has made measles start occurring in infants and adults instead of in children, and the death rate is more than three times higher.[221]

When diphtheria was still prevalent, parents whose children got the disease despite vaccination were fobbed off with the claim that the disease was less severe because the child was vaccinated, unless of course the child had died. In Vaccine Myth Number Seven I discuss a study done by the British Medical Research Council which sought an explanation for the failure of the vaccine to prevent diphtheria. The study doctors were expecting to find that vaccinated patients with diphtheria who had a high level of antibodies would have a less severe form of the disease than vaccinated people with a low level of antibodies. But they did not. "… there was no significant association, however, between severity and antitoxin content."[222]

"DIPHTHERIA DECLINED BECAUSE OF MASS VACCINATION"

Vaccine Myth Number Four: Diphtheria disappeared when mass immunisation of babies was introduced. Before then many children died from the disease. Nowadays it is still necessary to vaccinate all children against diphtheria, because if the vaccination rate falls below 95%, herd immunity will no longer protect the unimmunised.

Diphtheria has not disappeared, but it has become very rare. When singing the praises of the diphtheria vaccine, vaccine defenders fail to mention that diphtheria declined far more before the vaccine was introduced than it did after the vaccine was introduced. Its rarity nowadays has nothing at all to do with the vaccine, because the vaccine does not work. During the decades when diphtheria was still common, roughly half of the victims were adults, and half were children.[223] Mass vaccination commenced in 1940,[224] and neurological reactions were "reported occasionally".[225] The British Medical Research Council conducted a study on antibody levels to see whether the reason why vaccinated people got diphtheria was because they had failed to make enough antibodies.[226] This study is discussed in Vaccine Myth Number Seven.

Britain is one of the few countries in the world that has kept a record of infectious diseases for a long time. Deaths from diphtheria in England and Wales were recorded from 1866. The British Department of Health has this to say in a booklet that is aimed at promoting vaccination,

> The introduction of immunisation against diphtheria on a national scale in 1940 resulted in a dramatic fall in the number of notified cases and deaths from the disease. In 1940, 46,281 cases with 2,480 deaths were notified, compared with 37 cases and 6 deaths in 1957. From 1979 to 1986, 26 cases were notified with only one death.[224]

If you look at a graph of the drop that occurred after 1940, it appears that the vaccine was very effective at eliminating deaths from diphtheria. That is why health departments around the world use graphs of the British experience since 1940 to promote vaccination. The difference between their graphs and mine is that mine looks less posh because it is hand drawn.

Deaths from diphtheria since vaccine introduced

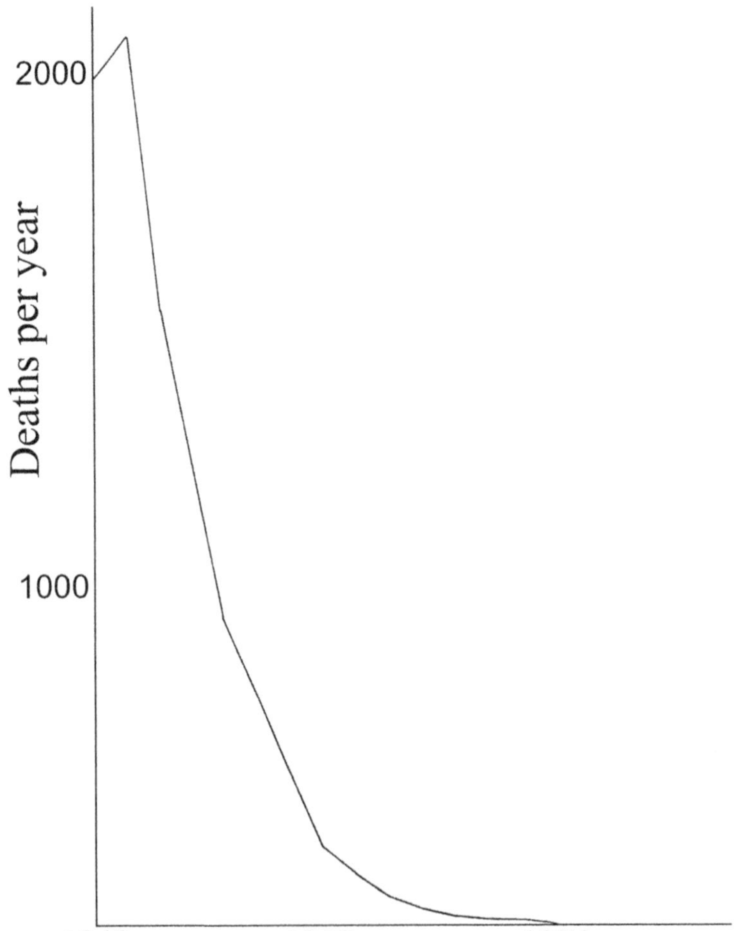

©Wendy Lydall

But the graph becomes a lot less impressive when you look at the history of the drop that occurred after 1902.

Deaths from diphtheria since 1902

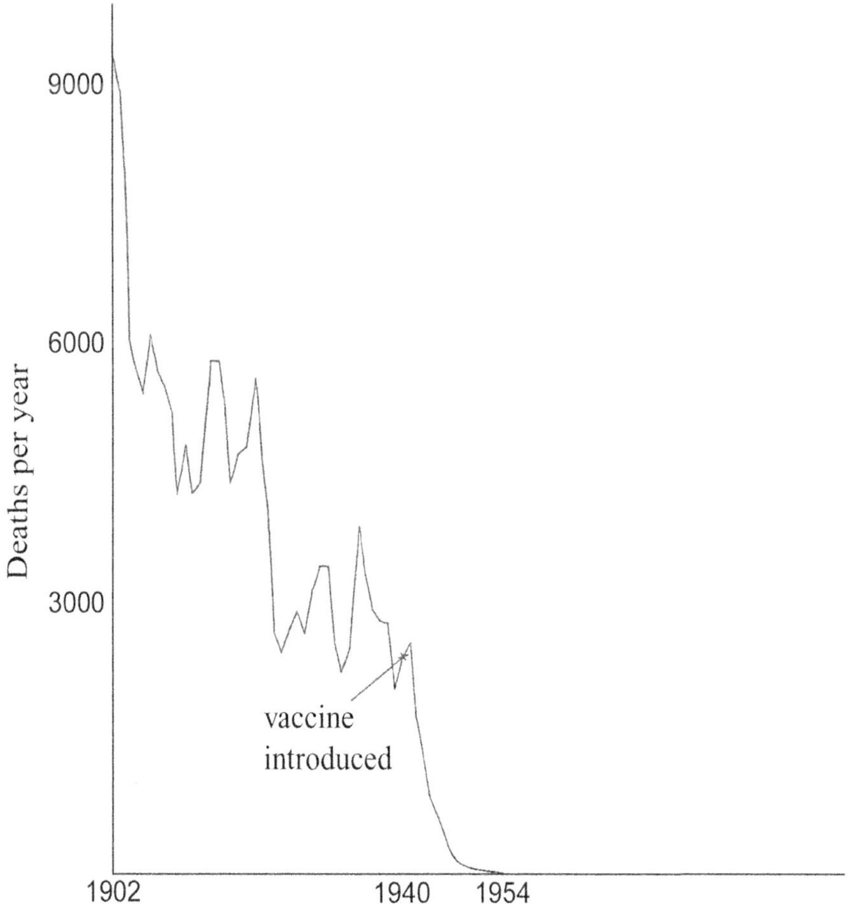

©Wendy Lydall

But this too, does not tell the whole story. From 1866 to 1893 there had been a huge increase in the number of deaths from diphtheria. It rose to a peak during the last decade of the 19th century, and then began to decline. The number of deaths from diphtheria in 1899 was three times as high as it was in 1869, while the population was only two fifths greater.

Deaths from diphtheria since 1866

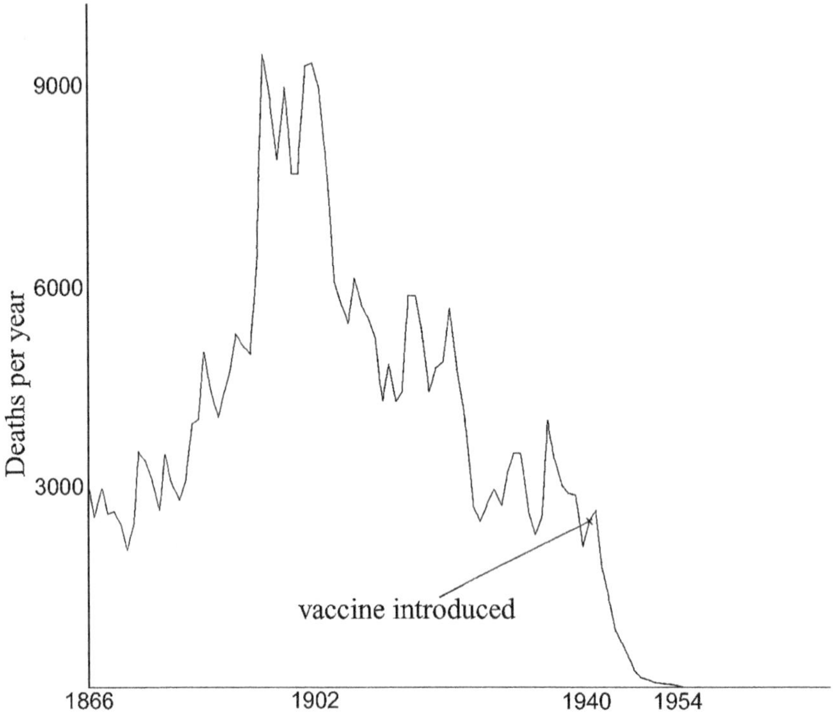

©Wendy Lydall

Should we give the people who compiled the British Department of Health's book on "Immunisation" the benefit of the doubt, and suggest that perhaps they did not know the history of diphtheria in their country? But if they did not know something as fundamental as that, then why was the British taxpayer paying them a salary? I believe that they deliberately tried to mislead the reader.

The idea that nutrition and hygiene made diphtheria decline is also without foundation. A look at the history of infectious diseases shows that nutrition and hygiene are irrelevant to the coming and going of germs. A hygienic lifestyle protects from waterborne diseases like cholera and typhoid, but it offers no protection against an airborne disease like diphtheria. Being malnourished does make a person more susceptible to a germ if the germ comes along, but what a person eats, and how much each person eats, does not make germs enter or leave the environment.

If the hygienists were correct, then the rise of diphtheria in Britain during the second half of the 19th century would have been caused by poverty and unsanitary living conditions. Living conditions in the cities had been very bad from the time of the industrial revolution, and the importation of wheat from North America caused more country folk to become destitute and to head for the cities. So there was a rise in the number of severely malnourished and poorly housed people during that time. Before declaring that this was the reason why the incidence of diphtheria rose at that time, we should ask ourselves why deaths from whooping cough and from scarlet fever were dropping sharply at the same time. Sometimes there is a coincidental correlation between the rise and fall of airborne infectious diseases, and the worsening or improvement of human living conditions, but overall there is no correlation.

In Victorian England most of the population lived in dire poverty, and the corrupt Relieving Officers and Guardians and cruel Taskmasters intended to keep it that way. A woman named Charlotte Despard decided to get the workhouses, and other institutions that entrenched poverty, abolished.[227] She realised that lack of nourishment caused ill health in poor children, which was contrary to the dominant social narrative of the time, and she forced the government to start school feeding schemes.[228] A street and a pub in London are named after her.

Rickets is a disease of the bones that is caused solely by the socioeconomic factors of malnutrition and lack of sunlight. It has no life cycle of its own because it is not caused by germs. In central London there was a permanent thick smog that blocked out the sun, and the impoverished people who lived there had deformed bones because of the smoke and the lack of food. Rich people chose to believe that poor people had rickets because they were inferior. The wealthy Charlotte Despard was considered to be extraordinarily stupid by her friends and relations for saying that rickets was caused by poverty.

Charlotte Despard also initiated the concept of officialdom checking up on the health of babies,[229] which has now degenerated into another way of selling pharmaceuticals. She was powerful because she was wealthy, and she brought about social reforms that triggered the elimination of rickets, and the end of some causes of child mortality. However, these reforms are not the reason for the decline of airborne diseases like diphtheria and scarlet fever. The virulence of those germs is not affected by housing and plumbing conditions. Like English sweating sickness and bubonic plague, they have dwindled because of natural forces which we do not understand, and which no one is researching. In 1963 Ethel Douglas Hume wrote,

> During the four years 1941-1944 the Ministry of Health and the Department of Health for Scotland admitted almost

> 23,000 cases of diphtheria in immunised children and more than 180 that proved fatal.
>
> In regard to the decline of diphtheria in Great Britain during 1943 and 1944, we are reminded that fifty-eight British physicians, who signed a memorial in 1938 against compulsory immunisation in Guernsey, were able to point to the virtual disappearance of diphtheria in Sweden without any immunisation. On the other hand, if we turn to Germany we find that, after Dr. Frick's order in April 1940 for the compulsory mass immunisation of children, this country in 1945 had come to be regarded as the storm-centre of diphtheria in Europe. From some 40,000 there had been an increase to 250,000 cases.
>
> An article in the number for March 1944 of a publication called *Pour La Famille* points out the rise in cases of diphtheria after compulsory immunisation. For instance, the increase in Paris was as much as thirty per cent; and in Lyons the diphtheria cases rose from 162 in 1942 to 239 in 1943. In Hungary, where immunisation has been compulsory since 1938, the rise in cases was thirty-five per cent in two years. In the canton of Geneva, where immunisation has been enforced since 1933, the number of cases was trebled from 1941 to 1943.[230]

When the germs that cause diphtheria become virulent in an area, most of the people who live in that area breathe in diphtheria germs. Some of the people who have diphtheria germs residing in their throats remain lively and healthy, while others get sick with the symptoms of diphtheria. This is because the immune systems of the former group are able to keep the germs under control. The ability of their immune systems to do this does not depend on whether or not they have been vaccinated, nor whether or not they have a lot of antibodies.[226] People who have diphtheria germs living in their throats but have no symptoms of sickness are called "carriers". Finding diphtheria germs in the throat of a person who is suffering the symptoms of diphtheria confirms that diphtheria germs are the cause of the sickness, while finding diphtheria germs in the throat of a person without symptoms confirms that diphtheria germs are present in the air at that time.

There was a time when carriers were considered a danger to others. *The Evening News* of 4th June 1920 reported that the medical authorities in a town called Alperton in Middlesex, England, took throat cultures from 700 children and examined them for diphtheria germs. They found that the germs were present in 200 of the children, so these children were accused of being "carriers", and were put in quarantine.[231] It appears that the authorities learned their lesson, and did not continue to round up and imprison "carriers". They realised that there are far too many "carriers" for them to lock up, and it is better not to seek them out.

Although diphtheria has become a rare disease, there are still sporadic outbreaks. In June 1992, a teenage girl who was in one of Hilary Butler's gym classes in a town south of Auckland, got diphtheria. At first it seemed to be just a nasty cough. She did not take a break even though she was overworking both academically and physically. When her condition became serious, she was admitted to hospital, where her aunt came to visit her. Her aunt had nursed diphtheria cases in Britain in the 1950s, and she said that her niece had the typical symptoms of diphtheria. The girl was flown by helicopter to a bigger hospital in Auckland, where they took a swab from her throat and confirmed diphtheria. When they learned that the girl was fully immunised, one of the doctors said to the mother, "Then it can't be diphtheria." They changed the diagnosis to bacterial tracheitis.

Many of the children in the same town had the same nasty cough, but only one other girl went on to get full-blown diphtheria. When she was hospitalised with the same classical symptoms of diphtheria, they took a swab which confirmed that she had diphtheria. Again they refused to call it diphtheria, because the girl was up to date with her jabs. This case was labelled epiglottitis and infected asthma.

We do not know how many other cases like this happened in New Zealand at that time. We only know about these two because they happened so close to Hilary. The medical people did not want to put it on paper that the two girls had diphtheria, because then there would have been an official record that the vaccine had failed. Hilary asked the medical authorities to take swabs from all the children in the region who showed mild symptoms of diphtheria, but they refused. It is probable that many of the children who were suffering from a "nasty cough" were actually battling against diphtheria germs. It is also probable that many of the people who lived in that area and had no symptoms at all, had diphtheria germs in their throats too.

The dishonest behaviour of the medical people involved in these two cases in New Zealand is probably replicated all over the world when diphtheria germs become active in the environment. Hilary said to me, "Just imagine if it had been my child that had come down with the symptoms. It would have been front-page news that I had caused an outbreak of diphtheria. But of course my children wouldn't get diphtheria because I give them enough vitamin C."

At the same time as this small outbreak occurred in New Zealand, there was quite a big diphtheria outbreak happening in Russia. The vaccine industry used the outbreak in Russia as an excuse for selling millions more doses of diphtheria vaccine. They persuaded their lackeys in health departments around the world to make it policy for diphtheria vaccine to be injected into teenagers and adults at intervals varying from 5 years to 15 years. They have combined diphtheria toxin with tetanus toxin, and most recipients think they are just getting a tetanus vaccination.

The vaccine industry claimed that the rear-guard diphtheria outbreak in Russia in the early nineties was caused by a drop in the vaccination rate. However, there was no drop in the vaccination rate, and when the rate was increased in response to the epidemic, it made no difference.[232,233] The World Health Organisation said that the reason for the epidemic was that the vaccine does not give life-long immunity like the disease does.[233] If that were the case, there would have been epidemics everywhere else too, because every other country in the world that used diphtheria vaccine had been giving it to babies only, and not to anyone who was older. Anyway, a natural dose of diphtheria does not give life-long immunity like a natural dose of measles does. Hygienists say that the epidemic was caused by the poverty that resulted from the break-up of the Soviet Union. It is true that widespread malnutrition will provide more victims for the virulent germ, but malnutrition does not make the germ become virulent.

Because the history of the disease has only been recorded for 150 years, we cannot predict what it is going to do next. It is possible that diphtheria is going to come back in a big way. We cannot assume that it is going to disappear entirely, just because English sweating sickness disappeared.

If the diphtheria germ decides to become virulent again, vaccinated people will get diphtheria, and the whole scenario of excuses and accusations will start up. If diphtheria does not break out again, they will continue to claim that their vaccine is the reason for the absence of diphtheria.

The history of scarlet fever in England and Wales gives some insight into the natural rise and fall of virulent diseases. In 1870 scarlet fever killed twelve times as many people in England and Wales as diphtheria did. Scarlet fever vaccine was never included in the vaccination schedule, yet scarlet fever declined so dramatically that it ceased to be listed in the British statistics from 1950.

During the 1930s and 1940s some articles that sung the praises of various scarlet fever vaccines were published in the medical literature. Despite the efforts of the manufacturers, no vaccine was ever introduced as part of any country's schedule. If it had become one of the routine vaccinations that babies are nowadays given, the vaccine industry and

Deaths from scarlet fever since 1866

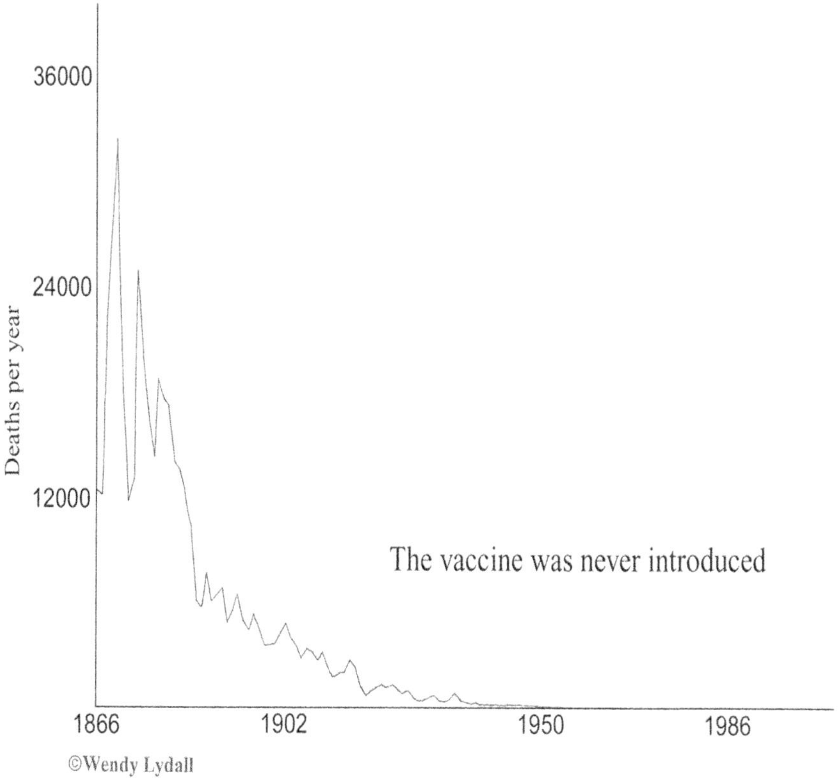

their lackeys in the media would constantly be telling us that it is because of vaccination that the world was saved from scarlet fever. They would be telling parents who refuse to accept the vaccine that they are irresponsible and a danger to society. I find it amusing that some people believe that a scarlet fever vaccine is on the infant schedule, and is the reason why scarlet fever has gone away.

Like diphtheria, scarlet fever has not entirely disappeared. Outbreaks are very rare, but they still happen. In 1989, when we were living in New Zealand, some cases of scarlet fever occurred in our suburb. In the IAS newsletter I asked if any readers knew of other cases, and people wrote in from all over New Zealand and told me that their children had had it. The 1989 flare-up of scarlet fever might have shown itself in other parts of the world too. Perhaps scarlet fever is going to come back, or perhaps it was just having a rear-guard action.

If vaccination against scarlet fever were routinely practiced, the cases that occurred would have either been explained away with the excuse, "the vaccine is only 99% effective," or the disease would have been labelled as something else, just like the diphtheria cases that Hilary witnessed. But because there is no vaccine for scarlet fever, the health department just kept quiet about the outbreak. If a vaccine had existed, they would have been telling parents that their children needed extra doses, and they would have been accusing parents of unvaccinated children of being the villains who caused the outbreak.

Here are the histories of the two diseases superimposed onto each other. Scarlet fever was so much more of a killer than diphtheria that I have had to squash down the diphtheria line.

Scarlet fever and diphtheria

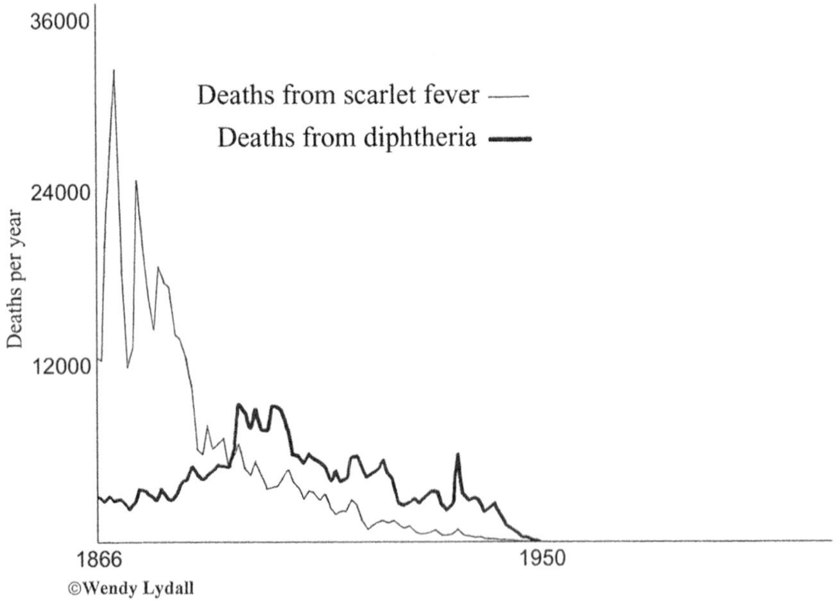

"WITHOUT VACCINATION THERE WOULD BE EPIDEMICS"

Vaccine Myth Number Five: Epidemics of killer diseases used to sweep across the land until vaccination put an end to them. If vaccination were to cease, these epidemics would start again.

No one knows what causes epidemics to start and end, nor why some remain in a certain locality, while others spread. The cause of the natural ebb and flow of epidemics is a topic that does not attract money for research because the drug companies would gain nothing by the answers being known. Some epidemics rise fast and then disappear suddenly, while others start slowly, stay at a peak for a long time, and then fade away slowly. Within the general rise and fall there are highs and lows that make the history of a disease look spiky on a graph. When an epidemic spreads across a large part of the world, it is called a pandemic. Human activity can make a difference to the number of people who get a disease during an epidemic, but humans have no power over the coming and going of the germ. The vaccine establishment wants people to think that if it were not for their intervention, we would constantly be threatened by terrible diseases. When there is no epidemic, they say that the reason that there is no epidemic is because some people have been vaccinated. When there is an epidemic, they say that their vaccine can make the epidemic go away. Sometimes the vaccination machine goes into overdrive when a disease breaks out, revaccinating the vaccinated and trying to put fear into the non-vaccinated, and then when the outbreak dwindles, the vaccinators claim credit for ending the outbreak. I have a dog who thinks that she defeats thunderstorms. If she barks long enough, the thunder goes away, and she has an air of satisfaction at her victory because she believes that she has successfully defended home and family from the threat. It suits the vaccine industry very well that medical bureaucrats choose to think in the same way as my dog thinks.

A prime example of dog-like thinking is the claim made by the vax pushers in New York state that their persecution of the Hasidic community resulted in the ending of the 2019 measles outbreak. Meanwhile the vax pushers had not succeeded in jabbing enough victims to create "herd immunity", and the outbreak dwindled of its own accord, as measles outbreaks always do.

Epidemics of infectious diseases come and go on a natural cycle, and the reasons why they come and go are not known. Some diseases have even disappeared completely, and the reason why they have disappeared is a mystery. At one time sweating sickness was a bigger killer than smallpox, yet it disappeared without a trace before microscopes were invented. Two and a half thousand years ago there was a contagious disease that killed a high proportion of people in North Africa and Greece. Two ancient Greek historians recorded the symptoms of the disease, and they do not match the symptoms of any disease that exists today. Bubonic plague has a history of breaking out suddenly and sweeping across the earth, killing millions in its wake. Why it does this is not known, and why it has long phases of dormancy in between is also not known. A pandemic of scarlet fever began in the 1820s, reached a peak in the 1870s, and then steadily declined of its own accord. I still encounter people who believe that scarlet fever was trounced by vaccination.

It is trendy among some anti-vaxxers to claim that modern hygiene is the reason why some diseases are no longer prevalent, but the theory does not stand up to scrutiny. Water-borne diseases like cholera and typhoid have been eliminated in the parts of the world where the water supply is chlorinated, and lice-borne diseases cannot thrive in the areas where people have enough resources to practice hygiene. However, airborne diseases like diphtheria and scarlet fever are not affected by hand washing and safe drinking water. Another trendy myth is that modern nutrition is the reason why some diseases have stopped being a problem. That is not correct. For a start, most human beings are not well nourished, but more importantly, nutritional factors do not affect the duration nor the locality of an outbreak. During epidemics of the diseases that need intervention, good nutrition does make a difference to an individual's chances of catching the disease, but it has no impact on the behaviour of the germ in the environment. The situation is different regarding the self-resolving childhood diseases. Good nutrition makes no difference to an individual's chances of catching the disease, but it does help to protect the individual from developing complications.

People who claim that hygiene and better nutrition caused smallpox and diphtheria to decline base their belief on the fact that the decline of these diseases coincided with the introduction of hygiene and better nutrition to

North America and Europe. They are confusing correlation with causation. Hygiene and nutrition cannot have been the reason for the decline because those diseases declined everywhere, not just in North America and Europe, and much of the world is still deprived of hygienic living conditions and nourishing food, yet does not suffer from those diseases.

Human beings have some quaint ideas about what causes epidemics to start and end. Bubonic plague broke out in China in the 12th century, and there happened to be a lot of earthquakes occurring at that time. Many people thought that the earthquakes caused the bubonic plague. In the new millennium there is still a lot of unscientific thinking about infectious diseases. The belief that the Great Fire of London made bubonic plague disappear from Europe is still prevalent, even though it is completely illogical. In 1665 London suffered from a bad outbreak of bubonic plague, and then in the following year the Great Fire burned down about a third of the city. The timing of the fire made some people believe that it wiped out the plague; the rationale being that the fire killed the rats that carry bubonic plague. However, the fire spread slowly, and eyewitness accounts describe how the rats ran away from the flames faster than the humans, who were carrying as many possessions as they could. The fire only burned on the north side of the Thames, so all of the rats on the south side of the river lived to a ripe old age. The fire did not make the plague disappear from London itself, let alone from the rest of Europe, yet books and websites for children teach that the Great Fire of London put an end to the plague.

Bubonic plague is a terrifying disease that is caused by a bacterium that lives in the stomach of a type of flea that usually resides in the fur of rats and other rodents. Infected fleas are found on rodents even when there is no epidemic. The fleas can survive away from rodents, so they are sometimes transported on cargo or on humans. The first symptom of bubonic plague is red spots in the groin and armpits. The spots swell and grow together forming big lumps called buboes. The buboes burst open when they are as big as eggs, and the victim either dies within five days, or recovers. Today a lot is known about this bacterium, but it is not known why it suddenly spreads among humans.

The pandemic of bubonic plague that has the greatest impact on modern thinking is the one referred to as the Black Death. This outbreak of bubonic plague started in central Asia, and moved eastwards into China, southwards into India, and westwards towards Europe. It took a jump from the Black Sea to Italy by ship, where it arrived in 1348. No one knows exactly what percentage of the population died during the Black Death. In places that kept records, the death rate from the disease varied between 12% and 66%, with the figures being higher near the sea. Historians estimate that roughly one third of the population of Europe died. This catastrophe had a significant social impact. It brought on the Renaissance, and it provoked insane persecution of minority groups like Jews, Arabs, widows, people with deformities, and people with leprosy.

Another pandemic of bubonic plague that killed millions and had a social and political effect was the one that started in 541 AD. It was called the "Plague of Justinian", and it had a profoundly negative effect on the economy of the Byzantine Empire.

After pandemics of bubonic plague break out they spread rapidly and kill most of their victims in the first few months, but they do not end abruptly. They linger on, and flourish sporadically. The outbreak that ravaged London in 1665 was at the tail end of the Black Death pandemic. During this revival of bubonic plague, a tailor in a rural English village ordered a cloth from London, and unfortunately the cloth was contaminated with bubonic plague bacteria. The tailor died soon after receiving the cloth, and then 267 of the 350 people who lived in the village died too.

Although orthodox medicine does not claim direct credit for the absence of bubonic plague, it uses the horror of bubonic plague for general fear mongering about infectious diseases. For example, a British made "educational" TV programme, which is repeatedly shown in Australia and New Zealand, tells the story of the village community that was devastated by the cloth that brought the plague from London, and then it tells the mythical story of how Edward Jenner invented a vaccine that wiped out smallpox, and then it shows schoolgirls lining up for their rubella jabs in order to be protected from germs. This is a classic example of manipulation by association. It conditions people to accept vaccination. When Chandra was a baby someone told me that in the old days one in every seven people died of the plague, and if it were not for vaccinations, that situation would arise again. "Just imagine what it would be like if one out of every seven of us died," she said, as part of her reason why I should allow Chandra to be injected with whooping cough vaccine.

Cholera is another disease that has a history of sweeping across the world and killing huge numbers of people. It originated in the delta of the Ganges River, where it had been in existence since the 7th century. In 1817 it suddenly took off and spread, travelling westwards across Europe and eastwards across Asia. News of the epidemic travelled ahead of it into Europe, and people became utterly paranoid in advance of its arrival. Cholera is a severe, fast-acting disease that causes cramps that make the victim writhe in agony, and makes the victim lose water quickly through violent vomiting and massive diarrhoea. Death occurs from dehydration unless the disease is stopped by homoeopathy, or the patient is continually rehydrated for five to seven days. Without treatment death can occur within 24 hours of infection.

During the 19th century orthodox medicine used all the usual remedies to treat cholera; mercury, bloodletting, opium, and laudanum. Arguments raged between those who believed that cholera came from the air, and those who believed that it was passed from person to person. It is now regarded as self-evident that cholera can be prevented by keeping the water supply free of sewage, but it took an awfully long time for anyone to work that out. When the people who discovered the connection between cholera epidemics and contaminated water published their findings, they were ridiculed and condemned. Dr. John Snow provided the most compelling evidence that cholera came from water that was contaminated with sewage, and he was viciously ridiculed by the establishment. He had previously been considered a weirdo by the medical establishment because he refused to do cruel experiments on animals while he was a medical student. (Nowadays people who refuse to vivisect are not allowed to become doctors.)

From 1817 to 1902 there were eight pandemics of cholera that spread like waves across large parts of the world. The first wave started in India and stopped its westward movement at Turkey. The second one covered Russia, Europe, and North America. In each place it struck suddenly, and with devastating results. In 1840 a third wave started in India, and it also reached North America. The fourth pandemic followed a different course; it went from the Mediterranean to Russia, instead of the other way round, and it did not reach America. The fifth one started in China, and travelled westwards across Europe, and then across the sea to America. America suffered badly during this one. The sixth one started in 1870, and spread more quickly than the others. Then there was a seventh one in 1891. It must have seemed to the inhabitants of Europe that cholera epidemics were going to pass over the land from east to west every few years for the rest of time. However, the eighth wave, which started in 1902, did not spread beyond southern Europe, and it claimed fewer victims as it went. In less than a hundred years, cholera had almost played itself out, and a sense of security began to settle in. But in 1961 cholera took off again, and epidemiologists were dismayed that none of their interventions, which included locking travellers up in dirty jails, could stop it from spreading into Western Europe.

No one knows why cholera stayed in one place for more than a thousand years and then suddenly took off, nor whether it will develop that sort of virulence again. Cholera still breaks out from time to time, and the reasons why it does that, and why it is absent from unhygienic regions for the rest of the time, are not understood. What is clearly understood is that it cannot spread when the water supply is clean. The Red Cross and other aid organisations are becoming increasingly successful at getting clean water to people who have lost their clean water supply due to political upheavals or natural disasters, and this saves lives. If they used homoeopathy as well they could save even more lives in these circumstances. When refugees fled from Rwanda in 1994, they had no choice but to drink water contaminated with cholera, so those of us who watch TV were subjected to the spectacle of lorry loads of bodies being dumped into pits. How different it would have been if homoeopaths had been allowed to come to the scene and save those people's lives. If the doctors who belong to Médecins Sans Frontières understood the principles of homoeopathy, they would be able to cure cholera, typhoid, typhus, E coli, and all the other infectious diseases that ravage impoverished and displaced communities. The medicine required to cure each patient would cost only a few cents, which is the main reason why the drug companies put so much effort into suppressing homoeopathy.

"IF ENOUGH PEOPLE ARE VACCINATED, THE DISEASE WILL DIE OUT"

Vaccine Myth Number Six: When enough people are vaccinated, the unvaccinated people are protected and most of them will not get the disease. If the infectious agent has no animal reservoir, the disease can be eliminated from this planet by vaccinating a high enough percentage of the human population. When enough people are immune to the disease, it cannot be passed on, and the germ dies out. This state of herd immunity is created when 55% of people have been vaccinated. Er, whoops that should be 75%. We now know that 95% have to be vaccinated to create herd immunity. Actually, 98% is not a high enough percentage, so we'll have to vaccinate everybody, and we'll have to give them booster shots every ten years. No, that will have to be every five years. Perhaps every three years will be more effective.

The theory of herd immunity has no scientific basis, but it is an excellent political tool for vaccine promoters to use when they want the public to believe that vaccine free families are a danger to everyone else. Research done in the city of Baltimore, USA, early in the 20th century, has been misused to promote the theory of herd immunity. The health department in Baltimore kept a record of every case of measles from 1900 to 1931. Dr. A.W. Hedrich, who lived in Baltimore, wanted to find out what proportion of children had already had measles at any one time. To do this he laboriously analysed the Baltimore measles data, month by month. He knew how many children under the age of 15 years there were in Baltimore each month from 1900 to 1931, and he worked out how many of them had already had measles. His analysis showed that the proportion of children under 15 who had already had measles never rose above 53%, and never dropped below 32%, during those thirty two years.[24,234] This means that every time an outbreak came to an end, at least 47% of the children in Baltimore had not yet had measles.

The vaccine industry misrepresented Dr. Hedrich's research by taking an absurd jump in logic. They said that when 55% of children are immune to measles, either through having had measles or through having been vaccinated against measles, epidemics cannot develop.[235,236] That is nonsense because there is a vast difference between a measles outbreak coming to a natural end when 53% of children have already been infected, and an outbreak coming to an end *because* 53% have been infected.

Since then the vaccination rate that is supposed to create herd immunity has steadily crept upwards from 55% to 95%, but the measles virus has not read the instructions. It becomes virulent whenever nature intends it to, and outbreaks occur even when there is a 98% or 100% vaccination rate.[219,237,238,239,240,241,242,243] During these epidemics, both vaccinated and unvaccinated people get measles.

A lot of claptrap has been written about herd immunity,[236,244] none of it grounded on actual scientific evidence. According to the theory of herd immunity, unvaccinated children are being protected from the disease by the vaccinated children, as long as enough children have been vaccinated. The vaccine enthusiasts produce elaborate mathematical formulas which they say are proof that herd immunity protected the unvaccinated. They also say that these mathematical formulas show that a high vaccination rate prevents outbreaks. However, in real life a high vaccination rate does not protect the unvaccinated, and it does not prevent outbreaks. When an infectious germ becomes virulent in the environment, and herd immunity is seen to fail, the vaccine enthusiasts make the excuse that a different mathematical formula should have been used for that type of population group. The myth of herd immunity is a political weapon, not a scientific fact.

The fact that measles vaccination creates temporary immunity leads to delusions about the possibility of eliminating measles. When the measles vaccine was introduced, it was with the promise that one shot would provide life-long immunity. Within the first year it was obvious that this was not so. Then they discovered that during pregnancy a mother who has had measles passes antibodies through the placenta to the baby, and in most babies these antibodies stay in the blood until the age of nine months. They thought that these maternal antibodies must interfere with the baby's production of its own immunity. So they declared that if a child were to be injected with the measles vaccine at the age of 10 months, it would build its own antibodies, and therefore have life-long immunity. But the vaccine still did not work. So they decided that at ten months a baby's immune system was not mature enough to develop enough antibodies, and they changed the dogma to say that the vaccine must be injected at 12 months.

When that did not work, the correct age for injection went up to 15 months. In most people this has the effect of postponing measles until the teenage years or later. When epidemics started breaking out among vaccinated teenagers, they decided that it was necessary for children to have a booster shot at the age of 11 years. New Zealand ran a decade behind the USA, following the same path of changes to policy as each policy was seen to fail.

Some countries have moved the second dose to the age of 4 years, while others are giving two doses during the early years, and giving a third dose at the age of 4. Finland is giving the first dose at 15 months, the second at 18 months, and a third dose at 4 years. This has not stopped children from getting measles.[245] Finland is one of the many countries experiencing an epidemic of autism.

Because the vaccine creates temporary immunity, there is always a period after mass vaccination is introduced in which it looks as though the vaccine is winning against measles. In the USA the vaccine was introduced in 1963.[235] The government said that its aim was to eradicate the measles virus from the USA by 1982.[235] They thought that 20 years of mass vaccination would make it impossible for the wild virus to survive. Mass vaccination at the age of 15 months caused a huge decline in the incidence of measles in the USA - at first. When the artificially induced immunity started wearing off, the graphs started going upwards again. The medicrats have a deceptive way of making it look like less of a failure. In some discourses, any person with measles who was vaccinated under the age of one, or who did not receive the booster jab at the age of 11 years, is classified as "unimmunised", even though their parents were told that they were "fully immunised".

The history of measles in Hungary shows that there is no such thing as "herd immunity". What happened in Hungary also shows that it will not be possible for humans to eliminate the measles virus. When Hungary was under communist rule, the medicrats there maintained a vaccination rate of 98% for 14 years, and they gave booster doses. But measles epidemics continued to occur.

The vaccine was introduced to Hungary in 1969. Although the "correct age" for vaccination was said to be 10 months, all children from 9 to 27 months were vaccinated during mass vaccination campaigns. In 1974 the vaccine became part of routine childhood vaccination, and mass vaccination campaigns were stopped. After that they kept up a vaccination rate of 98%.

In 1978 the "correct age" for vaccination was changed from 10 months to 14 months. Five years after the vaccine was introduced, the virus became virulent, and it was mainly unvaccinated 6-9 year-olds who caught measles. Six years later an epidemic occurred in which it was mainly 7-10 year-olds who caught measles. After this experience, they decided that as ten months had been the wrong age to give the vaccine, all children who had been jabbed at the age of ten months needed a booster shot.

In 1988 the measles virus became virulent again in Hungary, and an epidemic that lasted six months followed. During this epidemic the oldest people who had had the vaccine were 21 years old. Children who were 11-16 years old had had the booster shot. Seventy five percent of the cases for whom ages were recorded were aged 16 to 22 years. The age-specific attack rates were highest in 17-year-olds and second highest in 18-year-olds. From these figures it is obvious that the booster shot adds an extra postponement onto the original postponement in some individuals.

The Hungarian statistics are published in a report[246] from the Centers for Disease Control (CDC), which is based in Atlanta, USA. The compilers of this report comment, "Assessing waning immunity may be difficult because virtually all persons 17-21 years of age were vaccinated approximately the same number of years before the epidemic." This is a really strange statement. Do they think that artificial immunity will wane at the same rate in each individual? And do they really believe that the measles virus is present in the environment all the time?

In 1971 the World Health Organisation thought that measles had been eliminated from the African country of Gambia, because 96% of the population was vaccinated in 1967.[247] In 1972 measles was back in a big way, but they still thought that the strong faith that mothers have in modern medicine was going to help them in "the struggle to attain global control and eradication of measles by the year 2000."[247]

In the years before vaccine induced immunity wears off, measles vaccination does succeed in decreasing the number of cases of measles that occur, but it does not succeed in preventing measles in unvaccinated individuals. In 1984 an outbreak of measles in a Gambian village clearly showed that the background vaccination rate of 90% did not prevent unvaccinated children from getting the disease.[248] 30.1% of the unvaccinated children in the village got measles, while only 3.6% of the vaccinated children got it.[248] This shows that the vaccine prevents or postpones measles in the vaccinated, and that herd immunity does not exist. If there were a totalitarian state strong enough to force 100% of its population to be vaccinated against measles, they still would not be able to wipe out the virus. Dictators can regulate people, but they cannot bully the measles virus.

A typical opinion about measles is, "Measles is an eradicable disease. … humans are the only natural host and the epidemic spread … can only be maintained as a chain of serial direct transmissions of virus, involving acutely affected individuals."[249] This is errant nonsense. The measles virus is caught by humans in one of two ways. It is either caught from a person who has measles, or it is caught from the air. It does not need to be living in a human in order to survive. From time to time the virus becomes virulent and causes an outbreak of measles. In between these times it goes dormant, but it is still alive and well. Some outbreaks of measles are caused by an infected traveller coming into the region, while other outbreaks are caused by the virus coming out of its dormancy.

The person who gets measles first during an outbreak is called the "index patient". The vaccine zealots like to promote the idea that measles outbreaks are started by an unvaccinated person getting measles and passing it on to vaccinated people. These days they make the claim while making sure that the public cannot find out what the vaccination status of the index patient is. Back in 1983 there was an outbreak of measles in a school in which 100% of the students had been vaccinated, and the authorities not only investigated who the index patient was, they actually published the information.[237] There were four unvaccinated preschoolers in the community who got measles, so according to medical mythology, one of them should have been the first to get measles. However, the index patient was a 17-year-old boy who was "fully immunised". The authors say, "The source of his infection was not identified."[237]

I can tell them the source of his infection. It came from a virus that had recently entered a virulent phase, and was floating in the air. Simple. But they want to believe that measles can only be caught from another person with acute measles. Their point of view requires a traveller who is brewing an acute case of measles to enter the community before an epidemic can start. It negates the possibility that the virus goes dormant at times, and then gets virulent again. What happened in this outbreak is that the 17-year-old boy who was the index patient, was the first susceptible person to breathe in the virus when it changed from being dormant to being virulent.

The editorial note says, "This outbreak demonstrates that transmission of measles can occur within a school population with a documented immunization level of 100%. This level was validated during the outbreak investigation."[237] Not only does it demonstrate that measles can be transmitted within a fully vaccinated school, it also shows that measles can *originate* within such a school population.

When the Centers for Disease Control surveyed 93 outbreaks of measles in the USA, they found that 20 of the outbreaks had an index patient who came from overseas, while 73 of the index patients were local people, and no source of infection could be found. This shows that most outbreaks of measles are caused by the dormant virus becoming virulent. In these outbreaks 47% of the index patients were fully immunised.[250]

I can understand why the concept of a virus going into hibernation is foreign to mainstream thinking, because these days so many people live their entire lives separated from nature. I was fortunate enough to grow up on the African veld, where I witnessed the phenomenon of life resurging out of "nothing" in so many ways. For instance, a patch of land that is a dust bowl in the winter, turns into a big pond teeming with aquatic insects, eating each other mercilessly, when the summer rains come. When cattle walk across the spot in the winter, their hooves kick up the dust, and I wonder how the eggs of the insects can survive.

There are some parts of Australia where it does not rain for years at a time, and the creatures that live in these areas have to survive for long periods without water. There are frogs living in these regions, even though frogs need constant moisture to stay alive. When rain falls, puddles and billabongs form on the ground, and frogs abound. After a while the water dries up, so the frogs burrow 30cm down into the ground, where they slough off skin cells to form a watertight cocoon around themselves. They live inside these cocoons for several years, until it rains again. As soon as the next rain season begins, they scramble to the surface and start shouting for a mate.[251]

I suspect that germs that are not in evidence for fairly long periods of time, and then suddenly make their presence known, are able to go into some type of hibernation that is very hard for us to imagine. No one knows what the measles virus does between epidemics. Perhaps the technology needed to trace the measles virus between epidemics already exists. It is also not known what stimulates the virus to become virulent at the end of the dormant stage. The health status of the human host is not the trigger, nor is the movement of people, nor the size and density of communities. There is no space for a dormant measles virus in the thinking of people who want to sell measles vaccine. If research money were committed to exploring the matter, it might be discovered that measles viruses use epidemics to strengthen their DNA. Perhaps the virus can replicate itself while in the dormant state, but gains something extra when it causes measles cases in humans.

According to the theory of herd immunity, unvaccinated children are protected by the vaccinated children, as long as enough children are vaccinated. This is also errant nonsense. What about all the unvaccinated adults who are supposedly spreading germs?

In South Africa in 1980 I heard a doctor say that the Blacks were protected from disease because the Whites were all vaccinated. In effect he was claiming that a 20% vaccination rate is sufficient to create herd immunity. Even more ridiculous is the claim that Edward Jenner's cowpox vaccine made smallpox decline in Britain at the end of the 18th century. The vaccine supposedly did this with a vaccination rate of less than 1%.

People who want to bully health conscious families into vaccinating continually harp on the point that the unvaccinated are protected because the vaccinated create herd immunity. They want to influence public opinion to make people think that non-vaccinating parents are selfish people who exploit those who are vaccinated. In March 1992 the vaccine promoters in New Zealand started feeding the media with the idea that polio and diphtheria epidemics were going to occur because too many parents were not vaccinating. They could not seem to make up their minds exactly what percentage of people needed to be vaccinated to create herd immunity, but it wobbled around in the 80s and 90s. What they were careful not to tell the public is that the vaccination rate had been "too low" to prevent epidemics for ages, without any epidemics occurring. The existence of the vaccine is not the reason for the general absence of diphtheria.

Before the 1993 New Zealand general election, some candidates tried to win votes by saying that they would save the country from infectious diseases by promoting vaccination. This started the media and the medicrats into a frenzy of scaremongering about diseases, and the lie that the measles epidemic of 1991 was caused by unvaccinated children was repeated over and over again. By then they had made up their minds what percentage created "herd immunity", because they kept on saying that a 95% vaccination rate is necessary to prevent further outbreaks.

The World Health Organisation set the date for the elimination of measles at 2000, then moved it to 2007.[252] The new date is 2020, but they have changed the aim to be only for certain regions, not for global elimination.[253] The long term goal is to achieve global elimination by vaccinating nearly everyone on the planet at least twice. The myth of herd immunity is great ammunition for vaccine promoters, because families who do not "co-operate" immediately become cast as the villains of the piece.

People who think that they can control nature by large-scale interference, without causing unexpected consequences, always end up doing more harm than good. People with this mentality do not learn from the mistakes of others. A typical example of the results of this type of thinking happened in China during the rule of the megalomaniac named Mao Tse Tung. He introduced communist economic policies to China, which caused terrible hardship for the people. From time to time he staged "improvement" campaigns to distract his subjects from their real problems, and to boost levels of patriotism. One of these was an anti-sparrow campaign in which he persuaded the populace to use every means at their disposal to kill sparrows. The alleged reason why this was necessary was that sparrows eat crops, and consequently are a threat to human food supplies. The nation swung into action. Schools and villages vied with one another to see who could kill the most sparrows. Truckloads of dead sparrows were paraded up and down the streets. Dead sparrows were strung up on display, and the number of sparrows in China decreased drastically. The resultant imbalance in nature meant that insects ravaged the crops, and food shortages worsened. Of course the people did not manage to kill every last sparrow, and sparrow numbers have now returned to normal in China. The vaccinators are not thinking about what unforeseen consequences they may be unleashing by trying to eliminate measles. Increases in cancer and heart disease are some of the factors that they should be considering.

In June 1992 the New Zealand Health Department launched a mass vaccination campaign in schools that targeted 11-year-olds for MMR vaccine. The Immunisation Awareness Society (IAS) circulated a fact sheet about MMR vaccine in some schools. This incensed the Health Department. The medicrats in Wellington issued a press release saying that New Zealand has a chance of being the first in the world to eliminate measles, but the efforts of the health authorities are being undermined by the IAS, which is circulating information that is "misleading" and "quite wrong". "New Zealand has been the first in a number of fields, and there's no reason why we shouldn't be the first with measles," they complained. They said that measles was likely to be the next disease eliminated worldwide, after smallpox and polio. They were deluding themselves that they were on the verge of eliminating polio, because at that time the date for eliminating polio was set at the year 2000.[254] The World Health Organisation still claims that it is going to eliminate polio from the planet, even though the date for elimination has been passed.[254] Although polio is in a relatively dormant phase at present, (having run from the 1880s until the 1960s), accounts of it having occurred in ancient and medieval times suggest that it will come back. If the polio pandemic that is still petering out does come to a complete end, the vaccine defenders will say that it was vaccination that made it happen. On the other hand, if the polio virus has a resurgence of virulence, they will say it is because people did not have enough doses of the vaccine.

The last case of polio in Fiji occurred in 1959. Polio vaccination was introduced to Fiji in 1963, yet it is credited with ended the epidemic.[255]

In the city of Vellore in India there was a polio outbreak in 1991-92.[256] The vaccination coverage for those years was 98% for three doses, and in 1992 it was 90% for four doses.[256] What happened to herd immunity? All the children who got polio were "fully immunised".[256] There were no cases of polio in the 2% who were unvaccinated.

There was an outbreak of polio in the country of Oman, on the Arabian Peninsula, in 1988-89. It worried some officials from the CDC, UNICEF, and WHO, because it showed that it is not going to be possible to eliminate polio. The title of the CDC/UNICEF/WHO report was, *Outbreak of paralytic poliomyelitis in Oman: evidence for widespread transmission among fully vaccinated children.*[257] The report says, "Among the most disturbing features of the outbreak was that it occurred in the face of a model immunisation programme and that widespread transmission had occurred in a sparsely populated, predominantly rural setting, ... [and] a substantial proportion of fully vaccinated children may have been involved in the chain of transmission." They want to believe that vaccinated children cannot pass on the disease, so evidence that this is not true makes them uneasy.

Vaccinated children passing on the disease that they were vaccinated against happens all the time. In 1996 four babies died of whooping cough in New South Wales. Three of the four had caught whooping cough from a vaccinated person, and one from a person of unknown vaccination status.[258]

The belief in herd immunity leads to many delusions. One of them is that when the number of immune people in a community drops below a certain point, it will make the next epidemic come sooner. In 1976 there was publicity of bad reactions to the whooping cough vaccine in Britain, and as a result the vaccination rate for whooping cough dropped from 76% to 42%. The medicrats expected that the drop in the vaccination rate would make the next whooping cough epidemic be much worse, and they also expected it to make the epidemic come sooner. But the whooping cough bacteria paid no attention to human theories, and the disease followed the usual timing of its natural cycle of virulence. Whooping cough has a predictable cycle, unlike measles and mumps. It reaches a peak every 44 months,[259] and it continued to do so after the vaccination rate dropped to 42%. Medicrats expressed surprise that the epidemic did not start earlier because of the low vaccination rate.[260] There were also fewer cases and fewer deaths during this epidemic. The much lower vaccination rate of 42% made no difference to the timing of the peak in virulence, and it also made no difference to the long-term decline of whooping cough, which had been happening for a hundred years.

As part of their pro-vaccination propaganda, the vaccine promoters untruthfully claim that the drop in the British vaccination rate in 1976 caused an epidemic of whooping cough, with many deaths. The epidemic was not caused by the drop in vaccination, and also there were fewer deaths during this epidemic than during the previous epidemic.[261] The next epidemic started in 1981, and reached a peak in September 1982. The natural pattern of whooping cough was not at all affected by changes in the vaccination rate.

The Central Public Health Laboratory in London compiled a report on the difference between the epidemic that happened before the vaccination rate fell (1974 to 1975), and the one that happened after it fell (1977 to 1979). It says,

> Since the decline in pertussis immunisation there has been an unexpected fall in whooping cough admission and death rates – a fall that has affected children of all ages and vaccination status.[206]

If they had looked at the long-term history of whooping cough, they would have seen that the fall that occurred at that time was not unexpected. Officials who make the statement that a drop in vaccination in Britain caused a deadly outbreak of whooping cough are not telling the truth. Dr. Gordon Stewart says,

> The epidemics of 1977 - 1979 and 1981 - 1982 were in fact the expected cyclical recurrence of whooping cough every 44 months.[259]

The following graph shows that whooping cough has been in decline in Britain for over a hundred years.

Deaths from whooping cough

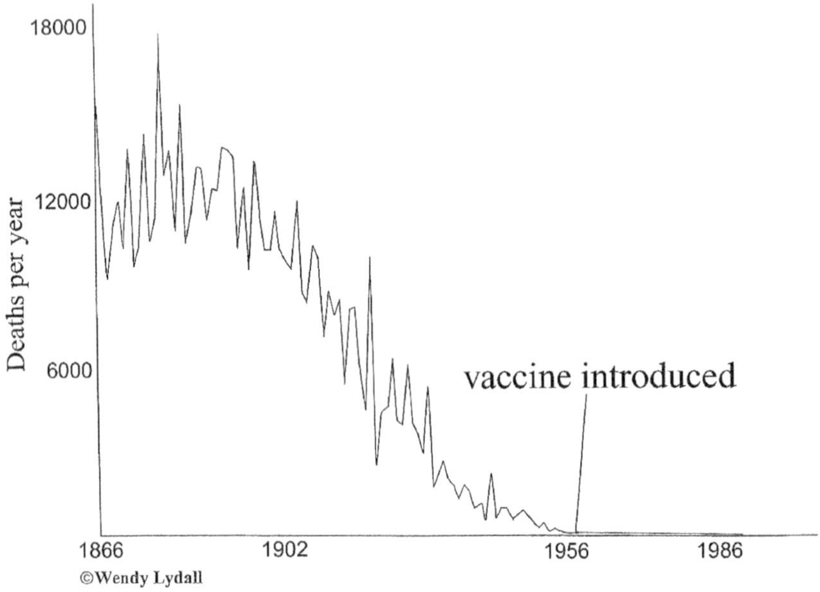

The same decline has occurred in other countries. Against the background decline there are minor ups and downs in virulence. It is the "ups" in virulence that we recognise as epidemics. The rises and falls in virulence occur at the same time all over the planet. Therefore it is not surprising that the two epidemics that Gordon Stewart is talking about followed exactly the same course in Sweden as they did in Britain. These epidemics started, peaked, and then dwindled at the same time in Britain as they did in Sweden, because the germ naturally increased in virulence, reached a peak, and then decreased in virulence, according to its predictable cycle. The first one peaked late in 1978, while the second one peaked in September 1982.[262]

The vaccination rates in Sweden and Britain were very different during the two epidemics under discussion, but that did not affect the behaviour of the germ. Neither did the fact that there was a dramatic difference in the Swedish vaccination rates during the first and second epidemic. During the first epidemic the vaccination rate in Sweden was 84%,[263] while it was 0% during the second epidemic. The first epidemic showed that the vaccine was 100% ineffective, because 84% of the children who got whooping cough were vaccinated.[263] So unlike other governments, the Swedish government stopped using the vaccine. The lack of vaccination in Sweden in 1982 made no difference to the behaviour of the germ that causes whooping cough. People who say that the vaccination rate in a particular area can cause or prevent epidemics are talking nonsense.

The natural decline in the incidence of whooping cough has become a rallying point for the vaccine promoters. They say that the fact that the incidence of whooping cough is declining in the unvaccinated as well as in the vaccinated shows that herd immunity is working.[264,265] This is flawed thinking as it does not show that herd immunity is working. Whooping cough is declining in the unvaccinated because whooping cough has been naturally declining for more than a hundred years, and it is still undergoing that decline.

The vaccine promoters are turning the natural decline in whooping cough to their propaganda advantage, by claiming that they are eliminating the disease from the planet. However, there have been times in the past when they have admitted the truth. When reading the following excerpt about the decline of whooping cough in the USA, bear in mind that the writer is a person who is very keen on promoting vaccines.

> There is little question that the natural history of some infectious diseases has changed spontaneously over the years, for reasons not entirely clear. An example of such a disease is pertussis [whooping cough], which exhibited a mortality rate

> of 12.2 per 100,000 population in the United States in 1900. By the late 1930's, prior to widespread immunization against pertussis, the mortality rate had decreased to approximately two per 100,000. In 1975 only eight deaths due to whooping cough were recorded in the United States.
>
> Whether this reduction prior to the development of widespread immunization (and even the change subsequent to immunization) is due to variations in the organism, changes in the host, or other undetermined factors is unclear.[266]

Whooping cough has become quite rare because of a natural decline that was in full swing for 80 years before the vaccine was introduced. It has small cycles within the big overall cycle. On the small cycle it peaks every forty four months, which is why the line in the graph wiggles so much. The regularity of the mini cycle is not so obvious from the graph, because the mini cycle is chopped up by the Gregorian calendar year. No one can predict whether whooping cough is going to disappear entirely, like English sweating sickness did, or whether it will reach a very low level, and then make a comeback.

The natural decline in whooping cough has been strong and steady, and it appears that some medicrats believe that it is going to disappear. They seem to have the intention of claiming that it has been "eliminated" by the vaccine. As I have described below, vaccinated children with whooping cough are often recorded as having something else, to hide the fact that the vaccine failed, but now there is a new development. Absurdly, some doctors and some laboratories will not test a child with the symptoms of whooping cough for whooping cough, because they say that the disease "no longer exists."[267]

Some vaccine pushers are doing the opposite. They are scaremongering that there is an increase in whooping cough, caused by the refusal of some parents to vaccinate. The real cause of the increase in reports of whooping cough is the introduction of the PCR test, which is able to identify cases of whooping cough that came up negative with previous less sensitive tests.

In 1991 there was an outbreak of whooping cough in Cape Town, South Africa, which showed clearly that herd immunity does not exist. Apartheid was collapsing, and resources were being directed at vaccinating black children. The outbreak occurred against a very high background vaccination rate, and the published commentary was refreshingly honest.

> [Vaccination] does not eliminate the circulating disease agents. As long as this is the case, the unvaccinated will

> remain susceptible even in the face of high or even very high vaccination levels.[268]

That rare admission has proven to be correct. However, the passing of time has shown that the vaccinated also remain susceptible in the face of high or very high vaccination levels.

"IMMUNITY CAN BE MEASURED BY THE DENSITY OF ANTIBODIES IN THE BLOOD"

Vaccine Myth Number Seven: When the germs that cause a particular disease are weakened, and then injected into the human body, the immune system builds antibodies, which are defences against that particular disease. If antibodies are present in the blood in sufficient quantities, the person will be immune to the disease. The number of antibodies that are present in each cc of blood reflects the level of immunity. A person who does not have antibodies will get the disease when exposed to the germ.

The idea that the density of antibodies represents immunity is treated as a scientific fact, because it is the marketing base for selling vaccines. The vaccine industry promotes the myth that antibodies are the most important part of the immune system, because vaccines create antibodies. The technology involved in measuring antibody levels has become increasingly sophisticated since antibodies were discovered, but the theory behind measuring antibody levels has never been scientifically sound.

When a natural infection occurs, the formation of antibodies is only a part of the immune system's response. As I will show, people with lots of antibodies can still get the disease, and people who lack antibodies can remain fit and well despite being exposed to the germs of the disease. The level of antibodies in the blood that is supposed to prevent a person from catching a disease is not determined by scientific investigation; it is just arbitrarily chosen. The history of the discovery of antibodies explains why the antibody threshold theory came to be accepted by the medical establishment.

Elie Metchnikoff was a Russian born zoologist[269] who discovered that there are cells within the bodies of humans and animals that fight invaders, and that these cells travel all around in the body, even in animals that do not have blood. He called these cells phagocytes. He went to work for the

Pasteur Institute in Paris, and he postulated the theory that phagocytes were the means by which the human body defended itself against germs. He experimented with a variety of bacteria, and published many papers and a book promoting his phagocyte theory.

This theory was not well received by the German scientists who believed that immunity was caused by something in the blood. Although Metchnikoff had been born in Russia, he had become a patriotic Frenchman, and at that time the Germans and the French were antagonistic towards one another, because it was not long after the Franco-Prussian War.

German scientists had evidence that there was something in the blood that killed germs, and they saw it as their patriotic duty to prove Metchnikoff's phagocyte theory wrong. A heated and not very polite debate carried on for many years. One side said that it was mobile cells that killed germs, and the other said that it was something in the blood that killed germs.

The Germans produced evidence that phagocytes do not always consume germs, and that the presence of blood makes phagocytes more effective, and that sometimes germs could be killed by the blood without phagocytes being present. The French, on the other hand, produced evidence that no matter how effectively blood could kill bacteria in a test tube, the owner of the blood would not necessarily be able to resist the disease.

The Germans and the French were both right of course, but the war of words did not end with them realising that their respective discoveries were equally important. The war of words ended with the Germans winning, because their theory was commercially profitable. The great breakthrough for the "something in the blood" theory came when Emil von Behring and Shibasaburo Kitasato discovered that blood can make antibodies to diphtheria toxin and tetanus toxin. They claimed that having antibodies to diphtheria toxin in the blood was the only thing that a human needed in order to be immune to diphtheria. The year after antibodies were discovered, Robert Koch made a public announcement that the phagocyte theory was dead. Paul Ehrlich published diagrams of how he thought antibodies operated, and these pictures captured the imagination of laboratory workers around the world. His theory of how antibodies function is now known to be wrong, but the pictures had a profound impact at the time.

Although scientists continued to talk about phagocytes, research work focused on antibodies. Antibodies were much easier to study than phagocytes, and they were also more exciting, because the blood can make antibodies in response to any substance. Blood can make antibodies to all naturally occurring substances, like germs or rabbit flesh or yeast, and it can make antibodies to man-made substances, like plastic and neomycin. All that has to happen is that the substance be injected into the blood stream, and the blood will make antibodies to it. The substance that is injected is called an "antigen". The most important reason why antibodies became regarded as the way to measure immunity, is that human beings can cause antibodies to be made. There is no commercial benefit to be gained from saying that phagocytes are of supreme importance to immunity, when you cannot make phagocytes.

Because the phagocyte theory became unfashionable in 1891, research into phagocytes was neglected for 60 years, although the technology to do this research already existed in the 19th century. In the 1960s research into phagocytes started in earnest again,[269] and now there is consensus that phagocytes and antibodies are of equal importance to immunity. But the vaccine industry is not about to abandon the antibody theory.

Diphtheria is caused by the toxins that diphtheria germs produce, not directly by the germs themselves. Antibodies to this toxin appear in the blood when a person is infected with diphtheria. The young vaccine industry called those antibodies "antitoxin", and they claimed that having antitoxin in the blood was the same thing as being immune to diphtheria.

When clinical experience showed that having antibodies in the blood does not necessarily make a person immune to a disease, Bela Schick came up with an idea to make the antibody theory sound plausible. Bela Schick was an Hungarian scientist who became an American citizen in 1923. He said that a person had to have a certain density of antibodies in the blood in order to be able to fight germs successfully. If the number of antibodies in a millilitre of blood was below that critical threshold, then the person would contract the disease. If the number of antibodies in a millilitre of blood was above that critical threshold, then the person would not get the disease. He even went so far as to declare that the critical threshold for diphtheria was one thirtieth of a unit of antitoxin. So now instead of the antibody theory, we have the antibody threshold theory.

In 1924 a vaccine for diphtheria was introduced to Britain, but it was not yet used for mass vaccination. The new vaccine was made from diphtheria toxin, and the idea was that the person who was injected with it would make antibodies to the toxin, and consequently be immune to diphtheria. Vaccine promoters wrongly claim that the existence of this vaccine is the reason why diphtheria is rare nowadays.

As the graphs in Vaccine Myth Number Four clearly demonstrate, vaccination has been irrelevant to the decline of diphtheria. When outbreaks of diphtheria do occur nowadays, it can be seen that vaccinated people are not protected. The ineffectiveness of the vaccine was more obvious in the early years of its existence, because diphtheria was still virulent in the environment.

In 1940 the Medical Research Council in Britain commenced a ten-year study to see if they could find an explanation for why vaccinated people get diphtheria. Nine doctors conducted the study, and it was published in 1950.[226] The authors of the study had expected to find that vaccinated people who were suffering from diphtheria had low levels of antibody, and that their contacts who did not catch diphtheria had high levels of antibody. They were hoping that they could explain to the public that the vaccinated people who got diphtheria were the ones who had failed to make enough antibodies when vaccinated.

> With a view to advancing the schemes for active immunisation then being initiated, and in order to encourage the more detailed investigation of cases of diphtheria which were being reported as occurring in inoculated persons, the Sub-committee offered to carry out certain examinations of pathological material from such cases. It was arranged that this service should consist of the examination of the bacterial flora of the nose and throat of the patient and the estimation of the circulating antitoxin of the serum separated from blood samples taken at the same time or, in any case, before diphtheria antitoxin had been administered as a therapeutic measure.[270]

The idea that there was an antibody threshold above which a person became immune to diphtheria had been accepted without question, and had become part of the medical dogma. In the preface to the Medical Research Council report, the authors state,

> Contrary to expectation it was found that quite a considerable proportion of cases of diphtheria occurred in inoculated persons who, judged by the antitoxin content of their serum, would normally be expected to be safe from attack.

They began the study by looking at the level of antitoxin in blood samples of 62 vaccinated people who were suffering from diphtheria in England and Wales. When the results were "paradoxical," they halted the investigation and reviewed their method.

> The paradox was this: on repeated occasions it was found that a sample of serum, taken from a patient with a clear history of inoculation, who had yielded diphtheria bacilli

> from nose or throat swabs, and who according to the clinical history exhibited some or other of the classical symptoms of true diphtheria, was found to contain quite large quantities of diphtheria antitoxin. Now according to Schick, persons whose serum contains not less than one-thirtieth of a unit of antitoxin per ml. or, according to workers in this and other countries, persons whose serum contains not less than one-hundredth of a unit of antitoxin per ml., should not contract diphtheria. Yet of 62 of the patients investigated prior to April 1942 no less than 25 (40%) were found to contain one-tenth of a unit, or more, of diphtheria antitoxin per ml. of serum; and of these, 5 contained 10 units or more, 7 contained 1 to 4 units, and 13 contained 0.1 to 0.8 units per ml. of serum; there was no significant association, however, between severity and antitoxin content.[222]

So not only had they found that high levels of antibody did not prevent diphtheria, they also found that it did not make the disease milder. The table they provide shows that according to the dogma of the "workers in this and other countries," 69.3% had enough antibodies to make them immune to diphtheria, and 8% had more than a thousand times the density of antibody that is supposed to confer immunity. So instead of being able to explain away vaccine failures to the public, the authors found themselves in the possession of evidence that the antibody threshold theory is false.

They decided that there must be some mistake in their method. They thought that perhaps the glass syringes that were used to draw the blood samples still had antitoxin clinging to them from the horse blood or human blood that had been in them during previous use. So they decided to set up a second investigation in which they would be sure that the syringe had been properly cleaned before the blood sample was taken from the diphtheria patient. The second part of the study focused on the geographical region of Newcastle and Gateshead, and they took great care to ensure that none of the equipment was contaminated with other blood.

> The primary object of the second part of these investigations was to determine whether it is a fact that true clinical diphtheria occurs in patients whose serum contains a concentration of antitoxin in excess of the level originally laid down by Schick as providing adequate protection against the disease, viz. one-thirtieth of a unit of antitoxin per ml. It was considered that an answer to this question could be obtained if rigid adherence to certain conditions relating to the selection of patients and

> the collection of pathological material and its examination was observed.[271]

Well an answer to that question was obtained, and the answer was that true clinical diphtheria does occur in people who have more antitoxin in their blood than the cut-off level "laid down" by Schick. They decided to keep the results from Gateshead and Newcastle separate, so that they would know there was a problem with their method if the results from the two regions were different. The results from the two areas were the same.

So this was really two studies, and they both proved the same thing. They both proved that being vaccinated, and having a high level of antibodies in the blood, does not protect a person from getting diphtheria. Some of these victims had one hundred and twenty times the density of antibody in the blood than that which was supposed to protect them.[272]

Another thing that perplexed the researchers was that they found that many of the nurses and family members who were in close contact with the diphtheria patients, and had very low levels of antibody in their blood, and also had live diphtheria germs living in their throats, did not catch diphtheria.[273]

On page 154 of the Medical Research Council report they give the results of a study done in Copenhagen. The Danish study was more thorough than the British one because it used controls. They measured the antibody levels of four groups of people;

* the vaccinated with diphtheria,
* the vaccinated without diphtheria,
* the unvaccinated with diphtheria,
* and the unvaccinated without diphtheria.

The Danish study found that vaccinated people who had diphtheria had the same spread of levels of antibody as vaccinated people who did not have diphtheria, and both of these groups had much higher levels of antibody than the third and fourth groups. So this study proved conclusively that vaccination does produce antibodies, but it does not produce immunity.

They also refer to earlier studies which showed that the antibody threshold theory was wrong.

> As long ago as 1920 Solis-Cohen et al. showed that the blood of some persons destroyed diphtheria bacilli whereas that of others did not and that the result was independent of the antitoxin content; others (Bloomfield, 1924; Arnold, Ostram and Singer, 1928) have emphasised the importance

> of the mucous membrane of the nose and throat in removing micro-organisms deliberately applied thereto, and Digby (1923) ascribed an important role to the tonsils and the subepithelial lymphoid tissue in effecting a similar clearance and destruction of micro-organisms.[274]

So as early as 1950 there already existed a weighty body of evidence which showed that vaccination against diphtheria is a useless procedure, and that the antibody threshold theory is false. Yet diphtheria vaccination is still forced on babies today. The Medical Research Council study of 1950 was done by nine doctors in a prestigious institution of orthodox medicine, yet it has been steadfastly ignored by the medical establishment. The lesson the medical establishment learned from this study is that they must not do studies on the relationship between antibodies and immunity, because maintaining the myth of the antibody threshold theory is essential for the promotion of vaccines. Subsequent evidence that the antibody threshold theory is false has emerged in anecdotal comments in reports on vaccine failure during epidemics.

In 1980 a vaccine promoter who was reviewing the history of measles vaccination in the USA, and making recommendations about future policy, had this to say,

> We must also acknowledge that questions remain about measles serology - for example, what titer shall we agree upon as the cutoff indicator of immunity?[235]

Serology means study of the blood, and titer, in this context, means density of antibodies. If achieving a certain density of antibodies in the blood actually means that the germs of that disease cannot replicate in the owner of the blood, then it should be possible, by doing research, to find out what that critical density is.

When a person's blood makes antibodies, the medical jargon used to describe the event is "seroconversion". Another phrase that crops up in vaccination talk is "immunogenic efficacy". This is medical jargon for "effectiveness at causing immunity". Before a new vaccine is marketed, it is tested to see whether it makes "enough" antibodies. The density of antibodies that is going to be accepted as "enough" is not decided by clinical experimentation. It is decided by sitting around a table and making a guess. If the vaccine creates "enough" antibodies in 80% of the test people, they then say, "The immunogenic efficacy of the vaccine is 80%."

Antibodies can do many different things. They can cover an invading germ to make it easier for the scavenger cells of the immune system to eat it. They can attract complement proteins towards a spot on the surface of a bacterium, and the complement proteins then punch a hole in the bacterium and make it explode. They can also immobilise a virus by grabbing hold of certain points on the virus and making it impossible for it to reproduce.[275] All of this is very useful, but the fact that antibodies can do these and other things does not automatically mean that having a certain number of antibodies in the blood will prevent the clinical symptoms of disease from developing in any particular human being.

There is a genetically inherited condition that makes a person unable to manufacture antibodies of any kind. Children who have this condition can have measles in the normal way, and acquire immunity, despite not manufacturing any antibodies.[276,277] This shows that something else is providing the immunity.

Many writers on the immune system accept the assumption that antibodies reflect immunity, and they do not question the validity of the assumption. Vaccine promoters like graphs which show the rise and fall of antibodies in the blood after a vaccine is swallowed or injected. The idea that antibodies are all that has to be considered in immunity has become so ingrained in the thinking of vaccine believers, that they consider the words "antibodies" and "immunity" to be interchangeable. In many articles in medical journals they use the word "immunity", when they are really talking about the level of antibodies. This skewed thinking leads to confusion in the minds of the bureaucrats who create vaccination policies.

An example of this skewed thinking occurred after the Immunisation Awareness Society compiled a fact sheet about the MMR vaccine for distribution in New Zealand schools. The Chief Medical Advisor to the Health Department wrote a rebuttal of our fact sheet that tried to convince parents that they should not believe what we had written. One of the points that our fact sheet made is that the measles vaccine does not prevent measles, it merely postpones measles till the person is older than the usual age for measles. The way that the medical advisor tried to refute that point was by saying that the vaccine "has been shown to produce antibodies in over 90-95 percent of those who are vaccinated." This indicates that he believes that manufacturing antibodies is the same thing as acquiring life-long immunity. What was especially amazing about this clumsy rebuttal was that it was made soon after an epidemic of measles in New Zealand had demonstrated that vaccinated children got measles as adolescents, while unvaccinated children got measles as pre-schoolers, or in the early years of school.

Shortly before the measles epidemic started, I gave a talk about the wrongs of vaccination to a group of nurses. This was followed by a talk on the virtues of vaccination given by a doctor. Instead of trying to refute the information that I had presented, the doctor spent her part of the talk drawing graphs on a blackboard showing what antibody levels do in the majority of people after the injections. She explained that live viral vaccines like the measles vaccine are given once only because they create "enough" antibodies at the first shot, while other vaccines are given three times because the first dose creates only a few antibodies, while subsequent doses create sufficient antibodies.

I was entertained by the body language of the audience while she spoke. My supporters from the Immunisation Awareness Society flopped with despondency. The young nurses who doubted the wisdom of vaccination looked bored because they had heard all this claptrap before, but the nurses who loved vaccination sat bolt upright, with their ears perked up and their eyes bright. They lapped it up because it justifies what they do all day.

On each of the graphs the doctor drew a line at the level at which immunity is supposed to be achieved. When she was discussing the polio graph, I asked her if she knew of any studies that confirmed that that particular level of polio antibodies really does create clinical immunity. She replied that she did not. I commented that I had been looking for such a study, and had not been able to find one. She was completely unperturbed by the lack of evidence to support the dogma. I suppose she thinks that because so many people in the medical profession believe the dogma, there must be some evidence to support it somewhere.

During the measles epidemic that started a few weeks after this gathering, half of the reported cases occurred in vaccinated children. This made the Health Department change its policy to saying that two doses of measles vaccine are necessary. So the dogma that says that live viral vaccine is needed once only was thrown out of the window, but they still love the graphs.

There are accounts of women with high levels of antibody getting rubella during pregnancy, and the baby being born with congenital rubella syndrome.[181,182,183,184,185,186] The myth that antibody levels reflect immunity will continue to be accepted by the government officials who buy vaccines from the manufacturers until consumer awareness brings about a change.

Before antitoxin and antibodies were discovered, the medical profession used a different but just as unscientific theory to decide whether or not a vaccine had caused immunity. If scratching smallpox pus into the skin caused a flare-up around the scratch, then it was said that the vaccine had "taken". If there was no reaction on the skin, then it meant that the vaccine had not taken, and it needed to be done again. They never had any scientific basis for this theory, they just made it up. Perhaps it originated as a way of pacifying people who were unhappy about the pain that the flare-up caused.

Some enlightening figures were collected during an outbreak of smallpox in Italy that ran from 1887 to 1889. Before the outbreak started, 98.5% of the general population had been vaccinated at least once, and many had been vaccinated more than once. All soldiers were vaccinated every six months. The Italian army kept a record of whose vaccinations had "taken" and whose had not. During the epidemic, 47,772 people died of smallpox.[278] Among the soldiers, the rate of smallpox was greater in those whose vaccinations had "taken", and out of those who got the disease, the death rate was twice as high in those whose vaccinations had "taken."[278] Clearly it is not true that a bad reaction to smallpox vaccination meant that the vaccination had created immunity.

"THE VACCINE FAILED BECAUSE ….."

Vaccine Myth Number Eight: The vaccine failed because the person had not had enough doses. We now know that you need two/four/five doses of that vaccine to become immune. The vaccine could not have been properly stored if it failed after so many doses. The vaccine did not work because it was given at the wrong age. The strain that made the disease break out must be different to the strain in the vaccine.

The vaccine industry claims that the reason why most people are not suffering from infectious diseases is because of vaccination, when in fact most of the time there is no virulent naturally occurring germ in the environment to test whether or not people are immune. A vaccine only gets an opportunity to fail when the disease comes into the environment. Very few people ever experience an infectious disease other than flu and the self-resolving childhood diseases. When an epidemic of one of the less common infectious diseases breaks out, only a tiny proportion of people actually come down with the prevailing malady. The exception to this is bubonic plague, which at the peak of its wave affected a high proportion of the population.

When a germ does become virulent and an outbreak of the disease occurs, vaccinated people get the disease. Medical doublespeak calls this "breakthrough disease". In some circumstances the medical authorities feel compelled to make excuses for the failure of the vaccine. I have encountered thirteen excuses to which vaccine promoters resort when they are confronted with evidence that a vaccine has failed. During outbreaks they often use more than one excuse at a time.

THIRTEEN EXCUSES FOR VACCINE FAILURES

Excuse number 1: "The cold chain must have been broken."

This is an excellent excuse because it is hard to prove that the cold chain was not broken. Each vial of vaccine is supposed to be kept at a temperature below 4ºC from the time it leaves the manufacturer until the time it is used. When a vial of vaccine is not kept at a temperature below 4ºC until the time it is used, it is said that the cold chain has been broken, and the vaccine may have lost its virulence.

In the absence of any investigation it is easy to say that someone in the transport line must have left the vial of vaccine out of the fridge for a while, and hence the cold chain got broken.

During the 1982 polio epidemic in South Africa, the medicrats said that polio was affecting the immunised because "the cold chain must have been broken". They collected 17 vials of vaccine from remote outposts, and brought them back to Johannesburg, making sure that the cold chain was not broken on the way back.[279] These were tested for virulence by seeing how much virus could be grown from the vaccine, and by being injected into children who had no antibodies to polio at all. The virus colonies grown from half of the vials were not dense enough to meet the internationally accepted "titre", but all of the children manufactured a satisfactory level of antibodies, so a conclusion about whether the cold chain had been broken could not be made. They then took strong measures to protect the cold chain, so this particular excuse was not available to explain away the failure of the vaccine during the next polio epidemic, which occurred in 1987 (see below).

One of the excuses for the failure of measles vaccination in New Zealand in 1991 was that the vaccine gets warm when it travels by ship from Europe. If that is so, then according to their dogma, there is no point in importing the vaccine. They might as well stop subjecting the children of New Zealand to the risk of adverse reactions.

Excuse number 2: "It must be a different strain."

This one amuses me because vaccination started off with the claim that cowpox causes immunity to smallpox, but when it suits them they say the opposite and claim that in order to create antibodies that will be effective, the surface antigen of the germ in the vaccine has to be exactly the same as the surface antigen of the invading germ. In other words, the germ that happens to come along years later and tries to cause disease, has to be the same strain as the germ that was in the vaccine, or else the antibodies will not work.

The "different strain" excuse is frequently used for whooping cough in vaccinated children, and now they are even beginning to use it for measles. It is not a popular excuse with the makers of measles vaccine, because they stand to gain financially from the introduction of repeated doses of vaccine. So they tend to support the idea that booster shots are needed.

The whole cell whooping cough vaccine contains a bacterium called bordatella pertussis. Whooping cough can be caused by bordatella pertussis, by bordatella parapertussis, or by an adenovirus.[280] A natural dose of whooping cough creates life-long immunity, no matter which of the three strains caused the disease. The vaccine promoters choose to ignore this when they blame a "different strain" for causing whooping cough in a vaccinated child.

A natural dose of measles is caused by only one strain, yet it confers life-long immunity to all the strains of measles virus. The reason why vaccines for childhood diseases do not confer life-long immunity, while a natural infection with the disease does, is not known. One theory is that because an injected vaccine bypasses the mucous membranes, the immune system does not process the germs in the vaccine in the same way as it processes the germs from a natural infection. The lining of the nasal passages, throat, and digestive tract contain different aspects of the immune system to what the blood contains. For example, there is Immunoglobulin A in the mucous membranes, but Immunoglobulin G and Immunoglobulin M in the blood. All the self-resolving childhood diseases are caused by germs that float in the air. They enter the human body via the mouth and nose, so they meet the immune system in the mucous membranes, and the germs spend a few days in this area before they move on to meet the different features of the immune system in the blood. It is theorised that something happens in those few days that makes the immune system able to mount life-long immunity after the encounter with the blood. The significance of different types of antibodies and different types of immunoglobulin is beginning to attract research. Another theory as to why a natural infection creates life-long immunity is that the process that causes the symptoms of each childhood disease also causes a process that has not yet been detected. The vaccine industry has no incentive to research how life-long immunity is generated, nor why vaccines for childhood diseases are incapable of achieving this.

Medical dogma says that a person who swallows the oral polio vaccine, which contains three strains of polio virus, can only make antibodies to one strain at a time. They also say that having antibodies to that particular strain does not make a person immune to the other two strains. They say that is why a person has to have three doses of vaccine, and cannot be considered "immune to polio" after swallowing only one or two doses. This is a useful excuse when children who have had one or two doses of vaccine get polio, but it becomes obsolete when children who have had three, four, or five doses of oral vaccine get polio.

When I first heard the claim that the human immune system can only make antibodies to one strain of polio at a time, I naively believed it, although I thought it was strange because the body can make antibodies to nine different diseases at the same time. This anomaly niggled in my mind, until I read the official report of the 1982 polio epidemic in Gazankulu, South Africa, in which the authors describe the tests they did to see whether vials of vaccine had lost their virulence. Thirty percent of the children who had no antibodies at all before vaccination, developed antibodies to all three strains after one dose. The report comments that this was consistent with previous observations made by the professor.[279] So we see that this excuse is not valid.

Excuse number 3: "Too few doses of vaccine were given."

For each vaccine there is a certain number of doses that is regarded as "scientifically correct". A plausible sounding reason is given for declaring that that particular number of doses creates immunity to that particular disease, but the number changes when the real world intervenes and demonstrates that the alleged magic number of doses does not cause immunity. When they change the number they also change the reason.

At the beginning of 1991 the dogma in New Zealand was that one dose of measles vaccine was sufficient to create life-long immunity, because it is a live virus vaccine. This was old-fashioned dogma that had already been discarded in the USA. When thousands of vaccinated children got measles in 1991 the dogma was changed to say that a second dose had to be given. Some governments are now adamantly claiming that two doses of measles vaccine will give life-long immunity. However, it has already been seen that children who have had three doses of measles vaccine can get measles.[245]

As mentioned above, the theory behind giving three doses of polio vaccine is that human blood can only make antibodies to one of the three strains of polio virus at a time, which sounds plausible enough until you know that this is not true, as blood can make antibodies to all three strains at the same time. When an epidemic of polio breaks out, and people who have had three doses of vaccine start getting polio, they increase the number of doses needed to create immunity to polio to four. As they have then run out of strains to blame, they stick to talking about "doses" and avoid mentioning strains.

The rationale behind giving whooping cough and diphtheria vaccine three times was that the first shot only creates a small number of antibodies, while the second and third shots greatly increase the density of antibodies in the blood. But now they give the vaccine four times, and five times in some countries, because three doses does not work. When the whole cell whooping cough vaccine was first introduced, it was given to babies of six months. At that age the first dose does make a lot of antibodies. When the age for the first shot was brought down to six weeks, it was found that such young babies could not make antibodies, hence the introduction of a second, then a third, and then a fourth dose. There was a complete disregard for the fact that the vaccine causes far more cases of brain damage at six weeks of age than it does at six months of age. The "not enough doses" excuse is being used for the failure of the new acellular whooping cough vaccine, even though it is given four times, and more often in some countries. However, some medicrats are saying that the new vaccine is failing because it is not as effective as the old vaccine. They have forgotten that the old vaccine was also not very effective.

Excuse number 4: "The victims did not create enough antibodies when they were vaccinated."

The antibody threshold theory is the commercial backbone of the vaccine industry, which is why I devoted considerable space in Vaccine Myth Number Seven to tracing its historical origins and exposing the myth. This excuse is not valid, because the level of antibodies in the blood is not a reflection of the level of immunity.

Excuse number 5: "It was given at the wrong age."

This excuse lasts until children who were vaccinated at the latest "correct age" get the disease. Then they have to change the "correct age" yet again, or revert to other excuses. I have described how after the measles vaccine had been used for a year in the USA, the "correct age" for vaccination was set at 10 months. Then it was moved to 12 months, then it was moved to 15 months, but children still got measles. Then they realised they would be making good and proper fools of themselves if they raised it to 18 months, so they opted for a booster dose at the age of 11 years, instead of altering the "correct age" yet again.

New Zealand went through almost the same scenario. When the vaccine was first introduced it was given at 10 months, but then they changed the "correct age" to 12 months. Then it was changed to 15 months, and then to 15 months plus a booster at 11 years. They lagged a decade behind the USA with each policy change. When a child gets measles before the first dose, or between the first and second dose, the New Zealand Health

Department still wants the child to have the two doses of vaccine.

Now the world-wide trend is to say that eleven years is the "wrong age" for the second dose, and giving the second dose much earlier will solve the problem. They are combining the "incorrect age" excuse with the "too few doses" excuse.

The Australian health department claims that administering the second dose at the age of 4 years will create life-long immunity. They are saying in their promotional literature that having the second dose at 4 years means the recipients will not need a third dose. We shall see.

It is not ideal for babies to get measles during the first year of life,[1] and when a woman has a baby before she has had measles, the baby is vulnerable to getting measles during the first year.[281] Now that the measles vaccine has existed for more than a generation, a new scenario is happening. Babies of vaccinated mothers who have not yet had measles are getting measles during their first year, and consequently suffering from a high rate of complications and death.[219,282] The ever resourceful vaccine industry is using this as an excuse for giving infants in impoverished regions an extra dose of MMR vaccine.[283,284]

Excuse number 6: "The vaccine was improperly handled."

This is a great excuse because it does not mean anything. It is used surprisingly often. People who are impressed by medical qualifications might think this statement has great import when it emanates from medically dignified vocal cords.

Excuse number 7: "The vaccine must have been overdiluted."

Do they mean that the total amount of the original substance was used but too much liquid was added, or that less than the total amount of the original was used before it was diluted? In the case of a live viral vaccine it is of no consequence anyway, because the virus starts to replicate once it gets into the body, and the result is an unpredictable "dose". With killed vaccines, dilution is also irrelevant, because the vaccine industry has never bothered to work out a "correct dose" per body weight. A six-week-old baby gets injected with the same amount as a five-year-old child.

In every instance where I have seen this excuse being used, there has been no mention of any investigation into whether or not the vaccine really was diluted.

Excuse number 8: "The vaccination rate in the community was too low to create herd immunity".

The brilliant logic of this excuse is that the unvaccinated children caused the vaccinated children to get the disease, whereas if there had only been a few unvaccinated children, they would not have been able to cause the vaccinated children to get the disease. The myth of herd immunity is used as a political weapon against health conscious families. Therefore I have discussed it in detail in Vaccine Myth Number Six.

Excuse number 9: "It must have been a bad batch."

This is usually an excuse made for serious adverse effects, but it is sometimes used for vaccine failures. I have never seen this excuse used in conjunction with an investigation into whether or not all the people who caught the disease when the germ became virulent had been injected with the same batch.

Excuse number 10: "He had not had time to develop immunity yet."

This excuse was introduced to explain away the failure of Louis Pasteur's rabies vaccine,[285] and it has been used ever since to reduce the figure of vaccine failures. An arbitrary length of time is chosen in which "immunity" is said to develop, and anyone who gets the disease within that time period after vaccination is not counted as a vaccine failure.

This is a particularly good excuse for them to use when a mass vaccination campaign is started up during an epidemic. Most of the vaccine failures can be excused away, because most of the vaccinated people who get the disease have been vaccinated "too recently". Epidemics always come to an end, and then they say that those who were vaccinated during the campaign, and did not get the disease, were protected by the vaccine, while at the same time saying that those who were vaccinated during the campaign, and did get the disease, were not protected because they had not had time to develop immunity.

This excuse is also used when the vaccine causes the disease it was supposed to prevent. A natural infection takes a while to incubate, so they say that the person must have been exposed before being vaccinated. The germs in the vaccine go straight into the blood, so in a person who is susceptible to getting the disease from the vaccine, the symptoms show up quickly. When this happens, the vaccinators say that the injected germs did not cause the symptoms. They say it was just that the person "had not yet had time to develop immunity." Doctors even sometimes say this when it happens in the absence of an outbreak.

Excuse number 11: "The wrong type of vaccine was used."

This is a useful excuse for those cases of measles that occur in the now older age group who were injected with killed virus measles vaccine, before live viral vaccine was invented. The converse does not happen. When a person who was injected with live virus vaccine gets measles, they do not make the excuse that killed virus vaccine should have been used, because killed virus vaccine is definitely out of favour.

The makers of oral polio vaccine and the makers of injected polio vaccine accuse each other of providing "the wrong type of vaccine." Although injected polio vaccine was ditched in most countries 50 years ago, it has made a comeback in some affluent countries, and is being used in some impoverished countries where infections of the digestive tract are common. The given reason for the latter is that when a person has diarrhoea, the oral vaccine passes out of the body too quickly for antibodies to be formed. So with each epidemic, the manufacturers of the type of vaccine that was not used in the affected area, can claim that the other type of vaccine is no good.

Excuse number 12: "The parents might have falsified vaccination certificates."

I have only seen this excuse used once, in a letter to the editor of a medical journal.[286] He was referring to a previous article about an outbreak in a high school with a 100% vaccination rate. His argument was that he had once come across a group of parents who opposed vaccination for nonreligious reasons, and he had "reason to believe" that some of them had falsified vaccination certificates. He apparently realises that this is a rather feeble excuse, because towards the end of his letter he says, "It is not likely that falsification of immunization records occurred to an extent sufficient to alter the results of the study."

Excuse number 13. "The vaccine was injected into the wrong part of the body."

The bloodstream carries the vaccine throughout the body, so the site of injection is irrelevant.

EXCUSES FOR THE FAILURE OF MEASLES VACCINE

Before the days of measles vaccination it was common knowledge that a natural dose of measles created life-long immunity to measles, and when measles vaccine was introduced the vaccine zealots expected that the vaccine would do the same. It was also common knowledge that there was a higher rate of complications of measles in people who got measles in adulthood compared to those who got it in childhood. The study on measles in Baltimore that was published in 1930 (and later used to concoct lies about herd immunity) found that 95% of people contracted measles before the age of fifteen.[234] It would have been ideal if someone had been able to follow the other 5% throughout life to see how many of them got measles during adulthood, and how many never got it.

In 1846 a Danish doctor was sent to the remote Faroe Islands in the Atlantic to investigate an outbreak of measles. There had been a gap of sixty five years since the previous outbreak on these islands, and the doctor found that people who were sixty five or older did not get measles if they had had measles as children, and that, "all the old people who had not gone through with measles in earlier life were attacked when they were exposed to infection".[287] He also found that there was a high death rate among infants who got measles when they were less than one year old, and a much higher death rate from measles in adults than in those under twenty.[287]

The vaccine industry's hope that measles vaccine would create life-long immunity was quickly dashed when they saw some children getting measles less than a year after being vaccinated. However, in most cases the vaccine postpones measles for more than a decade. *MMWR* is a weekly publication produced by the Centers for Disease Control in Atlanta, USA. It publishes articles about diseases in all countries, not only in the USA. In 1992 I read through all the data on measles epidemics in all the issues of *MMWR* published since the measles vaccine was invented, and they all showed the same thing; the bulk of vaccinated people with measles were in their teens or were young adults, while the bulk of unvaccinated people with measles were children. It made no difference what language the people spoke, nor at what age the first jab was given, nor whether booster jabs were given to try to bolster waning immunity.

In 1991 there was a measles epidemic in New Zealand which clearly showed that the vaccine failed. However, the vaccine zealots saw the epidemic as an opportunity to promote vaccination. They staged a brilliant campaign that succeeded in causing panic in many parents. Three months after the measles epidemic started, they conducted a five day blast in the media. On a Monday morning New Zealanders woke up to the "news" that a deadly virus had suddenly broken out and was sweeping through the population like a terrible reaper. Radio, TV, and newspapers made it a prime news story. Civil defence vans with loud-hailers built into their roofs cruised the streets of the poorer areas of Auckland, telling the population that a killer virus was on the rampage, and that children needed an injection to be protected. The vans reminded me of the Casspirs that used to patrol the black ghettos in South Africa, except that instead of spewing out teargas, they were spewing out lies. And just like in Soweto, children were the targeted victims. The existence of these vehicles in New Zealand is justified by the threat from earthquakes and volcanoes, but they were being misused to promote a pharmaceutical product.

The propagandists said that even if children were already vaccinated, they should be done again, or they could die. People flocked in droves to vaccination clinics. Even little children who had been done only a year before were done again. It did not seem to bother the parents that the first dose their children had been given was done with the promise of life-long immunity. Afterwards it was left to the committee members of the Immunisation Awareness Society (IAS) to give emotional support to the parents of those who were severely brain damaged by the vaccine during the campaign.

The high intensity part of the campaign ended on the Friday of that week, with the announcement that the vaccination campaign had been successful, and the epidemic was now under control. In the following week, more new cases of measles broke out than had broken out during the propaganda week, but the media kept quiet about it.

If the Health Department had been honest they would have said;

* a measles epidemic started three months ago, and it has not yet reached its peak,

* vaccinated and unvaccinated children are getting measles,

* if children are not properly cared for while they have measles, they can die,

* being vaccinated makes people vulnerable to measles at an older age.

IAS tried to get these four points across to the public, but the mainstream media was not interested in allowing the public to have access to the facts. The media only repeated whatever came from the Health Department.

Sociologist Kevin Dew wrote a thesis about the Health Department's fear mongering campaign, and about IAS's attempts to provide the public with factual information.[288] Kevin conducted his research without making the prior assumption that vaccination is safe and effective. He is in good company with writers like Herbert Spencer and Beatrix Potter. In his thesis he compared the claims made by the Health Department with the findings of scientific studies. He also showed how the Health Department created the "problem", and then presented themselves as having the "solution", due to their "superior knowledge". They then defined those who did not comply with the "solution" as deviants. He showed how the Health Department used the media as an agent of moral indignation, and how successful the campaign had been as a means of achieving social control. He described how the Health Department tried to use him as part of their propaganda exercise as soon as they knew that he was writing about them. He remarked that studying the Health Department felt like being embroiled in politicking, whereas studying the IAS felt like doing research.

The epidemic lasted another eight months, and everybody knew someone who got measles. People were talking about the fact that vaccinated children were getting the measles "very badly". Some medicrats started to mutter excuses for the failure of the vaccine. The chosen excuses were;

* The vaccine was given at the wrong age because in those days they did not know how to do things properly. (Half of the vaccinated children with measles had in fact been vaccinated at what was considered to be the "correct age" at the time of the epidemic.)

* The vaccine had been "wrongly handled".

* Unvaccinated children had caused the epidemic to break out and had made vaccinated children get it.

* The vaccine had baked in the sun on the ships on the way from Europe.

* and then finally they announced that one dose of vaccine was not enough, and a booster had to be given at age eleven, even to children who had already had measles as well as the vaccine.

A promising young Auckland gymnast was prevented from participating in the Olympic Games in Barcelona because she caught measles during this epidemic. New Zealanders had been very excited about her talent for gymnastics, because she was said to be the best in the world, and they were hoping that she would win a gold medal. First she had to participate in trials in the USA in order to qualify for the Olympics. She had no symptoms when she departed for the USA, but she came out in spots and a fever once she got there, and was unable to participate. Her father said,

> "It's just one of those things. Her Plunket records show she was vaccinated at 11 months and the experts now say it should be 15 months."[289]

What these self-proclaimed "experts" were not telling the poor man is that thousands of children who had been vaccinated at the "correct age" of 15 months were also getting measles. They also did not tell him that if his daughter had never been vaccinated, she would most likely have had measles when she was much younger, and it would not have been able to interfere with her career later on. To all the wrongs that the measles vaccine has done, we can add that it robbed New Zealand of the chance to win a gold medal in gymnastics at the Barcelona Olympics.

The measles epidemic lasted 11 months, with 8000 cases, which is a significant number in a small country like New Zealand. At the beginning of the epidemic, New Zealand Health Department dogma still adhered to the belief that one dose of vaccine at the age of 15 months would give life-long immunity, because it is a live viral vaccine. However, the statistics showed that half of the children who got measles were teenagers who had been vaccinated, and half of those had been vaccinated at the "correct age" of 15 months, while the other half had been vaccinated at 12 months. The unvaccinated children who got measles were all younger than teenagers, as nature intended it.

The official report of the Communicable Disease Centre[290] did not publish the figures. The report stated that the epidemic had occurred because not enough children aged 12 - 15 months had been vaccinated, and because only 82% of children had been vaccinated by their second birthday. Towards the end of the report an evasive admission was made,

> In addition to the failure to achieve high vaccination coverage levels, there is some evidence that primary and/or secondary vaccine failure also contributed to this epidemic, especially among older persons. To this end, the Department of Health recently announced a two-dose schedule for MMR vaccination, with the first dose to be administered at 12-15 months of age and the second to be given to *all* children at Form 1 [age 11].[290]

The term "primary vaccine failure" is used to describe a situation where a person does not make antibodies at the time of vaccination. "Secondary vaccine failure" is the terminology used when the person made antibodies at the time of vaccination, but the antibodies have either diminished in the blood or are presumed to have diminished in the blood before the disease was contracted. It is documented that people can get measles while they have a high level of measles antibodies,[291,292] but the vaccine industry is not keen on discussing this issue, and it is even less keen on labelling this type of vaccine failure. The term "tertiary vaccine failure" should be introduced into medical jargon to describe the situation when a person made enough antibodies at the time of vaccination, and the antibodies were still there when the person got the disease. Most cases of measles that occur in people with a high level of antibodies are automatically included in the category of "secondary vaccine failure" because their antibody levels were not recorded just before they got measles.

The term "waning immunity" was widely used by the New Zealand Health Department to justify the introduction of the second dose of measles vaccine, but now they avoid the term as it acknowledges that measles vaccine creates temporary immunity. At first they admitted that the jab for 11-year-olds was being introduced because measles vaccine does not confer life-long immunity, but only a few months later they stopped saying that, and started saying that it had been introduced purely as a catch up dose for the 40% of children who had missed out on the first dose. (Their own figures showed that only 18% had missed out on the first dose.[290]) From then on public health nurses and practice nurses were taught that the reason for giving the second dose is that 40% of children miss out on the first dose. Ten years later when New Zealand moved the second dose from 11 years to 4 years, the lackey level vaccinators still clung to the claim that one dose gives life-long immunity, and the second dose is only needed because some children miss out on the first dose.

The American Academy of Pediatrics has a different approach. It claims that when measles vaccine fails, it is because the individual did not make antibodies from the first dose, and therefore a second dose is necessary for everybody.[293] If this were true, the cases of measles in the vaccinated would occur during childhood, not later on. The American Academy of Pediatrics says, "The antibody response to a second dose of measles-containing vaccine in children who do not respond to the first dose of vaccine (primary vaccine failure) has been demonstrated to be sustained for long periods."[293] The "long period" of time to which they are referring is six years.[294] My idea of a long period of time is sixty years, not six. When they are once again shown to be wrong, they will introduce yet another dose. In medical doublespeak the second dose is now called "second opportunity".

In 1998 the Australian health department introduced a second dose of measles vaccine that was given at the age of four years. They sent out a press release saying that the two-dose schedule will give life-long immunity, and that children who have the second dose at this age will not need a third dose. Their confidence was not warranted as ten years earlier, during a measles epidemic in Finland, children who had received two doses of the vaccine, as well as children who had received three doses of the vaccine, got measles. None of the children had been vaccinated at the "wrong age".[245] It is known that people who are "fully protected" can pass on the measles virus without showing symptoms of measles.[295,296,297] What is not known is whether getting measles after vaccination protects against chronic disease, as natural measles does. Another thing that is not known is whether vaccinated people who get measles manage to acquire life-long immunity from the process. Whooping cough vaccine changes the immune system in a way that means that a vaccinated person who gets whooping cough does not acquire life-long immunity to whooping cough.[197,198] The same thing might happen with measles.

In eighty years' time it will be interesting to review the outcome of the policies of today. Most medical authorities might still be refusing to study the adverse effects of measles vaccine, but people who choose to make observations will be able to know the rates of chronic diseases. They will also know how many more doses have been added to the schedule, and what new "reasons" were given each time the dogma was changed. Despite all the failures there may be some people for whom two doses will be enough to prevent them from ever developing measles. Another possibility is that there may be something about being an adult that predisposes a person to not getting measles during adulthood, so that the wearing off of artificial immunity might be of no consequence in some people. Or we might see people who have had two, or three, or four doses getting measles in later life. Without naturally occurring measles there will be an increase in cancer and heart disease, but there are so many factors involved in the development of these chronic diseases that it will be difficult to pinpoint the role of lack of measles.

In the 1999 measles epidemic in Melbourne 84% of the reported cases were in people aged 18 to 30,[298] and in the 2001 epidemic in Melbourne 88% were aged 18 to 34.[299] The official figures do not include cases of measles in vaccine free children whose parents did not take the child to a doctor. Doctors are required to report cases of measles to the health department, but parents are not required to inform anybody when a child gets measles. The proportion of cases in young adults would have been lower if these home-treated children had been included in the data. Nevertheless, the cases in young adults show that vaccine-induced immunity wears off. After the 2001 outbreak, the health department put out a press release that urged young adults to be vaccinated again, as their age group had been injected with only one dose when they were children. The press release also said that people over the age of 34 did not need to worry, because they had not been vaccinated, and therefore had life-long immunity. The health department naively did not realise that they were admitting in their press release that vaccine induced immunity wears off.

An excuse for the failure of the vaccine that is beginning to pop up quite frequently is that in the old days people who had had measles in childhood received natural boosters to their immunity throughout life by repeatedly being in contact with children with measles, but now that measles has almost been eliminated, vaccinated people are not getting this natural booster. This is not a valid excuse because natural measles creates life-long immunity without any need for boosters. This was demonstrated by the fact that the people on the Faroe Islands who had had measles as children, and then had not been exposed to a case of measles for 65 years, were all still immune when exposed 65 years later, while the old people who had not had measles as children did get measles.[287] I predict that the myth that natural measles needs boosters will be used as a justification for repeated vaccination throughout life.

In many medical articles about measles the failure of measles vaccine is concealed by the use of dubious definitions of the words "preventable" and "non-preventable". The cases of measles are divided into "preventable" and "non-preventable" cases, instead of being divided into vaccinated and unvaccinated cases. The definition of "preventable" cases is those that occur in people who were not vaccinated, or who were vaccinated at an age that has since come to be called the "wrong age". The definition of "non-preventable" cases is those that occur despite the person having been vaccinated at the "right age", or being too young to have been vaccinated. So by dividing cases during an epidemic into "preventable" and "non-preventable", the authors avoid having to say what percentage of the cases occurred in vaccinated children. It makes it impossible for a reader to know how spectacularly the vaccine failed. If an article says, for instance, that 70% of the cases were "non-preventable", the reader does not know what proportion were vaccinated, and what proportion were below the age for vaccination.

The Australian medicrats also use this terminology. When a vaccinated person gets measles, they call it "non-preventable."[300] It is illogical to say that cases in the unvaccinated could have been prevented by vaccination, when the vaccine has not worked in what they call the "non-preventable" cases.

WHEN WHOOPING COUGH VACCINE FAILS

There is no need to make excuses for the failure of this vaccine when the condition is diagnosed as "viral whooping cough syndrome" or "croup", but when they can bring themselves to admit that it really is whooping cough, they often say that the child has caught a different strain to the one that was in the vaccine. Sometimes the doctor changes the diagnosis as soon as she or he learns that the child is "fully immunised".

"He's got whooping cough! You should have had him immunised, you silly woman."
"But doctor, I did have him immunised."
"Oh well, then it can't be whooping cough."

Where doctors are required to report cases of whooping cough to the authorities, they are more inclined to report cases in the unvaccinated than in the vaccinated.[301] My friend Jeannette took her two children to the doctor when they had whooping cough, because she wanted to get a certificate saying that they had had whooping cough. The elder child is vaccinated, while the younger child is not. This placed the doctor in a quandary because he wanted to say that the younger one had whooping cough, but the older one had something else. By the end of the consultation he grudgingly agreed that both children had whooping cough.

My friend Suzanne had a different experience. She was vaccinated and so was her son, while her daughter was not. All three got whooping cough at the same time, and the doctor had no qualms about announcing that the daughter had whooping cough, while the mother and son did not. The dad had had whooping cough as a child, which is why he could not catch it from his wife and children.

During the 1990-91 outbreak of whooping cough in New Zealand, I estimated that about half of the cases in our area were occurring in vaccinated children. I tried to get the local medicrats to collect some figures, but they were not interested. Of course knowing what percentage of the people who have whooping cough are "fully immunized" does not tell one the failure rate of the vaccine. To work that out, you need to know what percentage of the children and adults who live in the area are vaccinated, and how many of them have had whooping cough before. Another thing you need to know is how many of the children who do not get whooping cough during the current outbreak are going to get it when the disease comes back in about four years' time. So it is actually not possible to know the failure rate of the vaccine without doing a large demographic study over 20 years.

While I was dreaming of collecting statistics in Auckland, two medicrats in Wellington were collecting data in their area, and they obligingly published them in April 1991.[302] At that time the New Zealand schedule gave three doses of DPT before the age of five months, and considered someone who has had three doses to be "fully immunised". In this survey, only children who had proof of three doses of vaccine were classified as "immunised". Those who had had one or two doses, or were unsure of their vaccination history, were classified as "unimmunised". Of the 47 cases in individuals aged over 5 months, 30 were "immunised" and 17 were "unimmunised". Ten other cases were reported in babies under the age of 5 months. The number of doses of DPT vaccine each of these babies had had was not published.

So this means that 63% of the children with whooping cough, who were old enough to have had three doses, were "fully immunised". Now to some people these figures would imply that there is not much point in running the risk of a reaction to this dangerous vaccine, and it is a waste of time and taxpayers' money. But the medicrats said that the survey showed that it would be a good idea to accelerate the vaccination schedule so that babies are "fully immunised" by the age of three months, and to introduce a booster dose at the age of five years. One of the reasons they gave for this recommendation is that babies do not receive natural immunity from mothers who have been immunised.

In the USA they have a different definition of "fully immunised", with five doses of DPT being the required number for a pre-schooler. Sometimes the American authorities investigate and publish the details of whooping cough outbreaks. An outbreak that occurred in Oklahoma in 1983 was one that was investigated. Out of the cases with a known vaccination history, 36% were fully immunised according to the schedule, and another 46% had had some doses, with only 18% being unvaccinated.[303]

The chosen excuse for this Oklahoma epidemic was "low immunization levels in children appear to have been a major factor associated with this outbreak." But quite the opposite is true. The fact that there was a low background vaccination rate, and yet so many of the cases occurred in vaccinated children, is evidence that the low vaccination rate was not the cause of the outbreak. They did two surveys to find out what percentage of the background population was immunised. One came up with 65% and the other came up with 49%. If the latter figure is chosen (to be charitable to the vaccine believers), it can mathematically be said that this shows that the vaccine is 15% effective. That is without taking into account that those who were "protected" during this epidemic could still get it during a later epidemic.

The natural decline of whooping cough that has been happening since 1878 is a factor which the medicrats always choose to ignore when considering vaccine effectiveness.

An outbreak of whooping cough in a community in Massachusetts in 1992 was another one that was investigated and published.[304] The report does not give the background vaccination rate, but it says that 96% of the school students with whooping cough had had "four or more" doses of the vaccine. Some vaccine enthusiasts want to introduce "routine booster immunization throughout life."[305] I will not be among their customers.

They could not use the "low vaccination rate" excuse in the 1991 epidemic in Cape Town, South Africa, because the vaccine failed against a high background vaccination rate. At that time someone who had had 3 doses was regarded as "fully immunised". 94.9% of the child population had had at least three doses of DPT. In this epidemic, 45% of those with whooping cough who were old enough to have had at least one dose, had had three or four doses.[268] The excuse was made that the cases of whooping cough in the vaccinated may have been caused by other germs. What people are forgetting when they come up with this excuse is that a natural dose of whooping cough causes life-long immunity to all the germs that cause whooping cough, not only to the strain that caused the person to get the illness.

In Sweden they did not make excuses. From 1974 to 1978 the vaccination rate for whooping cough was 84%.[263] In 1978 the germ that causes whooping cough became virulent. 84% of children aged 1 to 6 who got whooping cough had been fully immunised.[263] As I said, the Swedish authorities did not make excuses. Instead they stopped using the vaccine. The end of vaccination did not cause an epidemic of whooping cough in Sweden.[262]

Although getting whooping cough twice was very rare, it was documented that it did happen in the days before vaccination.[306] In the era of vaccination it may happen more frequently because vaccinated people who get whooping cough do not create full immunity to whooping cough.[197,198] Both the old whole cell vaccine (DPT) and the new acellular vaccine (DTaP) do not prime the immune system in the same way as a natural dose of whooping cough does.[197,198] The result is that when a vaccinated person gets whooping cough, they are unable to create natural immunity, and are vulnerable to getting whooping cough again. So far there is not enough clinical data about repeated cases of whooping cough for a judgment to be made about the effect that vaccination is having on the incidence of repeat whooping cough.[307,308,309] In the future when data regarding repeated whooping cough is collected, it should not only record whether the patient was vaccinated before the first bout of whooping cough, but also whether the patient was treated with antibiotics and/or massive doses of vitamin C during the first bout of whooping cough. Massive doses of vitamin C can cut whooping cough short, and this may prevent the development of immunity. Giving antibiotics very early on in whooping cough does sometimes halt the progress of the disease, and the effect of this on the development of immunity should be assessed. As I have said elsewhere, when an infant has whooping cough, vitamin C should be given to prevent toxic shock, without concern that it may prevent the development of life-long immunity.

The idea that whooping cough vaccine cannot be expected to provide long lasting immunity because whooping cough itself does not create life-long immunity is beginning to appear in the vaccination propaganda. Estimates of the length of time that immunity from natural whooping cough lasts vary from 7 years to 100 years,[310,311] but the disinformation that is being spread around says that it lasts for 6 years. If that were true people would have been getting whooping cough every 6 years since 1866. In an article about the vaccination of teenagers, two vaccine promoters say, without giving a reference, "However, antibody levels do not correlate well with protection against pertussis, so proof of ongoing protection will have to come from epidemiological studies."[312] Among some vaccine enthusiasts there is still the belief that antibodies are the only important factor in immunity, and that people without antibodies will get whooping cough as soon as they are exposed to the germ. However, not all researchers adhere to this belief.[313]

The whole cell whooping cough vaccine (DPT) has been replaced in affluent countries with an acellular vaccine called DTaP, and the most common excuse made to the public for the failure of the new vaccine is that it is less effective than the whole cell vaccine because it is less toxic than the whole cell vaccine. This excuse ignores the fact that DPT vaccine was only 15% effective, and was not responsible for the natural decline in whooping cough.

EXCUSES FOR THE FAILURE OF POLIO VACCINE

The polio virus has been affecting humans for more than five thousand years, with the earliest evidence being found in Ancient Egypt. Two mummies show damage from polio, and an engraving shows an adult man with the typical withered leg. During human history polio came and went, and was recorded in various places. In the 1880s the virus entered a stage of virulence, and a worldwide pandemic followed. Some people like to believe that the polio virus does not exist and that the disease is caused by pesticide. The polio virus does exist and the symptoms of polio are different to the symptoms that are caused by every type of pesticide. Vaccinators become unhappy when the polio virus has a resurgence of virulence, and vaccinated people come down with polio. The excuses that they make for the failure of the vaccine can reach high levels of absurdity.

A prime example of absurd excuses occurred after the polio virus became virulent in the eastern half of Southern Africa in the summer of 1987-88. The eastern part of South Africa is lush and tropical, unlike the arid western half. In the 1980s millions of disenfranchised people lived in appalling slums in the area that is now called KwaZulu-Natal.

The previous polio epidemic had occurred in 1982. The excuses for the failure of the vaccine during that epidemic were that the vaccination rate had been too low, and "the cold chain must have been broken." After the 1982 epidemic, a concerted effort was made to increase vaccination coverage, and to ensure that the cold chain was not broken. The latter had required a tremendous effort because of the warm climate and the lack of electricity in far flung clinics. Their success meant that they could not use the "cold chain must have been broken" excuse, nor the "lack of herd immunity" excuse to explain away the failure of the vaccine in 1987-88, because they themselves had eliminated these excuses after 1982.

When the polio virus became naturally virulent again in 1987, the newspapers did some scaremongering about the extent of the epidemic, and the need for immunisation. There were the usual quotes from "medical experts" about the effectiveness of the vaccine. For example, "Dr. D. said once a person had been immunised, he was protected against the disease for life," and "If a child is immunised and lives in even the very worst conditions, he or she will not get the virus, even if there is polio in the area," and so on.

Officialdom had realised, during the smaller epidemic of 1982, that giving three doses of vaccine does not cause immunity, so they decided that four doses were needed to create immunity. On paper the figure remained three, but parents were being told to have four doses, "because three isn't enough to cause immunity". When the 1987-88 epidemic broke out, some individuals who had had four doses of oral polio vaccine got paralytic polio. At first the official line was that parents who said that their children had had four doses of the vaccine must be mistaken, because it is impossible to get polio after four doses of the vaccine. Two weeks later the official line changed again, and they said that it was necessary to have five doses of polio vaccine to become immune. The epidemic then came to its natural end.

In the official report they blamed the floods that had occurred two months earlier for the failure of the vaccine.[314] The south east coast of Africa is prone to floods. Until the 1960s the area nearest to the sea in KwaZulu-Natal had been covered with thick jungle, and about every thirty years flash floods would carry away everything in the valleys that lead to the sea. Despite the number of pythons and monkeys that drowned each time, life went on. By the 1980s a human population explosion had eliminated the jungle, and the area was covered with dense slums. Two months before the polio epidemic broke out there had been a terrible flood that had caused lots of people to drown, and had swept away the makeshift dwellings and meagre possessions of thousands of disenfranchised people. The flood occurred in only a small part of the area that was affected by polio, but that did not stop them from blaming the flood for the fact that the vaccine did not work. Floods are not blamed for the failure of the vaccine in areas that do not experience floods. For instance, the vaccine often fails in Namibia on the arid west coast, but its failure is not excused by floods, because floods never happen in Namibia.

A refinement of the flood excuse appeared in the Lancet two years later. "We speculated that the Natal epidemic was due to a high burden of wild type virus resulting from a breakdown in sanitation services which had followed the extensive floods in the area some months previously."[315] What nonsense! Millions of people had been living in slums without sanitation services for years before the flood. There had been no breakdown of sanitation services because there had been no sanitation services. Also, when a vulnerable person ingests polio virus from sewage, it takes only a few days for symptoms to appear, not two months. In any case, the vaccine is supposed to create immunity whether a person is exposed to a "high burden" or a "low burden" of wild virus. The real cause of the failure of the vaccine is that over the southern hemisphere summer of 1987-88, the naturally occurring polio virus underwent an increase in virulence in that region. Even at its peak the virus was not very virulent, as the hundred year-long pandemic was, and still is, naturally waning. The floods did not cause the wild virus to become virulent, and the floods did not cause the vaccine to fail. The vaccine failed because the vaccine failed. It failed in parts of KwaZulu-Natal that were not flooded, and in Qwaqwa, which is more than a hundred miles from the flooded area. Blaming the floods for the failure of the vaccine in this instance is absurd.

I emigrated from South Africa to New Zealand soon after this epidemic ended, and I met Hilary Butler a few weeks later. I mentioned the South African polio epidemic to her, and she wrote to the Centers for Disease

Control (CDC) in Atlanta, USA, and asked for details. The CDC did not answer her letter, so she telephoned Dr. Anthony Morris, the scientist who was fired by the FDA for warning the public not to accept the swine flu vaccine of 1976. He telephoned the CDC, and they told him that the only epidemic of polio in Africa at that time had occurred in Senegal. Senegal is in West Africa, more than four thousand miles north-west of KwaZulu-Natal. I thought that was an excellent way of denying the failure of the vaccine - just deny that the epidemic occurred. There had been hundreds of cases of polio, but due to limited resources only 196 could be laboratory confirmed. I had a Health Department print-out of the polio figures, region by region, and month by month, so Hilary sent the CDC in Atlanta a photocopy for their records.

The CDC's attitude made me curious about the World Health Organisation's view of the epidemic, so I wrote to them in Geneva and asked them how many cases of polio had occurred in South Africa during 1987 and 1988. I was amazed when they replied that there had been 54 cases. On the 27th December 1990 I wrote to the doctor at the World Health Organisation who had supplied me with the figure, and told him that according to the official South African figures there were 196 cases. I asked if he could explain to me why there is a discrepancy, and what source they use for their figures. I have still not had a reply to that letter, nor to a reminder.

I felt suspicious that the discrepancy meant that WHO were only acknowledging cases in the unvaccinated, so I wrote to the South African Health Department and asked them how many doses of vaccine each case had had. In response they sent me the vaccination status of each victim in KwaZulu/Natal, which was the region most affected by polio. This meant that I did not learn the vaccination status of the cases that occurred in the OFS, Qwaqwa and Transkei. (There was a huge patch of "Transkei" in the middle of KwaZulu/Natal because of the insane Bantustan policy that existed at the time.) In KwaZulu/Natal there were 49 confirmed cases in people who had had no doses of vaccine. So now I am even more suspicious, and wondering whether in the region for which I did not get the figures, there were 5 confirmed cases in the unvaccinated, making up the 54 that were acknowledged by WHO. If I had not been living in South Africa at the time, and been very interested in the whole affair because I had a new baby, I would not have become aware that the World Health Organisation's figure differed from the South African government's official figure.

While I was investigating the 1987 polio epidemic in South Africa, I discovered that the Minister of Health had revoked the law that made polio vaccine compulsory. The medicrats were dismayed by his action, and had asked all the newspapers not to report that polio vaccine was no longer compulsory. The newspapers had agreed to co-operate because they believed it to be in the public interest. (Radio and TV were state controlled, whereas newspapers were politically censored but not state controlled.) One day in 1988 the local state nurse and a doctor from Groote Schuur Hospital turned up on my doorstep to try to persuade me to vaccinate Kenny. It was a fun encounter, and one of the most entertaining moments came when I mentioned that I knew that the law making the vaccine compulsory had been revoked.

After an outbreak of polio in Israel in 1988, two groups of doctors were given the opportunity to make excuses for the failure of the vaccine.[316] Take a big breath before you read the next paragraph.

The one group said that the vaccine had failed because the oral vaccine that had been used 20 years previously wasn't potent enough against type 1 of the three strains of virus that you get in the vaccine, and because some children had been given only injected vaccine, which meant that they passed on the virus to susceptible people as they had no gut immunity. The other group said that the outbreak had been caused by long-term exposure to contaminated sewage, and by the fact that the strain of wild virus which caused the epidemic was sufficiently different to the strains in the vaccine to overcome the immunity created by a vaccine strain that wasn't potent enough. Meanwhile the first group had said that the antibodies that the vaccine produced were wide spectrum enough to have covered the different strain of virus.

What a lot of gobbledygook. Why don't they just admit that the vaccine did not work? As the long-term exposure to contaminated sewage had been going on for some time, why had the victims not had polio before? And isn't being vaccinated supposed to protect one from germs no matter whether you catch them from the air, other people, or open sewage?

All these excuses are made in the context that polio was undergoing a natural decline, and the vaccine industry was claiming credit for that decline.

In the town of Vellore in India there was a polio outbreak in 1991-92.[256] The vaccination coverage for those years was 98% for three doses, and in 1992 it was 90% for four doses. All the children who got polio were "fully immunised."[256] There were no cases of polio in the unvaccinated. The three doctors who wrote to the Lancet about this outbreak say, "We believe it was due to sub-optimum vaccine efficacy and inadequate herd effect." Now I like those excuses. They are getting closer to the truth. It's a pity they cannot just come clean and say, "The vaccine did not work and herd immunity does not exist." They make the suggestion that seven doses of vaccine should be given, "with high coverage to achieve eradication."

The promise that polio vaccination will cease once polio is eradicated is still floating about, but some are saying that vaccination has to continue forever because a live polio virus can be created through genetic engineering.[317,318]

COVER UP OF THE FAILURE OF RABIES VACCINE

Louis Pasteur said that his rabies vaccine would work as long as it was given to the victim of a bite before any symptoms developed.[285] Once use of the vaccine became widespread, it was seen that vaccinated people often got rabies. These failures were excused away by saying that anyone who got rabies within a month of starting the treatment was not protected by the vaccine, and could not be counted as a failure.[319]

This technique drastically reduced the number of failures that had to be acknowledged. So, for instance, the official failure rate of Pasteur's rabies vaccine at the Kasauli Institute in 1910, was given as only 0.19%. They arrived at this figure by excluding all the deaths that occurred during the course of fourteen injections, and all those who died within fifteen days of completing the course. Out of 2073 people who were injected after being bitten or licked by suspected rabid animals, 26 died of rabies, but 14 died during the treatment, so they were not counted, and 8 died within 15 days of completion of the treatment, so they were not counted. Only four died after the 29-day cut-off. Those four are the only ones counted for the statistic.[320]

Vaccine believers like to view the 26 deaths as evidence that 2047 people were saved. What they overlook is that the cases that do not get rabies are not necessarily vaccine successes. We would only know how many of the vaccinated people were saved by the vaccine if we had statistics of rabies in people who were not injected with the vaccine after being licked or bitten by a suspected rabid animal. It was not in the interests of the newly founded vaccine industry to gather such information.

When a person gets rabies from the germ in the vaccine, the symptoms are usually not exactly the same as rabies that has been acquired naturally. The old-fashioned word for rabies is hydrophobia, so they called the rabies-like syndrome that occurred after vaccination "paralytic hydrophobia". A more recent word for the condition that is often caused by rabies vaccine is "neuroparalysis". Sir Graham Wilson has this to say about neuroparalysis,

> It was not long after the pasteurian method of protecting against rabies was taken into routine use that attention was drawn to cases of neuroparalysis occurring during or just

> after the course of treatment. Little was said about them in print. Among the directors of the Pasteur Institutes there was a conspiracy of silence, caused by a fear partly of bringing Pasteur's method into disrepute and partly of bringing blame upon themselves. Their position was not an easy one. Though little was acknowledged publicly, rumour was active and each fresh case furnished the occasion for local conversation and gossip. The poisonous atmosphere of covertly expressed criticism in which they moved reacted on the morale of the staff and made them miserable.[321]

He forgets that only people with a conscience feel miserable under these circumstances. Most people can stop themselves from being miserable by indulging in pathological denial. Denying reality is the way to stay happy if you are part of the vaccination machine. It is also the way to stay employed.

However, a certain group of doctors decided not to indulge in pathological denial, nor to suffer the misery of guilty consciences. They gathered together data about adverse effects, and they testified against their colleagues who were dishonestly suppressing data about adverse reactions.[321] In April 1927, the director of the Pasteur Institute in Morocco, Dr. Remlinger, reported to the International Rabies Conference,

> We were impressed with the discrepancy between the number of observations published by directors of institutes and the number of cases orally acknowledged by them to have occurred … We have come to the conclusion that certain institutes conceal their cases. On various occasions we have found in medical literature observations concerning paralysis of treatment, and we have afterwards failed to find in the report and statistics of the institutes concerned any mention of these unfortunate cases.[322]

When the people who stand to gain financially from favourable statistics are in complete control of the raw data, it is easy for them to omit to mention failures and adverse effects of their product. Although Dr. Remlinger came clean about rabies vaccine adverse effects and vaccine failures in 1927, the industry continued to foist Pasteur's vaccine onto the public, until they had a new rabies vaccine that they could foist onto the public instead.

EXCUSES FOR THE FAILURE OF BCG VACCINE

The first vaccine for TB was invented by Robert Koch, and it was made with human TB germs. Its use was discontinued because it killed too many babies. The commercial void that this left was filled by two Frenchmen who thought of the idea of making a vaccine from the strain of germ that causes TB in cows. This vaccine is called BCG. It does kill a lot fewer people than Robert Koch's vaccine did, and it has been raking in money for the vaccine industry ever since 1921.

When I lived in Cape Town I associated with a lot of medical people and medical students, and I often heard them muttering about the fact that BCG vaccine does not work. TB was rife in the black ghettos because of malnutrition and lack of proper housing. Most houses were made of pieces of corrugated iron that had been propped up next to one another in the mud, and Cape Town has a cold, damp climate.

The official stance of the South African Department of Health was that "BCG vaccine is 79% effective." This claim was based on a study that had been started in 1950 by the Medical Research Council in Britain, and had followed up the participants for ten years.[323] The study found that out of the 12,699 unvaccinated participants, 213 got TB, and out of the 13,598 vaccinated participants, 48 got TB. The study authors say, "... this represents a reduction of 79% attributed to vaccination."[323] A doctor pointed out in the British Medical Journal that those who got TB from the vaccine were not included as cases of TB, and if they had been, there would have been no difference in the incidence of TB between the vaccinated and the unvaccinated.[324]

This vaccine is not only useless, it is also harmful. It has some serious long-term adverse effects, and it kills some babies and some teenagers outright. Homoeopathy cures TB very effectively and cheaply, so there is no excuse for using this dangerous vaccine, even in cold, damp slums. Despite the fraudulent finding that "the protective efficacy of this vaccine was thus substantial," the international muttering about the uselessness of BCG vaccine continued.

It was decided that the World Health Organisation should do a large study in a malnourished area to ascertain once and for all whether or not the vaccine was effective. The study involved two hundred and sixty thousand children, which made it large enough to ensure that there would be no quibbling afterwards about whether or not the study was representative. Well of course if the study had found that the vaccine decreased the incidence of TB, there would have been no quibbling afterwards, but the study found that BCG vaccine actually increases the risk of catching TB,[325,326] so the quibbling continues. In 1980 the editor of the Lancet wrote,

> Thirteen years ago, D'Arcy Hart reviewed the conflicting evidence on BCG effectiveness and spoke of the need for a fresh field trial to clarify outstanding controversies, particularly in the face of increasing use of BCG in developing countries. There followed the latest Indian field trial with 260,000 participants, organised with the collaborative skills of the Indian Council of Medical Research, the World Health Organisation, and the United States Public Health Service. But it has not clarified - just the opposite. Though the 7½ year follow up results reported in the Indian Journal of Medical Research are incomplete, they are negative - in fact, slightly more tuberculosis cases have appeared in vaccinated than in equal-sized placebo control groups. It looks like another zero effect.[327]

A negative effect is not a zero effect. It is dishonest to call it a zero effect. Furthermore, he says that the result has not clarified the situation, when it has clarified it very well. This editorial also lists eight excuses that have been put forward by others as reasons for the failure of the vaccine, then the editor says, "but there is no compelling evidence for any of them." Well, at least that is honest. The editorial ends off with a call for "clarity of judgment and courage to match the challenge." If the medicrats had any clarity of judgment and moral backbone, they would have ceased using the vaccine as soon as the study result came out.

A year later there was another editorial in the Lancet which dragged out eight feeble excuses as reasons why BCG vaccination must be continued, despite the result of the World Health Organisation's study in India.[328]

A leading article in the medical journal called *Tubercle* had this to say,

> The widely publicised results of a large, controlled trial of BCG vaccination in South India showed, after 7½ years of follow up, no evidence of a protective effect against pulmonary tuberculosis. This unexpected result, which has given rise to much discussion and speculation, has led to doubts about the value of BCG vaccination in general. Against this background a conference of experts was convened in Delhi … So far there has been no satisfactory explanation of the negative result of the Indian trial, despite an intensive search in every direction …[329]

It makes me chuckle to visualise teams of scientists with their heads down, conducting an intensive search in every direction - in every direction that is except the obvious one - which is facing up to the fact that the vaccine does not work. The *Tubercle* article goes on to suggest yet more possible excuses for the failure of the vaccine. Maybe these batches of vaccine were not potent enough. Maybe the wrong strains were used. Maybe the protective effect of the vaccine was masked by the fact that the whole population had been exposed to the wild germ before being vaccinated. Maybe the solution is to vaccinate "early in life" so that the recipients do not have a chance to meet the wild germ and become immune before they get vaccinated.

The vaccine industry knows that suppressing information about vaccine failures is the best way to avoid having to make excuses. On talkback radio in Auckland I heard a lady describe how she had been a teacher when teenagers were mass vaccinated with BCG in New Zealand schools. She said that 15 of the pupils at her school had contracted TB despite vaccination, and the Health Department had suppressed the information. "I believe in immunisation," she said, "but I don't think they should have done that."

We will have to wait until a new vaccine is introduced to replace BCG before they will admit that BCG does not work. The new vaccine will not work either, but it will make a lot of money. BCG causes osteitis (bone inflammation) in 1 in 3000 well-nourished babies,[330] and lots of other horrible reactions, including death.[331] TB is easily cured by homoeopathy, and TB germs do not become resistant to homoeopathic remedies like they do to drugs. There is no excuse for using BCG anywhere in the world.

HOW HOMOEOPATHY WORKS

Homoeopathy, like electricity, was always there, it just needed to be discovered. The discovery was made in 1790 when Dr. Samuel Hahnemann was trying to figure out how quinine poisons the body. He observed that when quinine is homoeopathically potentised, it cures both malaria and quinine poisoning, without causing any side effects. He then realised that all toxic substances can cure a wide range of diseases, without side effects, when they are homoeopathically potentised. The chemical drug industry, which in 1790 was already very powerful, tried to silence Dr. Hahnemann, as they realised that the new discovery made their treatments obsolete. They have been trying to extinguish homoeopathy ever since.

Homoeopathy is completely different to herbalism and naturopathy. Homoeopathic remedies are made by diluting a toxic substance and then shaking it, and then diluting it again, and shaking it, over and over again. This procedure, which is called potentisation, can be applied to any poisonous substance. Simply diluting a substance does not make it potent – the shaking is essential for the release of the energy that gives the remedy its potency. After the poisonous substance has been potentised it is no longer poisonous, and it becomes a remedy that interacts with the electromagnetic field of the body. When a remedy is being chosen for a sick person, the symptoms that the patient is showing have to be carefully observed. Once all of the symptoms have been observed, a remedy that would cause those symptoms in its crude, unpotentised form is chosen. It is of no consequence whether the symptoms that the patient is suffering are caused by the poison from which the remedy is made, or by something completely different. The reason why homoeopathically potentised quinine cures malaria is that the symptoms of quinine poisoning and the symptoms of malaria are the same.

When a substance is made into a homoeopathic remedy by potentisation it is given a Latin-sounding name so that people of every language will be able to refer to it without confusion. The number that appears on the label after the name is called the potency, and it tells you how many times the substance has been diluted and shaken. Being repeatedly diluted and shaken converts the substance from matter into energy, and when the medicine touches a mucous membrane in a person, the energy is released. It does not work chemically, like a drug or herbal remedy does. The medicine should not be swallowed, but should be placed under the tongue, or held in the mouth, so that it is in contact with mucus membranes. One of the ways that the pharmaceutical industry tries to denigrate homoeopathy is by saying that there is nothing in the remedies, and that they are only effective because of the placebo effect. Homoeopathy is effective on babies, on adults in a coma, and on animals, and many published studies have shown that homoeopathy is not a placebo effect.[332] The way that the energy in the remedy stimulates the change is not known, but there is a difference between not understanding how something works, and something not working. The people who control the pharmaceutical industry know that along with vitamin C, homoeopathy is the biggest threat to its profits, so they are strongly motivated to convince people not to try it.

Homoeopathic medicines are not toxic and have no side effects, but they will have a detrimental effect if they are taken many times a day for a few weeks by someone who does not have the corresponding symptoms. If an inquisitive child manages to get into the first aid cupboard and swallow a whole bottle of *arnica 30*, nothing will happen. However, if a person with no symptoms repeatedly takes *arnica 30* over a period of time, he or she will start developing the symptoms of arnica poisoning. The resulting condition would be the same as the symptoms that would appear if someone were foolish enough to consume soup made from the arnica plant.

Homoeopathic medicine is very fragile. It loses its potency if moisture gets into it, or if particular pungent aromas come into contact with it. Eucalyptus oil, citronella oil, T-tree oil, mint, camphor, wintergreen, menthol, and peppermint are some of the substances that make homoeopathic remedies lose potency. (Curry, garlic, chilli, and spices like cinnamon do not have this effect.) If a homoeopathic remedy is stored in the same cupboard as a substance that has a strong smell, some molecules of the substance will sneak in through the lid of the bottle and depotentise the remedy. When a person has taken a homoeopathic remedy, it continues to work in the body for a period of time. If the person makes contact with an aroma that de-activates homoeopathic remedies, the remedy "switches off" and stops working.

Diseases that take a long time to develop need a few months of homoeopathic treatment to be fully cured, while diseases that take a short time to develop are cured very quickly by the right remedy. Homoeopathy can treat both chronic and acute diseases, and is very effective at curing the infectious diseases that need intervention. Homoeopaths sometimes make the mistake of trying to "cure" the self-resolving childhood diseases, when they should only use homoeopathy to cure the complications of these diseases, if complications arise.

There is no single remedy for each disease, so we cannot say that A is the cure for cholera, and B is the cure for arthritis. Each patient has to be individually assessed so that the right remedy can be given for their particular set of symptoms. The symptoms of cholera differ slightly from one person to another, while the symptoms of arthritis can be very different from person to person. There are many remedies that can be used to cure tuberculosis (TB), but *tuberculinum 200* is the one to consider first. Millions of people die each year because this cheap remedy is not used. If the TB patient has the unusual symptom of being weaker in the mornings, and gaining strength during the day, then *acalypha indica 200* is the appropriate remedy.

An amateur can practice homoeopathic first aid quite safely, but needs to get outside help if there is a life-threatening condition. The concept of a first aid kit takes on a new meaning when homoeopathic remedies are included in the kit. *Arnica 30* is one of the primary first aid remedies. It eliminates pain that is caused by physical trauma, it speeds up healing, and it helps with the emotional shock that accompanies some injuries. Potentised *arnica* works instantly, but it only defeats pain that is caused by physical trauma; it has no effect on pain caused by illness. It makes sprains heal quickly, and if taken soon after a knock it prevents a bruise from developing. *Ledum 30* antidotes insect and spider bites, *pulsatilla 30* cures conjunctivitis (pink eye), *aconite 30* given soon enough prevents a chill from turning into flu or a cold, and there are a host of other first aid remedies that are safe and effective. Dr. Hahnemann encouraged his patients to keep first aid remedies at home.

The remedies that are commonly used in first aid situations can also be used for chronic conditions, but a greater level of knowledge of the remedies is needed for the treatment of chronic conditions. Homoeopathy can seem confusing at first because each remedy can be used for a wide spectrum of conditions, and each condition can be treated by a wide spectrum of remedies, and yet there is only one remedy that has the optimum fit for the presenting symptoms.

The amount taken each time is not important; one pill has the same effect as three pills, and one drop has the same effect as three drops. However, the number of doses and the timing of subsequent doses are important. A remedy that is prescribed by a homoeopath will come with instructions about the frequency of the doses, but when you are choosing a first aid remedy yourself you need to be guided by how long the effect of each dose lasts. If the right remedy has been chosen there will be an immediate improvement in the condition, and when the improvement stops, it is time for the next dose. This could be after a few minutes or a few hours, depending on the condition. The length of time before the remedy stops working gets longer after each dose. *Arnica 30,* for example, will make the severe pain that results from slamming a finger in a door fade quite quickly, but the pain might return after only half a minute. A second dose is needed as soon as the pain comes back. The pain will be gone for longer after the second dose, and so on. If a second dose is given too soon, it can stop the first dose from working. The length of time a remedy keeps on working depends on the potency used, the severity of the condition, and the vitality of the patient.

The choice of potency is not crucial, but a general guide is that the low potencies like 6, 12, and 30 are suitable for conditions that are largely physical, while the higher potencies like 200 or 1m are suitable when there is a stronger emotional side to the condition. 1m means that the remedy has been potentised a thousand times. Most injuries have a shock component, and potentised *arnica* treats both the physical trauma and the emotional shock. Dropping a heavy book on a foot causes a low level of emotional shock, so *arnica 30* is suitable for removing the pain in the foot, preventing a bruise from developing, and countering the small amount of shock. The high potency of 1m is suitable when physical injury is combined with deep shock, like that from a traffic accident. If *arnica 1m* is not available, *arnica 30* will also help an accident victim recover from the shock, but it will need more doses to complete the recovery. In German they call the high potencies the "deep" potencies, which is a better choice of word.

Remedies that are in the 6th potency have been diluted and shaken only six times. When the French government investigated homoeopathy they found that remedies in the 5th potency contained a few atoms or molecules of the original substance, but in the 6th potency there were no longer any atoms or molecules of the original substance in the remedy.[333]

Arsenic is a very poisonous substance, but the homoeopathic remedy *arsenicum,* which is made by potentising arsenic, is non-toxic. A person who is unfortunate enough to suffer acute arsenic poisoning will experience vomiting, diarrhoea, and stomach cramps, and will bend forward, eventually lying down in the fetal position, and dying if there is no intervention. *Arsenicum 30* is an excellent first aid remedy for stomach upsets that are caused by germs. One of the advantages of homoeopathy is that when choosing a remedy you do not have to know which germ has caused the problem. You just look at the presenting symptoms, and you choose a remedy that matches them. So when a person is suffering from vomiting, diarrhoea, and stomach cramps, and feels inclined to bend forward, *arsenicum 30* causes a rapid recovery. It makes no difference whether the symptoms are caused by a germ like rotavirus that floats in the air[334] and causes what is often called "gastro", or "a tummy bug", or is caused by germs on food that has gone rancid, or that has been contaminated with fecal matter, and cause what is called "food poisoning". There are a number of first aid remedies for stomach upsets; *nux vom*, *ipecac*, *carbo veg*, and *arsenicum* are among the remedies to consider, but you know that *arsenicum* is the right choice if the patient starts to bend forward.

Stomach upsets are one of the situations in which homoeopathy often works astonishingly fast. One day Kenny's teacher telephoned me and told me that Kenny and a friend were in the sick room with stomach ache. I took along my homoeopathic first aid kit and found the two boys on the floor of the sick room, both curled into the fetal position, moaning and groaning as if they thought they were dying. The fetal position was the clue for selecting *arsenicum*. I managed to get some into each groaning mouth, and within minutes the two boys were sitting up and talking. Another dose after ten minutes made them bounce up and go back to the classroom. A teacher who had been with them all along was astounded, but the school principal believed that they had been faking it, because of the fast recovery. Homoeopathy is easy to learn as you go along, and once you have seen a remedy do a "miracle" cure, you tend to remember it for next time. *Arsenicum* is not limited to first aid situations, and qualified homoeopaths sometimes prescribe it for chronic conditions.

Ledum 30 is the first aid remedy for any puncture wound, like a prick from a needle, a thorn, or a sharp animal's tooth. *Ledum 30* removes the pain, and if it is given soon after the injury it trounces infection, including an infection with tetanus germs. If tetanus germs have entered the wound, and treatment is only started after symptoms of tetanus have appeared, *ledum* is not the correct remedy. Also, if the wound is not a puncture wound, and tetanus germs are in it, *ledum* will not prevent the development of tetanus.

Bites and stings from small creatures that inject poison into the flesh are also puncture wounds, and *ledum 30* is the remedy to use for these, if treatment starts soon after the bite or sting has occurred. *Ledum* antidotes the poison from insect and spider bites even when the poison has provoked an allergic reaction. Spiders are a hazard in Australia. In 1999 Chandra was bitten on the hand by a large spider that was hiding on the back of a towel. It took me ten minutes to find the *ledum 30*, and by then her hand was red, swollen, and paralysed. This was three hours before she had to write an exam. The remedy halted the swelling, and then the swelling subsided and the redness disappeared. Mobility returned slowly. By the time she left for her exam, her hand was back to normal, except for two huge fang marks. This is what the pharmaceutical industry does not want you to know how to do. Under "orthodox" treatment she would have suffered for quite a few days, and her exam would have been postponed.

When Chandra was eight she had an allergic reaction to a wasp sting at school. Her teacher telephoned me and said, "Chandra has been stung by a wasp on her hand and the swelling is going up her arm, and she says you have some medicine for it." I zoomed to school with *ledum 30*, and found that her whole hand was red and swollen, and the red swelling had engulfed her wrist and most of her forearm, and was spreading upwards as I watched. As soon as the remedy made contact with the mucous membrane under her tongue, the redness and swelling stopped where it was, and spread no further. After an hour the swelling had gone, but it took a few days for the redness to disappear completely. This is not welcome news for the makers of antihistamines.

When a child wakes in the night and screams from earache, *kali bich 30* can eliminate the pain and have the child sleeping again in a matter of minutes. Treating chronic earache is more complicated. When a chronic ear problem is permanently banished by homoeopathy, "orthodox" medicine loses customers for its antibiotics, pain killers, and grommets.

The remedies come in the form of little white pills, white powder, or clear liquid. The white stuff is lactose or sucrose, and the liquid is distilled water and alcohol. The active ingredient is not a chemical, it is a vibration. Powder is the best form for a baby, because pills can slip into the lungs, and the alcohol in the liquid tastes horrible. If you don't have the remedy that the baby needs in powder form, try crushing the pills between two desert spoons, or with a mortar and pestle. The hard type of little white pills tend to fly across the room when you try to crush them between two spoons, but the soft type crush easily. In a baby's mouth the powder does not need to go under the tongue. As long as it goes into a mouth that has no food in it, the vibration will be absorbed.

With some conditions it is easy to know when the remedy has stopped working, and when the next dose is required. When Kenny was pushed off a climbing frame by another child he cried with pain, and for a moment I thought that one of the bones in his forearm was broken. *Arnica 30* switched off the pain instantly, but it wore off quickly. It was like a light being switched on; suddenly the pain was back. *Arnica 30* once again removed the pain instantly. The effect of this second dose lasted longer than the effect of the first, but suddenly the pain was back again. The effect of the third dose lasted even longer, and the fourth dose lasted over two hours. I decided I had made a mistake in thinking that a bone was broken, because he was playing happily with his train set on the floor. Then I noticed that when he leaned on his arm to reach a train, the broken bone stuck out sideways, so he did need to have it put in plaster. Potentised *arnica* is a very effective pain killer, but only when the pain is caused by physical trauma.

If a person is undergoing drug treatment of any kind, homoeopathic remedies can be taken without them interacting with the drugs. However, homoeopathic remedies do interact with each other. Some remedies reinforce each other, while others counteract each other.

One night at a restaurant my husband and I had the "seafood special" as an entree. The next morning Chandra suffered an injury that required stitches, and we needed *arnica* for shock because the injury had come close to being very serious. As the hours passed we began to suffer nausea, and we took more *arnica*, thinking that the shock had caused the nausea. By midnight we were vomiting, and we realised that we had food poisoning. The "seafood special" had been old fish with strong tasting mayonnaise piled on top of it. We took *arsenicum* and started to improve immediately. We were up all night with Chandra, who was wide awake after spending some of the day under general anaesthetic. We took more doses of *arsenicum* each time we began to slip back into feeling queasy again, and later I started taking *arnica* again for shock. By daybreak my husband was fully recovered from the food poisoning, but I was still sick, having ceased to progress when I restarted the *arnica*. Later I looked up the clinical relationship between the two remedies, and discovered that *arnica* prevents *arsenicum* from working.

Homoeopathic remedies continue working for a long time in the body, as long as they are not de-activated by an antagonistic aroma. Some homoeopaths are very slack about warning their patients to avoid strong smelling oils and mint toothpaste. Another homoeopathic story about Chandra arises from when she broke a metatarsal bone while on a teenage camp. Her foot swelled up like a balloon, but soon after the injury occurred she took *arnica 30,* which made the swelling subside so rapidly that the camp director thought no bone was broken. The camp ended the next day, and her lower leg was put in plaster. Over the next six weeks she took a dose of *arnica 30* whenever the break began to ache, which happened less and less frequently. There was one setback, however, when the pain returned dramatically. A few days after the bone had been broken she accidentally brushed her teeth with mint-flavoured toothpaste, instead of our usual mint-free toothpaste. Within seconds of the toothpaste entering her mouth the break became intensely painful. The toothpaste had de-activated the *arnica 30,* which had been silently working in her body. Once the mint taste had disappeared from her mouth, another dose of *arnica 30* was able to again stop the pain. The toothpaste industry is obsessed with putting mint or pungent Australian plants into toothpaste, so it requires an effort to find a brand of toothpaste that is compatible with homoeopathic remedies.

The way that Dr. Hahnemann discovered the phenomenon of

homoeopathy was quite fortuitous. The sequence of events began when he gave up practicing medicine because he was unhappy about the fact that the treatments he had been taught to use always harmed, often killed, and never cured his patients.[335] He was fluent in eight languages, so he turned to translating medical writings as a way of earning an income. In this way he became familiar with the views of ancient doctors like Hippocrates and Paracelsus, as well as with the beliefs that were current in his own time. In 1790 one of his tasks was to translate an 1170 page book that had been written by Dr. William Cullen, who was a high profile pharmaceutical man in Edinburgh at the time. One of the things that Dr. Cullen had written was that quinine cures malaria because of its "tonic action on the stomach". That of course is complete nonsense. Quinine does not cure malaria, and its action on the stomach has nothing to do with its ability to temporarily suppress the symptoms of malaria. However, reading what Cullen had written prompted Hahnemann to think about what quinine actually does. He experimented on himself by taking a dose of quinine twice a day for several days, and he developed the symptoms of malaria for a few hours after each dose. This convinced Hahnemann that Hippocrates and Paracelsus had observed something important when they had said that the effects of a medicine should be similar to the effects of the sickness. When a healthy person takes some quinine, he or she temporarily develops the symptoms of malaria, but when a person who is suffering from malaria takes quinine, his or her symptoms disappear for a while. The same principle applies to other herbs which are used for other conditions.

The most important part of the discovery was still to come. Hahnemann decided to dilute the quinine because it is toxic, and as he was a trained chemist as well as a doctor, he ensured that there was an even distribution of the substance in the liquid by banging the vial of liquid on his desk a hundred times between each dilution. To his surprise he found that the diluted substance had a more powerful medicinal effect than the original substance. By shaking the vial to distribute the quinine he had unwittingly released some kind of energy that is still not understood. Repeated diluting and shaking makes the remedy able to bring about a permanent cure, instead of just temporarily suppressing the symptoms. For the next twenty years Hahnemann experimented on himself with hundreds of medicinal plants to see what effect they had on his healthy body, and then he used them in their potentised form on patients who presented with those symptoms.

Hahnemann called his new discovery "homoeopathy", from the Greek words "homoios" (similar), and "pathos" (suffering). His definition of the word "cure" is, "To restore health rapidly, gently, permanently; to remove and destroy the whole disease in the shortest, surest, least harmful way, according to clearly comprehensible principles."[336] Hahnemann soon realised that he could make remedies from toxic substances that were not recognised as medicines. For instance, people who worked in the copper mines exhibited symptoms of copper poisoning. He used potentised copper to cure these symptoms, whether or not they arose from exposure to copper. First he had to find a way of diluting non-soluble metals. Modern homoeopaths use all the old remedies as well as new ones made from modern toxic substances like naphthalene and petroleum.

Samuel Hahnemann wrote a lot about the principles and philosophy of homoeopathy. The book in which he summed it all up is called *Organon of Medicine*. He also documented the case histories of his own patients. A book that lists the symptoms that can be caused/cured by a number of substances is called a "materia medica". The modern materia medicas contain some substances that were not available to the early homoeopaths, but the early materia medicas are just as useful now as they were when they were compiled. Medical textbooks become obsolete and have to be replaced, but homoeopathic books always remain valid. Knowledge about homoeopathy can increase, but homoeopathy does not change.

Homoeopaths are curing malaria in Africa and India, and treating patients for the toxic effects of anti-malarial drugs, but some medicrats want them to stop. The war cry is that there are no randomised double-blind placebo-controlled trials of homoeopathy for malaria, and the evidence is all based on case reports. Drugs that kill the malaria parasite are expensive and toxic. They can cause symptoms like psychotic behaviour, blurred vision, cold sweats, fever, confusion, ringing in the ears, blood in the urine, fainting, seizures, comas, rash, shakiness, cardiac dysrhythmia, cramps, nausea, diarrhoea, vomiting, swelling, and kidney failure, to name but a few. The malaria parasite can hide away from the drug, making it look as though the patient is cured, but then re-emerge later. The parasite can become immune to a brand of drug, so that it does not even work temporarily. None of these problems occur with homoeopathy. Millions of people with malaria do not have access to drugs, so when the pharmaceuticalists say that these people should not be allowed to receive homoeopathic treatment for malaria they are demonstrating that they are not concerned about the welfare of the people. They have the same heartless attitude towards victims of cholera in remote places who could be cured quickly and cheaply.

The latest round of attacks on homoeopathy are focused on misrepresenting the research that has been done on homoeopathy so far. Homoeopathy will survive this latest onslaught just like it has survived all the others. The pharmaceuticalists will not succeed in killing off homoeopathy, but they do succeed in killing off millions of people whose lives could be saved by homoeopathy.

SOME POINTERS REGARDING THE PREVENTION AND TREATMENT OF INFECTIOUS DISEASES THAT NEED INTERVENTION

While the self-resolving childhood diseases cannot be prevented by healthy living, steps can be taken to prevent the infectious diseases that need intervention, and should be taken, because these diseases are harmful and have no long-term benefits. These diseases can only be caught when the germ that causes them is present in the environment. In some geographical regions the germs that cause typhoid, cholera, and amoebic dysentery are present in the water, and a traveller can get very sick, or even die, from drinking the water. The airborne diseases that need intervention cannot be avoided through good hygiene, and it cannot be predicted when nor where they will put in an appearance. Avoiding eating empty calories is the first step towards protecting oneself from the airborne diseases that need intervention. The germs that cause AIDS, hepatitis B, and hepatitis C live in blood and in semen, and avoiding them is more complicated than avoiding waterborne germs.

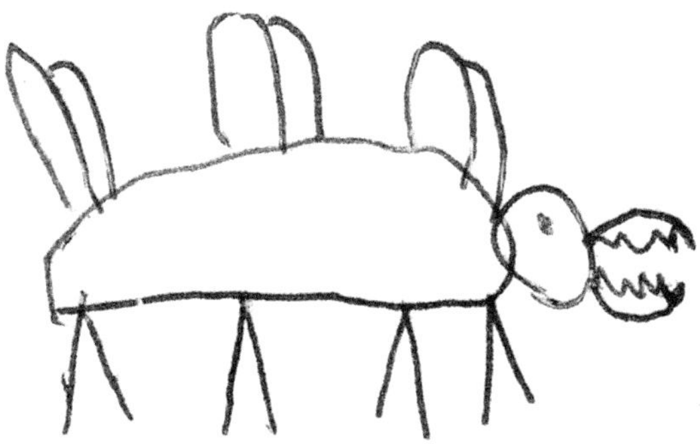

A fierce germ setting off to attack an innocent child

Sufficient rest is essential for preventing some diseases, boring though it may sound. Unfortunately it is not always possible to obtain wholesome food, because the food industry prefers to sell products with a long shelf life. Furthermore, our immune systems are under strain from all the pollutants in the air and water, the pesticides and additives in the food, and the poisonous metals in our teeth. On the other hand, we have many advantages that our ancestors lacked. Vitamin and mineral pills made of natural extracts go a long way towards compensating for modern food, and they can help one to survive if germs do manage to cause symptoms of disease.

Vitamin C has become such a cliché in the health field that it is easy to overlook how important it is to take extra doses of vitamin C when we are under attack from germs. The amount of vitamin C needed daily varies from person to person. The amount needed is affected by things like the genetic legacy, what damage has been done to the immune system in the past, and what poisons the bureaucrats add to the water. When germs come into the environment, the need for vitamin C increases dramatically. Vitamin C gets used up quickly in germ wars, so it needs to be replaced every few hours. Too much causes diarrhoea, so it is easy to know when the limit has been reached. Dr. Linus Pauling says,

> Vitamin C is not a wonder drug, a drug that cures a particular disease. It is instead a substance that participates in almost all of the chemical reactions that take place in our bodies, and is required for many of them. Our bodies can fight disease effectively only when we have in our organs and body fluids enough vitamin C to enable our natural protective mechanisms to operate effectively.[337]

The most enlightening part of the book from which that quote is taken is chapter 12, entitled *The Medical Establishment and Vitamin C*. Knowing the lengths to which the medical establishment goes in order to suppress information about vitamin C is sufficient to convince the health conscious reader that vitamin C supplementation is beneficial. Dr. Linus Pauling won the Nobel Prize in Chemistry in 1954, but now the drug company shills are attacking him on Wikipedia and other sites because they don't want people to know about the benefits of vitamin C. Vitamin C has a direct effect on bacteria and viruses, it breaks up the toxins produced by germs, and it helps the phagocytes in the immune system eat germs faster.[338] It also helps wounds to heal, it reduces the symptoms of allergic reactions, and it helps addicts who are fighting addiction.[339]

Each spring I receive phone calls from young people who are planning to spend their long student vacation travelling in foreign countries. They want advice because they are scared of travel vaccines, and they are also scared of the infectious diseases that might be lurking at their destination. They have good reason to be scared of both. Only a fraction of deaths from travel vaccines make it into medical journals.[340,341,342] The fraction is so small that it is not even the tip of the iceberg, nor is it the penguin on the tip of the iceberg. It is the flea on the penguin on the tip of the iceberg.

Prospective travellers are often told that certain vaccines are "required" for entering the country that they intend to visit, when vaccines are not required. Yellow fever vaccine is the only one that is required by any country, and only a few countries require it. Furthermore, it is only required by those countries if the traveller is arriving directly from a country that is considered to be a yellow fever zone, and even then it is not required if the traveller has a letter from a doctor saying that the traveller must not be vaccinated. The letter can be addressed, "To whom it may concern", and it does not need to give a reason why the traveller must not be vaccinated, but it must be written by a registered medical practitioner. Sometimes travel itineraries can be arranged to avoid the hassle of finding a doctor who will write such a letter. For instance, Egypt considers Kenya to be a yellow fever zone, so if you go to Egypt first, and then to Kenya, no letter is necessary.

It is common for mongers of travel-vaccine in Australia to lie to prospective travellers that if they do not purchase the product they will not be allowed back into Australia.

Although there are no simple solutions for avoiding infectious diseases while travelling, there are many protective measures that are worth taking. It is particularly difficult to obtain nourishing food while travelling, so a good supply of non-acidic vitamin C pills is advisable, even for healthy youngsters. Vitamin C powder is impractical for travellers, as it can easily be spoiled by moisture. It is better to use pills, but of course they must be good quality pills, in a matrix that does not hinder absorption.

It is difficult to avoid waterborne germs when travelling in unhygienic countries. A good present to buy for a loved one who intends to travel to dubious areas is an electrical gadget that boils a small amount of water at a time, along with the relevant electrical connections for the countries they intend to visit. In remote areas where there is no electricity, the people use fire to cook their food, so a traveller can use the fire to boil water. Some hotels and restaurants in unhygienic places do not boil the water when they make tea or coffee. Plush carpets and a grand reception hall are no guarantee that the water supply is not contaminated with typhoid, cholera, or amoebic dysentery. Nasty germs can survive in very little water. They may, for instance, be present on salad leaves, if you are in a place that permits the use of unchlorinated water. Even unpeeled fruit and bottled liquids can be contaminated. Those stories about fruit being injected with river water to make them heavier are not fairy tales. I bought a mandarin on the banks of a famous river that doubles as a sewer, and when I opened the skin, brown water came bursting out. When I looked at the skin carefully I could see where the water had been injected in. In another country that undervalues hygiene, I bought a bottled fizzy drink from a respectable looking shop, and there was a cockroach sealed inside it.

In theory homoeopathy can cure every disease, but homoeopaths are scarce in many countries. The pharmaceutical cartel has systematically worked on eliminating homoeopathy in every country, starting in the USA with the *Flexner Report* of 1911. So far their tentacles have failed to gain control of India. Homoeopathy can only save your life if the right remedy can be prescribed, and then obtained in time. Diseases like cholera, typhoid, and typhus respond rapidly to the correct potentised remedy, even when the patient is almost dead. But if you do not have the right remedy with you, and you cannot get it in time, you are in danger of dying. So doing your best to avoid the germs of these diseases is well worthwhile.

Medical doctors are trained to think of each medicine as a cure for a particular disease. In homoeopathy there are many cures for each disease, but only one is suitable for a particular individual. Unless the right remedy is chosen for the specific symptoms of that particular person, the remedy will not work. This means that when an epidemic of a disease that needs intervention breaks out, each sick person has to be assessed by a homoeopath in order to achieve a high or 100% cure rate. Although most cases of cholera respond to potentised camphor (*camphora*) or potentised copper (*cuprum*), and most cases of polio respond to *gelsemium* or *lathyrus sativa*, you cannot call *camphora* and *cuprum* the remedies for cholera, nor can you call *gelsemium* and *lathyrus sativa* the remedies for polio, because they are not appropriate in every case. If a wrong remedy is chosen, it does not cure the disease.

Another disadvantage to homoeopathy is that the potentised energy in the medicine is very fragile. The remedies can be depotentised by being near something with a strong smell, or by being zinged with metal detectors. When travelling it is best to pack toothpaste that does not contain mint, and deodorant that does not contain eucalyptus oil or tea tree oil. Insect repellent that has a pungent smell should be packed in a different bag.

POLIO

Polio is not a childhood disease. It is a very serious disease that needs intervention to make it go away. The medical establishment considers polio to be a childhood disease because it occurs more frequently in children than in adults, and because they do not understand the difference between self-resolving childhood diseases and diseases that need intervention.

There are three main strains of polio virus, with over 250 subtypes. The virus is more inclined to become virulent in warm weather than in cold weather. It can float through the air, as well as being able to survive in water. When the virus is virulent it can be caught both from infected sewage, and from the air. Waterborne diseases like typhoid and cholera can be prevented by keeping the water clean, but polio germs are not dependent on water for survival. The pandemic of polio about which we hear so much began in the 1880s, reached a peak in the 1920s, and abated during the 1960s. In the 1920s it was overshadowed by the "Spanish" flu epidemic, which might be why it is not well remembered from that time. Polio is occasionally mentioned in historical documents, and it is known to have occurred in Ancient Egypt. It is not known whether historically recorded outbreaks were just localised outbreaks or part of a world-wide pandemic, but it is known that the disease was not present all the time. There is no reason to believe that the polio virus will not become virulent again in the future.

Some people believe that the polio pandemic that started in the 1880s was caused by the introduction of hygienic disposal of sewage in Europe and North America. They believe that before hygiene was adopted, children were automatically exposed to polio germs when they were very young, and they developed immunity, and that when hygiene was adopted, children were no longer exposed at a young age, and therefore were not immune when they got exposed later on. For this to have been possible it would have been necessary for polio germs to have been virulent all the time, to ensure that every child was exposed at an early age. But polio germs were not virulent in the environment all the time. The polio virus changes in virulence, and most of the time it is absent from the environment. This means that most children who live in unhygienic surroundings do not encounter the virus while they are very young, and that in historical times most children were not rendered immune by lack of hygiene.

The polio pandemic that started in the 1880s affected both communities that had recently introduced hygiene, and those that had made no change to the way they handled sewage. Chimpanzees in the wild are affected by polio when the virus becomes virulent in the air, and they have not changed their lifestyle habits for two million years.

When the polio virus enters the body of a human, or of any primate, it multiplies in the throat and intestines. Most people who are infected with the virus experience no symptoms at all, while some experience symptoms that get no worse than flu. These two groups of people do not realise that they have been infected with the polio virus. It is only if the virus moves from the gut into the nervous system that the symptom of paralysis occurs. During the early part of the infection the virus is breathed out into the air. About a week after infection it passes through the intestines into the faeces. Saliva and mucus contain polio viruses during the first part of the infection, but as polio does not cause sneezing, this is not a major means of spreading infection.

When the wild virus becomes virulent, cases of polio begin to appear. As the virulence of the virus increases the number of cases of polio also increases, until a peak is reached. Then the virulence starts to decrease, and so do the number of cases. Cases cease to occur when the wild virus completely loses its virulence. Nowadays the beliefs that, "polio is caused by hygiene," and, "polio is caused by lack of hygiene," run side by side in medical dogma. The idea that the polio virus changes in virulence is not popular with the medical establishment. Even less popular is the idea that when the polio virus goes through a stage of virulence, the small percentage of individuals who get the disease do so because they have a particular susceptibility. The polio virus went through a stage of virulence in Australia in the 1950s, as it did in many other countries. There was one remote rural town in which only one child got polio. When the child asked the doctor why he had been the only one to get it, the doctor told him it was because he had breathed in at the wrong moment. This shows that the doctor believed, as many doctors do, that exposure to the polio virus inevitably results in polio, and that all the other children in the area did not get it because they did not breathe in the virus.

Polio can easily be mistaken for flu during the early stages, as the initial symptoms are a sore throat, fever, tiredness, and a headache. When it is known that there is a polio virus in the environment, it is safer to regard every case of flu as suspected polio, and to treat it homoeopathically and chiropractically or osteopathically so that it is cured before it does damage. A feature of polio is that the early symptoms sometimes clear up, and the patient seems better, but then the symptoms come back again a few days later, and quickly progress to full-blown polio.

If polio progresses beyond what looks like flu symptoms, there will be nausea or vomiting, the headache will be severe, and there will be stiffness in the neck and back. Once these symptoms appear there is great danger that parts of the body could become paralysed. The paralysis can cause death, especially if it affects the lungs. Nerves get damaged by the polio virus, and some get destroyed. When this happens the victim suffers a degree of disability for the rest of his or her life. If the victim is not fully grown when the nerves are damaged, the affected limbs will not grow properly afterwards, so that the person ends up with one or more limb that is small and withered.

Survivors of polio are also afflicted with the onset of new symptoms 30 or 40 years after they have had the disease. This is because the nerves that were not damaged by polio get worn out over the decades, by having to do the work of the damaged nerves as well as their own work. This problem is called post-polio syndrome.

The key to avoiding polio when the virus is virulent is avoiding the things and situations that increase individual susceptibility. You cannot avoid breathing in the virus when it is floating in the air you breathe, but you can adopt measures that make yourself better able to fight off the infection. Polio is a very bad disease that can lead to permanent physical disability or death, so it is important for parents to be wary of the virus. If an epidemic of polio breaks out in the region where you live, there are five lifestyle factors that need careful attention. These are;

* Obtaining sufficient rest,
* Avoiding chills,
* Avoiding refined foods,
* Avoiding vaccines,
* and keeping the tonsils intact.

REST

Tiredness makes people vulnerable to polio. Avoiding tiredness during polio outbreaks is as important as avoiding sugar. Children get tired more easily than adults, and they need a good sleep routine to keep their immune systems working well. Just going to school is enough to make some children tired, especially if they are under 10. Children who get tired from the normal school day should be kept at home when the polio virus is virulent in the environment. Missing lessons is not as serious as getting polio. Back in the 1950s when the polio virus was virulent in the environment, the authorities would sometimes close schools. Their reason for doing this was to prevent children who were brewing the disease from breathing out the virus onto their classmates. That was a good reason, but it had the secondary benefit that children were less vulnerable to the virus, because they were able to rest and play at home, instead of having to keep up with schoolwork and school activities.

Children can be chronically tired if they have difficulty sleeping, or if they have bad bedtime habits. Most cases of insomnia can be cured by organic calcium supplements, or by homoeopathic treatment for inability to absorb calcium. Bad bedtime habits are much harder to cure, especially when the parents are overworked and tired.

In 1991 I chatted to an elderly lady who had had polio in 1956. At the time she was mother to a toddler and a baby, so she was generally tired. One morning she woke up with "flu", and she was feeling really rotten. Her mother offered to come around and help with the daily chores, but she refused the offer because she did not want to burden her mother. She felt that she must hang the nappies on the line before she had a rest. Her mother had a feeling that something was wrong, and came to the house without telephoning again. She found her daughter collapsed on the ground under the washing line, and called an ambulance. The woman, who is now a granny herself, spent a long time in hospital with polio, and when she was discharged she could only walk very slowly. She still cannot walk at a normal pace. She told me that all the other polio victims that were in the hospital at the same time as she was, had also been very tired at the time that they contracted the disease. She now regrets that she tried to do too much on that morning, because it was by over-exerting herself that she made the "flu" reach the paralytic stage of polio.

When polio was prevalent everyone in the community was exposed to the virus, and it was an observable fact that physical activity increased the risk of a polio infection progressing to paralysis. This has been confirmed by studies.[373,374,375,376]

CHILLS

During childhood diseases, getting chilled can bring on complications, but with polio, a chill can be the factor that makes the person catch the disease in the first place. A classic example of how polio can be caught is the way that Franklin D. Roosevelt caught it in 1921. He was an adult with

5 children. His biographer, Allen Churchill, writes,

> Although Franklin seemed outwardly healthy, he had suffered an unusual number of serious illnesses as a man. Following his five week attack of typhoid in 1912 he had had acute appendicitis, lumbago, tonsillitis, pneumonia, double pneumonia, and influenza, together with frequent sinus attacks and head colds which may have been caused by the overdose of chloroform at birth. In December, 1919, his tonsils had been removed, and after that he seemed less prone to sickness.[377]

This sets the scene. Taking the tonsils out made him "better", because it pushed the illness inward.

> On the afternoon of August 9, roughhousing with his boys on the deck of the Black Yacht, he toppled off into the freezing Bay of Fundy. He laughed this off as a great joke, but the icy waters dealt his body a severe shock.
>
> The next afternoon he took Anna, James, and Elliot out in his small sailboat Vireo. On an island close to Campobello they spied a forest fire. The four landed, cut evergreen boughs, and spent several hours vigorously fighting it. Back on Campobello, a hot weary Franklin suggested a refreshing dip in Lake Glen Severn, a mile and a half away. With the children after him, he ran at dogtrot to the lake. The swim failed to invigorate him - the only time in his life this has happened, he told Eleanor on his return to the cottage. So he suggested another dip into the colder waters of the bay. In wet bathing suits, the four finally jogged back to the house.
>
> Here Franklin found his daily mail and newspapers. Out of doors, still wearing the damp bathing suit in air turning chill, he sat and read for thirty minutes. All at once a shattering chill and sharp pains shot through him. He went to bed. Next morning he was feverish and still in pain. He also complained that his right leg was weak. When he tried to get up, the right knee buckled. Next, both legs became affected. By the third day the paralysis had spread to nearly every muscle from the chest down.[377]

Remember that this happened at a time when the polio virus was virulent in the environment. Sitting around in a cold wind after a swim not make you get polio if there is no polio virus in the air. This tragedy and many others like it made it obvious to health authorities that chills are a major risk factor in catching polio. In 1948 the New Zealand Health Department warned parents of the danger with this poster;

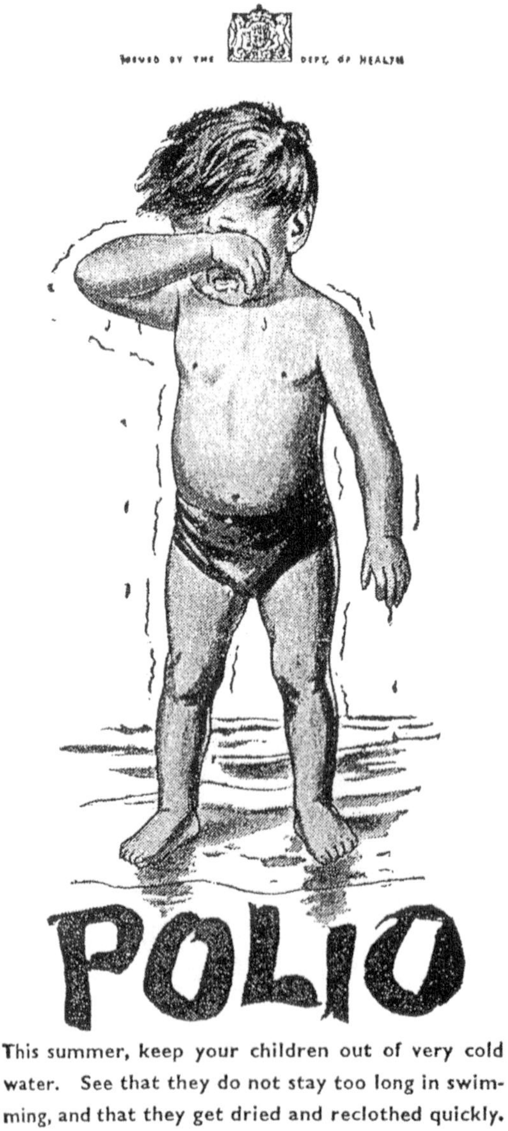
POLIO
This summer, keep your children out of very cold water. See that they do not stay too long in swimming, and that they get dried and reclothed quickly. Chills and fatigue are allies of the poliomyelitis virus.

Why did they know that then when they do not know it now? It reminds me of the way the Ancient Greeks knew so much about mathematics and astronomy, yet their knowledge was forgotten, and had to be rediscovered all over again during the Renaissance.

During the 1940s some cruel experiments were done which showed that chilling monkeys made them more likely to become paralysed after having polio germs injected into their brains, but there are no studies of the effect of chilling on human susceptibility to polio.

REFINED FOOD

When the polio virus becomes virulent, eating a nutritious diet is crucial for protection. Providing the family with wholesome food during a polio epidemic requires time and effort. Take a careful look at what you eat over the next 48 hours. If the wild polio virus suddenly became virulent, would your family's diet be good enough for them to breathe in the virus and suffer no ill-effects? You need to be sure that children are properly nourished when there is a polio virus in the environment, and the first step is cutting out all refined foods. When foods like wheat or rice are refined, the outer layer of the grain is removed. The outer layer contains vitamins, minerals, amino acids, and fibre, while the inside contains only starch. Eating starch on its own makes the immune system unable to function properly. The food industry removes the outer layer of grains because pure starch has a much longer shelf life than whole food. The bacteria and moulds that spoil stored human food are not attracted by food that lacks nutrients. Apart from affecting immunity, the loss of the vitamin B in the outer layer of grains is a major contributor to the modern epidemic of heart disease. Many people should not eat wheat at all. Wheat allergy is more common than coeliac disease, and for those people whole wheat is even more damaging than refined wheat.

Sugar is the worst of the refined foods. The sugar industry has managed to make people believe that consuming sugar is necessary for survival, but sugar has only been a part of the human diet for a short while. In ancient times a few people had access to sugar cane, but most of the world's population survived happily without it. Sugar was introduced into the western diet as a result of the slave trade that operated across the Atlantic Ocean,[358,359] and has been wreaking havoc with the health of the population ever since. The slave trade and the sugar trade worked hand in glove – enriching a few and enslaving millions. The sugar industry in Australia was also founded on slavery.[360,361] Wealthy Queenslanders paid "blackbirders" to fetch slaves from the Pacific Islands, by force or by trickery. By then slavery had been made illegal in the British colonies, so the slaves were described as "indentured labourers". Social activists encouraged people to boycott sugar because of the means of production, perhaps not realising that people who took their advice would be healthier. Sugar suppresses the immune system,[157] weakens the bones and teeth,[362,363] leeches vitamins and minerals from the body,[364] causes heart disease [365,366] and it is fattening.[367] After sugar is eaten, the immune system is depressed for at least five hours.[157]

Eating sugar makes the blood sugar level rise quickly, and then drop quickly, causing bad behaviour in children. These fluctuations eventually exhaust the body's ability to manufacture insulin, and the result is type 2 diabetes. In the olden days type 2 diabetes was known as "sugar diabetes". Brown sugar and "raw sugar" are no better than white sugar. Sugar is addictive, so some adults find it difficult to withhold it from their children because they themselves are addicted.

Perhaps you do not add sugar to your food, but are you eating packaged foods that have had sugar added by the manufacturers? Flour is added to many products, which of course is refined flour, because it has a longer shelf life than whole flour. Naturally you do not eat white bread, except for now and then – more often than you think. And then there's pasta and pizza and pies. Well of course you only eat the whole grain kind, except when you're in a hurry - which is most of the time. We kid ourselves that we eat a wholesome diet, but we often cheat because it is difficult to organise wholesome food for the family all of the time. Under normal circumstances we get away with cheating, but during a polio epidemic the risk is too high to be negligent about children's food. Ensuring that only wholesome food is consumed can be a hassle at first, but polio is a worse option. Most children like melted cheese on whole grain bread, and sausages made of pure meat, and unpolished rice flavoured with miso, and stir-fried vegetables. In my experience most children hate boiled vegetables.

The second nutritional step towards ensuring that children are not vulnerable to polio is to make sure that they eat enough protein. Protein enhances the immune system,[368] and a lack of protein causes a craving for sugar. When children are whining for sugar they can usually be fixed by being given a protein snack. Beware of "health bars" that say they contain protein, but are actually made of starch and sugar. Protein is made up of amino acids that are joined up together, forming long chains. The order of the amino acids in the chain determines what type of protein is formed. For instance, the cells in the muscle in your arm and the cells that make up your kidneys contain the same amino acids, but the tissue has a different texture because the amino acids are joined up to each other in a different order. Every cell in the human body is built out of protein, including the cells of the immune system. Our bodies can manufacture some of the amino acids we need to build cells, but there are some amino acids that we cannot manufacture, so we need to eat them. They are called the essential amino acids. When these amino acids are all together, they form what is called a complete protein. It is necessary to eat all of them at the same time in order to be healthy. Animal proteins, like those in meat, fish, eggs, and cheese, contain all the essential amino acids, and are therefore called complete proteins. Almonds and soy beans are also complete proteins. Whole grains contain some of the essential amino acids, and so do legumes. If you eat whole grains and legumes at the same time, you get all the essential amino acids, so you get a complete protein. It is interesting that many traditional foods around the world consist of a combination of the local grain and the local legume. Combining unpolished rice, lentils, spices, and tasty vegetables all in the same dish is a favourite modern way of eating complete protein.

If a product contains some amino acids it is not fraudulent for the label to say that it contains protein, because amino acids are proteins. But the product will only have the effect of building cells if it contains all the essential amino acids. Vegetarians and vegans can get enough protein if they eat soy beans or soy derivatives, almonds, or foods that are combined so that the amino acids complement one another and form a complete protein. Many meat eaters do not eat enough protein, and they fill themselves up with white bread, white pasta, and white rice. A non-vegetarian diet does not automatically provide enough protein. You may have heard that too much protein harms the kidneys. That is a lie that was first told in 1972 at a press conference that had been called to discredit an American doctor who was making people healthy by recommending a nutritious diet.[369] Eating lots of protein does not harm the kidneys.

If you run a sugar-free home you will have the problem that people in the outside world will try to pressurise your children into consuming sugar. Some children are good at resisting this pressure, while others cannot. You can help them resist the temptation of accepting the offer of junk food by ensuring that they are not deficient in protein. To feel good we need to have a steady amount of glucose in our blood. The liver and pancreas are designed to work co-operatively to keep this amount steady. Eating sugar sabotages the body's balancing mechanism. It makes the amount of glucose in the blood rise rapidly, and then fall to an uncomfortably low level. This makes the person feel unhappy, and makes them crave more sugar. The manifestation of this in children is that they start whining or being naughty about twenty minutes after eating the sugar. Some adults think that the solution is to hand out more sugar. This not only sets a child on the path to type 2 diabetes, it also suppresses his or her immune system.[157]

Eating complete protein makes the blood sugar level stay at a healthy al for a long time. If a person's blood sugar level is badly out of balance, eating small amounts of complete protein three or more times a day is more helpful for keeping the blood sugar level stable than eating a large amount once a day. Some people need to eat small amounts of complete protein as much as seven times a day for more than a year before they can maintain a stable blood sugar level by having protein only once a day. A child whose blood sugar level is stable will not be drawn towards sugary junk. Advertisements recommend giving children a breakfast that is composed of starch and sugar. A child who has eaten complete protein instead of starch for breakfast will be better able to cope with school work and emotional challenges.

Both adults and children who are addicted to sugar can feel emotionally threatened when they encounter someone who does not partake of the habit, and their retaliation against the sugar-free offender can be quite unkind. They don't necessarily restrict themselves to attacking adults, so health conscious parents sometimes find themselves not only counselling their children about nutrition, but also counselling them about how to cope with the nasty behaviour of a sugar addict. Just seeing a child decline to eat something sugary can set the addict off on a round of verbal abuse. It is also not unusual to see an adult berating the parent of a sugar-free child for depriving the child of fun. In fact children are far more able to enjoy themselves and have fun when the amount of glucose in their blood remains stable.

There is a theory that a deficiency of calcium makes a person more vulnerable to polio, but there are no studies on the matter. The need for calcium increases during pregnancy, and the risk of polio increases during pregnancy.[370,371,372] There might be a relationship between the two.

RECENT VACCINATION

When the polio virus is naturally virulent in the environment, injecting vaccine material into a person increases the risk of him or her contracting polio. After a vaccine has been administered, there is a period in which a person has lower resistance to infections. Usually this is not a problem because there seldom are the germs of an infectious disease in the environment, but when the germs are present, the likelihood of succumbing to them is greatly increased by being vaccinated against another disease. As early as 1901 the period of suppressed immunity that follows vaccination was described as the "negative phase of diminished bactericidal power."[378] In 1967 Sir Graham Wilson labelled disease that occurs as a result of this suppressed immunity "provocation disease."[379]

When the polio virus still had global episodes of virulence, it was an empirically observable fact that children were more likely to come down with polio if they had recently been vaccinated against diphtheria, whooping cough, or with the combined diphtheria and whooping cough vaccine. An official investigation into the 1949 epidemic in Britain found that the risk of contracting polio was greatly increased for 28 days after vaccination, and that the period of greatest risk was from 8 to 17 days after.[380] The chief medical officer in Britain then told the regional medical officers to use their own discretion, and vaccination was suspended in many areas until the natural virulence of the polio virus abated.[381,382] In 1951 the Health Department of New York City suspended vaccination against whooping cough and diphtheria from June 15 to October 1, in order to avoid cases of provocation polio.[383] Sir Graham Wilson says,

> Working on the London County Council figures, Benjamin and Gore (1952) calculated that during 1949 the risk of contracting poliomyelitis [polio] was nearly four times as high in children of 9 - 24 months who had received an injection of combined diphtheria and pertussis [whooping cough] vaccine within the previous six weeks as in a control uninoculated group.[384]

The injected polio vaccine also increases the risk of contracting polio shortly after vaccination. An interesting point that emerges from Graham Wilson's collection of data is that the injected polio vaccine causes provocation polio when used during an epidemic, while the oral polio vaccine does not. Also of interest is the fact that the brands of vaccine that contained aluminium had a worse provocation effect than the brands without aluminium.

The polio virus was not globally virulent during the later part of the 20th century, but it has become virulent in limited areas from time to time. When this happens, recent vaccination increases the risk of catching polio. For instance, the polio virus put in an appearance in the country of Oman in 1988. A study found that 35% of the cases of polio in babies aged from five to eleven months had been provoked by injection of DPT vaccine.[385] Of course a vaccine can only provoke polio when there is a polio virus in the environment, but it is clear that one way of protecting yourself if the polio virus becomes virulent in your area is to avoid all vaccines.

TONSILLECTOMY

Having had one's tonsils removed increases the risk of catching polio.[371,386,387,388,389] Studies from 1910 to 1953 found that when tonsils ecently been removed the risk was very high, but there was still increased risk after ten years.[388] Some health departments instructed doctors to refrain from removing tonsils while the polio virus was virulent.

The tonsils are the first line of defence against airborne infections. They are made of lymphoid tissue, and this tissue is swarming with immune system cells. If the tonsils become sore and inflamed, it is because they are being overloaded with toxins and underfed with nutrients. Massive doses of vitamin C will fix them, as I learned in 1977. I was living in South Africa near a hospital called Settler's Hospital, and there were lots of severely poverty-stricken, disenfranchised people living in the same town. I was approached by a woman who asked me to give her five rand so that she could have her tonsils out at the hospital. Five rand was two weeks wages for a black person who was employed, and this woman, like the majority of Blacks in the town, was unemployed. I did not feel like parting with five rand, so I shone a light on her tonsils. The sight was revolting. The flesh had split into canyons that were filled with green and yellow pus. This condition is called quinsy. I looked it up in one of the books written by the nutritionist Adelle Davis, and vitamin C was recommended. I had an unopened bottle of vitamin C on the shelf which had cost two rand. The bottle had been sitting there ever since I had bought it with the intention of doing the right thing and taking a pill every day. So I gave her the bottle and told her how much to take, and how often. I was really trying to save myself three rand. A few days later the woman came round and I looked at her throat again. The flesh of her tonsils was smooth and healthy. And it stayed healthy. I had not only saved myself some money, I had also inadvertently saved her from losing an important part of her immune system.

Weleda's *Zinnober D6,* taken alternately on the hour with *Erysidoron 1*, rapidly converts struggling, overloaded tonsils into healthy, hardworking tonsils. There are many single homoeopathic remedies for tonsillitis, which are chosen according to the way the tonsillitis manifests. The barbaric act of removing the tonsils lowers a person's immunity for the rest of his or her life.

TREATING POLIO

Paralytic polio has been cured in a number of different ways. If someone in my family came down with polio, I would have them treated by a homoeopath right away, and by a chiropractor or osteopath as soon as possible. I would also give them large doses of vitamin C to help their immune system fight the virus. Polio is a fast-acting disease, and there is no time to waste. The appropriate potentised remedy, selected by a properly trained homoeopath, will cause an improvement in the patient in a matter of minutes.

Don't be tempted to try choosing the remedy yourself. A good homoeopath knows the materia medica well, and can select a remedy that corresponds to all the prevailing symptoms, not just to some of the symptoms. You can afford to experiment with treating flu yourself, because if you do not succeed in choosing a remedy that makes the patient's body kill the virus, then the patient is only left with flu, or post viral fatigue syndrome. But polio is a much more serious disease. Failure to kill the virus can result in life-long paralysis or death.

Modern medicine calls polio an incurable disease because they cannot cure it, but intensive care in hospital can prevent victims from dying during the acute phase. Artificial ventilation prevents death from lung paralysis, and intravenous fluids help to sustain life, but modern medical treatment cannot prevent nerve damage.

I was a child during the fifties when the polio virus was virulent, and I remember the unlucky ones with their callipers hobbling around at school. For them the effect was going to be life-long. One classmate was in a wheelchair as a result of polio when we were only six. At playtime he sat in his wheelchair and did French knitting with a wooden cotton reel that had four tacks nailed into it. He made a brightly coloured rope that seemed miles long. He coiled it and made it into a big carpet. He had time on his hands because he could not run around the playground with us. It was all quite unnecessary because there were a lot of properly qualified homoeopaths in Johannesburg. One of them, Dr. Archie Taylor Smith, is mentioned by Dr. Dorothy Shepherd in her book on how to treat infectious diseases homoeopathically.[390] She quotes the remedies he recommends for the different types of onset "to break up the disease in its early stages." Treatment in the next stage prevents paralysis, while treatment during paralysis prevents nerve damage and death.

I remember my mother telling her friends that homoeopathy was the way to treat polio, and I remember her mentioning the name of Dr. Archie Taylor Smith, among others. My mother also spoke about Archie's success at treating a girl from Bulawayo in Zimbabwe for brain damage from DPT vaccine. The girl's parents drove the 550 miles from Bulawayo to Johannesburg on very underdeveloped roads once a month to see Archie. The child did not recover fully, but Archie's choice of remedies accomplished a remarkable improvement. In another suburb in Johannesburg there lived a batch of little boys who were destined to become my brothers-in-law two decades later. They were treated successfully by Archie for a number of ailments, and he cured their father of a life-threatening condition. The

.at homoeopathy can do seem amazing to people who have no .nd experience of it.

The polio virus does damage when it moves from the gastro-intestinal .act into the cells and attacks the nervous system, so it is a good idea to keep the skeleton free of subluxations. Subluxations are minor displacements of the bones. (Pharmaceutical medicine only acknowledges subluxations that are severe enough to show up on an X ray.) When the vertebrae of the spine are out of position, they impede the flow of information along the nerves. An adjustment to correct the position of the bones in the neck is particularly helpful to stop giving flu or polio germs an advantage.

It surprised me to learn that chiropractic and osteopathic care can help to alleviate residual paralysis after the acute stage of polio has passed. The first time I heard about this was in 1972, when my mother and I went on a bird club camp in the Magaliesburg mountains. A woman who walked with a peculiar gait started putting up a tent next to ours. Her body was crooked, and her movements were rather awkward. My mother, with her usual tact, said, "Let me help you. You look as though you have a crick in your neck." The lady was not fazed by that, and she told us that she had had polio at seventeen, and the specialist had told her she would never walk again. At twenty-one she had started chiropractic treatment, and was up and about in a matter of weeks. Some years later she was walking up Adderley Street in Cape Town when the specialist came walking down the street. He was astounded to see her walking, and when she told him that a chiropractor had done it, he was furious, and reprimanded her for going to a "quack".

When the polio vaccine was being developed there was a fund raising effort called the *March of Dimes* that used posters to advertise their cause. One of the posters showed a photograph of a little girl called Winifred Gardella who had lost the ability to walk because of polio. In the photo she is standing supported by crutches, with her legs in callipers. Medical treatment was unable to improve her condition, but later a chiropractor named Lewis Robertson got her walking again.[391]

Good old vitamin C comes to the rescue again when the polio virus is wreaking havoc in the body, but it has to be injected. A person with polio is too sick to swallow megadoses of vitamin C. An experiment published in 1935 found that vitamin C inactivates the polio virus in a test tube.[392] That was followed by controlled trials on monkeys that did not replicate natural circumstances, but did show that vitamin C prevents paralysis. Nobel Prize winner Dr. Linus Pauling says,

> Dr. Fred R Klenner, a physician in Reidsville, North Carolina, was the first person to report the successful treatment on polio

patients by injecting large amounts of ascorbic acid.[393]

The great nutritionist Adelle Davis says,

> Some years ago it was my good fortune to visit with Dr. Klenner and hear him lecture ... Dr. Klenner told of an eighteen-month-old girl suffering from polio. The mother reported that the child had become paralysed following a convulsion, after which she soon lost consciousness. When Dr. Klenner first saw the child, her little body was blue, stiff and cold to the touch; he could neither hear her heart sound nor feel her pulse, her rectal temperature was 100 degrees F. The only sign of life he could detect was a suggestion of moisture condensed on a mirror held to her mouth. The mother was convinced that the child was already dead. Dr. Klenner injected 6,000 milligrams of vitamin C into her blood; four hours later the child was cheerful and alert, holding a bottle with her right hand, though her left side was paralysed. A second injection was given; soon the child was laughing and holding her bottle with both hands, all signs of paralysis gone. Dr. Klenner quite understandably speaks of vitamin C as "the antibiotic par excellence." A physician who later obtained striking results at the Los Angeles County Hospital by treating severe infections with vitamin C matched Dr. Klenner's enthusiasm with the remark, "if anything should be called a miracle drug, it is vitamin C."
>
> With his extremely ill patients, Dr. Klenner found that no vitamin C whatsoever could be detected in the blood only a few minutes after massive doses were injected; nor was any vitamin C found in the urine. It is his belief that this vitamin combines immediately with toxins and/or virus, thus causing the fever to drop.[394]

You can see why the makers of paracetamol/tylenol, who happen to control the curricula at medical schools, do not want doctors to know about vitamin C. Drugs that reduce fever do so by crippling the immune system, not by helping the immune system fight the invader. I wonder how many millions of children have died when an injection of vitamin C could have saved them. Dr Klenner himself says,

> Many physicians refuse to employ vitamin C in the amounts suggested, simply because it is counter to their fixed ideas of what is reasonable, but it is not against their reason to try

.ie new product being advertised by an alert drug firm. ‹ is difficult for me to reconcile these two attitudes. On the other hand, many physicians who have been willing to try vitamin C against the virus of poliomyelitis have obtained the same striking results as we reported.[395] Scores of letters from practitioners here in the United States and in Canada could be presented in evidence. In some instances doctors have cured their own children of poliomyelitis by giving vitamin C and in other cases doctors themselves have been cured.[396]

In 1955 a doctor in Illinois published a report of his success with small doses of vitamin C,[397] but no controlled trials on humans have been done, and they are unlikely to be done anytime soon.

TETANUS

Tetanus germs can exist on anything in the environment, but they are most prolific in soil that is contaminated with animal dung. They can only cause disease in a human if they enter the bloodstream through a wound. They do not cause disease when they are breathed in or swallowed, and they cannot be caught from another person. Even a tiny wound like a pin prick can allow tetanus germs to enter the bloodstream. Tetanus germs thrive if they get into blood that lacks oxygen, which is why tetanus seldom occurs in fit, healthy adults. Most deaths from tetanus occur in babies who are born in communities that live in close proximity with animals, because the umbilical cord is often cut with an implement that is contaminated with cow dung.

Even though the blood of most healthy individuals is an unfavourable environment for tetanus germs, everyone should take steps to avoid tetanus after a wound. It is a fast-acting and potentially fatal disease, and the conventional medical treatment for it, which just aims to keep the patient alive while the disease runs its course, is not always successful. Non-conventional treatments, however, are very effective, and can save the life of the person even when the disease is advanced. The two most effective treatments for tetanus are vitamin C and homoeopathy. Curing tetanus with vitamin C sounds simplistic, but it actually works, as I will show. First let's talk about prevention.

Cuts and open wounds should be disinfected with an antiseptic liquid, and any bits of dirt or wood in the wound should be removed. Washing with water does not kill germs, and if the water is not sterile it can cause infection. It flabbergasts me that some health departments tell parents tha water is sufficient to cleanse an open wound.

Puncture wounds that have been made by something like a pin, a thorn, or an animal's tooth are problematic wounds because tetanus germs can be delivered deep into the flesh, out of the reach of disinfectants. The homoeopathic remedy *ledum 30* should be taken after all puncture wounds. If an innocent looking little splinter gets under the skin, it is worth taking a dose of *ledum 30,* because there can be tetanus germs on wood. After a bite from an animal the patient should take *ledum 30*, even if it looks as if the flesh was torn open enough for effective washing. *Ledum 30* should form part of the home first aid kit.

Tetanus bacteria and tetanus toxoid can be inactivated by vitamin C,[398] so it is a good idea to take megadoses of vitamin C after any kind of wound. If there happen to be no tetanus germs in the wound the money spent on the vitamin C will not have been wasted, because vitamin C helps the immune system kill any other types of germs that might be lurking in the wound.

Vitamin C is not only useful as a preventative of tetanus; it also cures the full-blown disease. A medical experiment was done in a hospital in Dhaka, Bangladesh, to see if vitamin C helped in the treatment of tetanus.[399] The subjects consisted of one hundred and seventeen people who were hospitalised with tetanus. They were divided into two age groups; those up to 12 years and those over 12 years. Each group was then divided into those who received the conventional treatment plus vitamin C, and those who received only the conventional treatment. Unfortunately they did not create a group that was given vitamin C but no conventional treatment.

The amount of vitamin C that was given was only 1000 mg of ascorbic acid, which is not a high dose. However, it was given intravenously, not orally, which made it more effective. Dr. Archie Kalokerinos discovered that vitamin C is five times more effective when it is injected instead of being swallowed.[159] The injection of vitamin C saved the lives of all the children, but it only saved 40% of the adults. No deaths occurred in the children who were given this small amount of vitamin C, while 74.2% of the children who were not given vitamin C died. 37% of the adults who were given 1000 mg of vitamin C died, while 67% of those not given vitamin C died.

These results show that the amount of vitamin C given to the adults was too small for their body weight, as it only saved 40% of them. The adults should have been given more than one injection, because vitamin C gets used up quickly in a person who is fighting a serious infection.[159] Nevertheless, the injections of vitamin C made a significant difference to the survival rate of the adults. This experiment was published in a medical

984.[399] It clearly shows that injections of vitamin C save the ...ople with tetanus, yet no public hospital in the world has started ...itamin C injections as a treatment for tetanus.

...harmaphiles get angry when I mention vitamin C for tetanus, saying ...at there is only one study on the matter, and a treatment cannot be based on only one study. They are such hypocrites. There are no studies which show that pharmaceutical treatments cure tetanus, which is not surprising as pharmaceutical treatments do not cure tetanus. However, the ideal treatment would be a combination of vitamin C, homoeopathy, and life support at a hospital. In the distant future that may be how it is done.

As I have said, homoeopathy is great for preventing the development of tetanus, and homoeopathy can cure tetanus. But if vitamin C injections are available, there is no need for homoeopathy to cure tetanus, because the vitamin C alone is sufficient. If homoeopathy is to be used it needs to be accessed quickly, because tetanus is a fast acting disease. The correct remedy needs to be given in the right potency, and with the right frequency. Potentised *hypericum* is often mentioned as the cure for tetanus, but tetanus is not something for amateurs to experiment with. The symptoms of tetanus are not exactly the same in every patient, and the chosen remedy should match all of the symptoms that the patient is exhibiting. There are over forty possible homoeopathic remedies for tetanus, so the remedy should be chosen by someone who knows the materia medica well.

Pharmaceutical medicine says that there in "no cure" for tetanus, and that the patient has to be "managed" to keep him or her alive. They use muscle relaxing drugs to control the spasms, antibiotics to try to kill the germ, drugs to keep the heart beating and lungs moving, a ventilator to help the person breathe, and immune serum globulin to tackle any toxin that has not yet attached itself to a nerve. They are not supposed to give a drug to suppress fever, but sometimes they do, and this works against the patient's chances of survival. The modern drugs they use to deal with the symptoms of muscle tightening are much safer than curare, which is the old-fashioned one that they used to use. Old statistics on tetanus are meaningless because many of the patients actually died from curare poisoning, not from tetanus.

After the 2004 Boxing Day tsunami thousands of doctors and nurses from around the world rushed to help the survivors. In Aceh 127,000 people were killed by the wave, while 100,000 survived being tossed by the wave and hit by debris. Of the latter, 100 died in hospital because tetanus had infected their wounds. The doctors and nurses just had to watch helplessly as their tetanus patients died. If those doctors and nurses had known the rudiments of homoeopathy, or been able to use injections of vitamin C, they could have saved their patients. The reason why they had not been taught how to cure tetanus is that vitamins and homoeopathic remedies do not bring in profits for the pharmaceutical industry.

TB (Tuberculosis)

TB is caused by a bacterium that can attack any part of the body, but most commonly attacks the lungs. Damp housing, malnutrition, and chronic tiredness are risk factors that predispose a person to TB, and nowadays being infected with the HIV virus also makes people vulnerable to TB. TB is associated with overcrowding because poor people usually live in crowded conditions, but overcrowding in itself does not cause TB. Rich people who live in big houses are also at risk of coming down with TB if they do not eat sufficient nourishing food. A king of Sweden and a Hollywood star have died of TB.

The bacteria live in the throats of a high percentage of the world's population, but the germs are unable to cause sickness in people with adequately functioning immune systems. One third of the world's population has a latent infection of TB, but they are not spread evenly over the world.[343,344] A latent infection can become active at any time during an infected person's life,[345] and the cause of activation can be alcoholism, diabetes, kidney disease, cancer, drugs that suppress the immune system, malnutrition, tobacco smoke, lung damage from sandblasting (for instance in workers who shoot sand particles at denim jeans to give them the "faded" look), or HIV infection.[346,347]

The disease has existed in humans for thousands of years, and for most of that time people did not realise that it is contagious and that malnutrition plays a crucial role in allowing the germ to harm the body of the host. Robert Koch isolated the bacterium that causes TB in 1882,[348] and after that people began to make the observation that malnutrition is the primary risk factor for TB. The role of malnutrition has more recently been confirmed by studies.[349,350,351,352]

A perfect diet of organically grown, unprocessed food is not necessary to prevent TB. If that were the case, most people in the world would be suffering from TB. Eating things like mincemeat, unpolished rice, pumpkin, and apples prevents TB. Some people are too poor to buy enough of such simple fare, while others have been influenced by disinformation that tells them to eat sugar and refined grains. In the old South Africa, radio and TV aggressively promoted sugar as the greatest benefit to health. Many people were illiterate because apartheid kept them out of school, and they believed that bright coloured sugary drinks were better for them than milk. Whole wheat bread was cheaper than white bread, but people were told that white bread was better. So not only did they have very little money because their labour was exploited, but what little they had was wrongly spent. The results were things like high infant mortality, and rampant TB. BCG vaccine was compulsory, and was given to newborn babies and to children without parental consent. It is possible that the vaccine increased the incidence of TB, as it was shown to do in India.[325,326] No record was kept of how many infants died from BCG vaccine, although sometimes deaths caused by the vaccine were reported.[353]

You do not need a first class diet to avoid TB. You need sufficient calories laced with some vitamins and minerals, and you need to be housed in an abode that is dry and warm. Affluent people who have sugar with every meal do not get TB, because they dilute the sugar with protein and minerals. TB dwindles when a society becomes more affluent, and it resurges when the economy slumps. The USA and New Zealand both experienced great affluence after World War II. As a result, TB declined dramatically in both countries. BCG vaccine was used in New Zealand, but not in the USA. Medical mythology has it that the vaccine caused the decline in New Zealand, and antibiotics caused the decline in the USA. When the New Zealand economy collapsed in 1987, the incidence of TB began to rise dramatically. An economic downturn in the USA also caused an increase in TB in that country, and this was aggravated by the spread of the HIV virus, which lowers resistance to TB.

Some of the symptoms of TB include; continuous cough that lasts more than four weeks, loss of appetite, night sweats, pains in the chest, breathlessness, tiredness, weakness, and loss of weight. Coughing up blood is a sign that the disease is well advanced. Not all of these symptoms are present in each case, and there are other symptoms as well.

The drugs that are used in an attempt to cure TB can have serious side effects, and they have to be taken every day for six to nine months. When the TB germ mutates, new drugs or combinations of drugs have to be tried out. Enormous amounts of money and effort are put into trying to deal with the problem of TB, but these well-intentioned people are barking up the wrong tree. Most cases of TB can be cured by *Koch Tuberculinum 30*, which is made by homoeopathically potentising a vaccine that was invented by Robert Koch. This vaccine was made from human TB germs, and it killed so many babies that it was withdrawn. Websites that glorify Robert Koch tend to omit this ignominious detail. Once the vaccine is homoeopathically potentised, this deadly vaccine saves lives. It has the potential to save millions of lives, because enough medicine to cure one person costs less than a dollar. If governments were to introduce homoeopathy to treat TB, the most expensive part for them would be maintaining clinic buildings in poor areas, and paying the salaries of the people who administer the remedy. Trained homoeopaths would be able to cure all the cases of TB for which *Koch Tuberculinum 30* is not the correct remedy.

In the 1950s two French scientists showed that when vitamin C is added to a test tube that contains TB germs, the vitamin C kills the TB germs.[354,355] Naturally this news was not received with enthusiasm by the pharmaceutical industry. In 2012 some scientists in New York who were trying to make a vaccine for TB found that when they put a bit of vitamin C into the test tube that contained the germ culture, it killed the TB germs, including drug resistant TB germs.[356] In 1938 an Austrian doctor reported great improvements in his TB patients when he administered vitamin C.[357] A trial needs to be done to see whether high doses of vitamin C can cure active TB.

DIPHTHERIA

When diphtheria was still prevalent, homoeopaths successfully cured patients by choosing the correct potentised remedy for each individual case. The symptom picture of diphtheria differs from patient to patient, but it always includes the symptoms of weakness, increased heart rate, and a membrane growing on the back of the throat. When diphtheria has a fatal outcome, it is usually because of cardiac arrest, or because the membrane has grown across the opening of the throat and caused suffocation. This membrane changes in appearance as the disease progresses, and the colour and thickness of the membrane at the time that the homoeopath takes the case is one of the most important factors in choosing the right remedy. When the illness starts suddenly and progresses rapidly, the appropriate remedy is *mercurius cyanatus*. This remedy is particularly useful for saving the lives of babies with diphtheria.

Pharmaceutical medicine has three treatments for diphtheria. Antibiotics are given to kill the bacteria and to prevent the patient from infecting others. Horse serum that contains diphtheria antitoxin is injected to neutralise any toxin that has not yet caused damage. Thirdly, a surgical cut called a tracheotomy can be made through the membrane that is blocking the throat to enable the patient to breathe. The CDC website proclaims that antibiotics and antitoxin are the treatments for diphtheria, and then adds, "About 1 out of 10 people who gets diphtheria will die." Someone should tell them that is not exactly a glowing endorsement of their treatments.

The death rate under orthodox treatment was higher when they used mercury to treat diphtheria. A doctor who was a strong advocate of the mercury treatment[400,401] made a beautifully ironic attack on both homoeopathy and on doctors who disapproved of using mercury to treat diphtheria. He accused homoeopaths of being hypocrites because they "have so bitterly railed against it" while using it themselves under the name of "mercurius dulcis".[401] The homoeopaths did use mercury for diphtheria, but the writer is too arrogant to inform himself of the fact that they used it in a non-toxic, potentised form, and only for patients who presented with the appropriate symptoms, not for every case of diphtheria. The irony comes when he ends his promotion of mercury with, "Happily, the day of bigotry and intolerance in medicine is rapidly passing away," meaning that all doctors are soon going to start using mercury for diphtheria. He is the bigot, not the doctors and homoeopaths who wisely cautioned against the use of mercury.

Diphtheria has not disappeared, although it underwent a considerable natural decline during the 20th century (see graphs in myth number four). No one can predict what it is going to do in the future. If it were to return in a big way, homoeopaths would once again be able to treat it successfully.

MENINGITIS

Meningitis is inflammation of the membranes that surround the brain, and it can be caused by bacteria, viruses, toxins, drugs, vaccines, and some chronic diseases. Meningococcal meningitis is the most dangerous type of meningitis, and it is caused by a bacterium, so it responds really well to antibiotics. There are thirteen strains of the bacterium that can cause meningococcal meningitis, and vaccines have been invented for some of them.

Infectious meningitis is rare, but when it happens it is an emergency, and treatment must be started right away, or the patient can die within hours. One of the features of meningococcal meningitis is that it starts suddenly and progresses rapidly. Meningococcal meningitis can be difficult to diagnose because symptoms vary with each case. Symptoms can include a sudden high fever, a stiff neck, collapse, nausea, aversion to light, severe headache, and a rash of little red spots that grow in size and begin to look like bruising. The rash does not appear if the germs concentrate on attacking the brain and do not enter the blood. If the rash does appear, waiting to see if it starts changing into purple blotches could be a fatal mistake. If meningococcal meningitis is suspected, an antibiotic should be given right away, otherwise the patient could be dead before any tests come back from the lab. Doctors usually undermine the good effect of an antibiotic by giving a drug to suppress fever at the same time, so if a loved one has meningococcal meningitis, or is suspected of having it, try to prevent the doctors from giving a drug to suppress fever. They should also use injections of vitamin C along with the antibiotic, because the benefits of warmth, fever, antibiotic, and vitamin C augment each other when combined.[48,49] Hopefully in the future doctors will comply with this best practice. A person with meningitis is usually too ill to swallow vitamin C pills, so vitamin C powder should be stored in the home in an airtight container in case of this type of emergency. The biggest danger is that the doctors might not treat the meningitis at all. They sometimes send the patient home saying nothing is wrong, and then the patient dies, or the disease progresses to a point where it does permanent damage.

A qualified homoeopath could nip the condition in the bud, even after collapse, but this is not a situation for experimentation by an amateur. Viral meningitis cannot be helped by antibiotics, so a correctly chosen homoeopathic remedy, combined with injections of vitamin C, is ideal.

As is the case with all vaccines, vaccines for meningitis were not properly tested for adverse effects before they were licensed for use on the public, and reports of severe adverse reactions are simply ignored.

HEPATITIS B

Hepatitis refers to inflammation of the liver, and the inflammation can be caused by toxins or by germs. Confusion about how the various types of infectious hepatitis are caught helps the vaccine industry sell hepatitis B vaccine. Hepatitis A, hepatitis B, and hepatitis C are all caused by viruses that attack the liver, but these viruses do not all enter the body in the same way. Hepatitis A can be caught from another person's saliva, from cutlery and crockery that has not been properly washed, from food that has been prepared by someone who has not washed their hands, or from shellfish that is harvested from water that is contaminated with sewage. Hepatitis B and C are different in that they need to enter a person's blood in order to cause infection. As with HIV, the virus that causes AIDS, the viruses that cause hepatitis B and C can be caught from contaminated needles, contaminated blood products, or by having sex with someone who is a carrier.

The symptoms of hepatitis B include nausea, jaundice (skin turning yellow), tiredness, loss of appetite, pain in the liver, sore joints, sore muscles, a skin rash, and dark coloured urine. Not all symptoms are present in all cases, and some people get infected without displaying any symptoms at all. Once a person has been infected, the virus can continue to live in his or her body for a long time. This can happen whether or not the virus causes any symptoms when it first infects the person. So a person who has been exposed to one of the risk factors for catching hepatitis B may be carrying the virus in his or her body, even though he or she has never experienced the acute symptoms of hepatitis B. In some carriers the virus causes liver damage, and in rare cases, liver cancer. Drugs that are used to treat people who are carriers of the hepatitis B virus have the problem that they do not work very well, and they have unpleasant adverse effects.[402]

As for adverse effects of the vaccine itself, in 1999 The Association of American Physicians and Surgeons submitted a statement to the U.S. House of Representatives saying that, based on reports to VAERS, the risk of a severe reaction to hepatitis B vaccine is a hundred times greater in most children than the risk of the disease, that the adverse effects of the vaccine have not been properly determined, and that the system behind the use of the vaccine is financially corrupt.[403] VAERS is the American database to which doctors are supposed to report vaccine reactions that they witness. Only a tiny proportion of severe reactions are reported to VAERS, so in reality the risk of a severe reaction to the vaccine is about a thousand times greater than the risk of the disease.

In 1994 France launched a mass hepatitis B vaccination campaign, which was followed by a huge increase in cases of multiple sclerosis. There was discussion and there were denials, and a whole lot of "studies" were rushed out to prove that the vaccine does not cause MS. A study that found that hepatitis B vaccine does cause MS had trouble getting published, but it finally was published.[404] Twenty years after the mass vaccination campaign, an epidemiological study confirmed that the vaccine was the cause of the increase in MS.[405] It was closely followed by a study that found that hepatitis B vaccine does not cause MS, it just accelerates it in people who already have MS.[406] The vaccine industry loves it,[407] but Dr. Marc Girard has written a brilliant critique on PubMed Commons, showing how completely unscientific the methodology is, and that the study does not prove that hepatitis B vaccine does not cause MS. Dr. Girard has presented evidence that the known risks of hepatitis B vaccine are greater than the risk from the disease, and that studies that have unfavourable results are not published.[408] For instance, studies that found that hepatitis B vaccine causes lupus and Graves disease were not published.[408]

If a mother is a carrier of hepatitis B, the virus can be transferred to her baby during pregnancy or birth, and injecting the baby with hepatitis B vaccine soon after birth reduces the risk of the baby becoming a carrier.[409] A Cochrane review of the practice found that in most of the studies, effectiveness of the vaccine was judged by the creation of antibodies, rather than by long-term clinical outcome,[409] and none of the studies made a sincere attempt to assess the frequency of adverse effects.[409] Naturally the vaccine industry wants every baby to be injected with the vaccine at birth, even if the mother is not a carrier of hepatitis B. I know mothers whose tests for the hepatitis B carrier state came back negative, but the doctors still tried to bully them into vaccinating their baby soon after birth.

Michael Belkin's five week old daughter was killed by hepatitis B vaccine in 1998, when hepatitis B vaccine was still given on its own. The autopsy found that her brain was swollen, which is a common reaction to vaccinations of all kinds. The New York City Coroner tried to report the death to VAERS, but was blocked from doing so. Two months later Michael attended a workshop about reactions to hepatitis B vaccine that was presented by the National Academy of Sciences. Doctors from around the world expressed their concerns about the vaccine, but the FDA and CDC made disparaging remarks about the evidence that had been presented. By 1998 VAERS had received 17,497 reports of severe reactions to hepatitis B vaccine, which included deaths, central nervous system damage, and liver damage. The FDA and CDC know that only a small fraction of reactions ever get reported, yet they declared the number of reports to be acceptable. Using his expertise in statistics and econometrics, Michael testified to Congress in 1999 about the fraudulent way in which the vaccine had been approved for infants by the Advisory Committee on Immunization Practices, and about the failure of the FDA to act upon the reports they had received, but the vaccine juggernaut rolls on.

The vaccine industry drums up fear of hepatitis B in order to promote their product, and they fudge the background facts about how hepatitis B is caught. In Australia there was a campaign to persuade all teachers to accept the vaccine. Teachers were told that they could catch hepatitis B from the children they teach. The truth is that the only way teachers can catch it is by having sex with the children, or by sharing needles with them during recreational drug abuse. This type of dishonesty has appeared all over the world in the promotion of the vaccine. My daughter's teacher had a severe reaction to the first dose of hepatitis B vaccine, but the bullies still wanted him to accept more doses. He was furious when he learned that he could not catch hepatitis B from the children.

The Australian pamphlet that promotes hepatitis B vaccination on the day of birth is typical of the way that the vaccine pushers misrepresent the facts. The pamphlet is given to mothers when they are already in labour, instead of being given out during pregnancy. A woman who is in labour is usually not able to think clearly, be assertive, think of the right questions to ask, nor go to the library to do some research. This is precisely why the pamphlet is given to mothers at this time. The pamphlet contains four blatant lies, six clever half-truths, lots of omissions, and 2 serious omissions. The first serious omission is that it does not mention that the vaccine is made from genetically engineered yeast. There is a public outcry in Australia about the fact that the government subsidises genetically engineered crops, while not supporting sustainable agriculture. Yet the media will not talk about the fact that the government injects genetically engineered yeast into babies on the day they are born.

The other serious omission on the pamphlet is that it does not mention that if the mother's blood has not been exposed to hepatitis B infection, the baby cannot catch hepatitis B from her. A baby is not old enough to be promiscuous or to share needles with other drug addicts, so the only way that he or she can become infected with hepatitis B is through contaminated medical products or instruments. That is not likely to happen in a country that screens blood products and cleans medical instruments. In any case, catching an acute infection of hepatitis B is not nearly as dangerous as being injected with genetically engineered yeast on the day that you are born.

One of the clever half-truths on the Australian pamphlet is the statement that the risk of becoming a hepatitis B carrier is highest during infancy and early childhood. This is half true, because if the baby's blood is exposed to the hepatitis B virus during infancy or early childhood, the risk of him or her becoming a carrier is higher than it is from blood exposure when he or she is older. However, what the pamphlet does not mention is that the risk of the baby's blood being exposed to hepatitis B during infancy and early childhood is much lower than it is during adolescence or adulthood.

In the blatant lie category the pamphlet says, "Serious side effects of hepatitis immunisation are rare." Serious side effects are not rare, however, they are rarely acknowledged. When a severe reaction to hepatitis B vaccine is presented to a doctor or nurse, they usually just deny that the vaccine is the cause. A baby born at Box Hill hospital in Melbourne in September 2002 was doing well. He was contented while awake, and feeding and sleeping well. When he was two days old he was injected with hepatitis B vaccine at 4 pm. He immediately stopped feeding, and he cried constantly. The mother was very concerned, but the nurses were not. He continued crying until he died at 7 am. The newspaper published the death notice, but not the cause of death. The package inserts of hepatitis B vaccines say that vaccination is contraindicated for persons with a history of hypersensitivity to yeast. How are you supposed to know, on the day of birth, whether or not a person is allergic to yeast?

In 1988 the hepatitis B vaccine made with human blood was introduced into New Zealand. The policy was that newborns were to be vaccinated a few days after birth, and a nurse had to stand and watch the babies for 20 minutes so that if one had a bad reaction to the vaccine, she could inject the baby with adrenaline. After a few months a nurse telephoned Hilary Butler and told her that the policy had been changed. Nurses had now been instructed to carry adrenaline and a syringe at all times, because some babies were going into shock more than 20 minutes after the vaccination, and some were dying in the time that it took for the nurse to gallop to the store and fetch adrenaline after she noticed the reaction. A normal brain would think that the policy should have been changed to suspend vaccination, but bureaucratic brains are not normal.

Hepatitis B vaccine was introduced to both Australia and New Zealand with the claim that a child could catch hepatitis B in the playground from the scabs or open wounds of carrier children. The New Zealand government employed Saatchi and Saatchi to make a terrifying TV advertisement that promoted fear of the disease and trust in the vaccine. The advertisement featured empty playground equipment and a doll that fell to the ground. Saatchi and Saatchi have great talent. The advertisement was so chilling, bordering on spooky; it sent a shudder down one's spine. After the vaccine was introduced, the theory that children could catch hepatitis B from other children was put to the test by a study in Sydney, and it was found that hepatitis B is not passed on from child to child.[25,26]

Some institutions that employ nurses make hepatitis B vaccine compulsory for their staff, and I know nurses who have chosen to make a career change rather than have the stuff injected into their bodies.

Homoeopathy can cure hepatitis B.[410]

CHOLERA

Cholera is a waterborne disease, so unboiled water should be avoided when travelling in countries where cholera is endemic. Even if you are young and fit and healthy, don't make the mistake of thinking that you would be immune if you swallowed some cholera germs. Try to oversee the cooking of all food that you are going to eat. Don't assume that an expensive hotel has an hygienic kitchen just because there are plush carpets on the floor of the dining room. Salad may have been washed with contaminated water. Also, don't assume that tea and coffee are made with boiled water. It is safer to make your own hot drinks with a gadget that you immerse in a cup of water. Some travellers carry with them an assortment of homoeopathic remedies for diarrhoeal type diseases, just in case.

Cases of cholera cannot occur in regions where the water supply is kept free of contamination, even if someone who is a carrier of the disease moves into the region. The ideal treatment for cholera is a combination of homoeopathy, antibiotics, rehydration with an electrolyte solution, and zinc supplementation. As described in myth number five, the cholera germ changes in virulency, sometimes sweeping across the world, felling thousands as it goes, while at other times just lurking about in contaminated water. When people get the less virulent form of cholera, antibiotics and rehydration are usually sufficient to prevent the patient from dying. A study done in Bangladesh in 2008 found that giving a zinc supplement to children with cholera reduced the length of time that the diahorrea lasted, and reduced its severity.[411]

In 1826 a wave of cholera started in India and spread steadily towards Western Europe. Homoeopaths were the only people who were successful at treating this disease as it crossed Europe. Dr. Frederick Hervey Foster Quin was an English doctor who had become seriously ill while in Italy in 1825, and had been rapidly cured with homoeopathy. This experience had made him curious about homoeopathy, so in 1826 he had gone to Germany to learn from Dr. Samuel Hahnemann.[412] By 1831 cholera was afflicting much of Europe, but it was particularly bad in the part of Eastern Europe that was then called Moravia. Dr. Quin travelled to Moravia to study the epidemic, and soon after his arrival, while eating his dinner, he was suddenly struck down with the violent form of cholera. (Cholera often strikes suddenly. During one of the waves that crossed Europe, scores of people at a grand ball in France suddenly fell down with the sickness.) Dr. Quin was carried to a bed, and when he came out of the coma he treated himself with a remedy. He began to recover, and then he started treating others while still sick and weak. Later he wrote, "I was overworking from morning to night treating cases of cholera, all the other doctors being bedridden."[413]

Cholera is one of the diseases that strikes very fast and can kill within a day. In response to these fast-acting diseases, homoeopathy works very quickly to effect a cure. Onlookers are stunned by the rapidity with which a patient reverts from being at death's door to being well. Diseases that take a long time to develop, like arthritis, take much longer to be cured by homoeopathy.

After Dr. Quin left Moravia, the mayor of the town where he had worked sent him a letter of gratitude for starting to work before he was fully recovered. In the letter he mentions that from the time that Dr. Quin started treating the victims of cholera, no patient died.[414] Dr. Quin founded the British Homoeopathic Society in 1844.[415,416] At one time Dr. Quin was personal physician to the bloke who later became the King of Belgium. Homoeopathy still remains available to the privileged few, while the inhabitants of Belgium's former colonies die in droves from cholera. The World Health Organisation (WHO) should arrange for homoeopaths to enter refugee camps during cholera epidemics and treat each affected individual with one of the three remedies that cure cholera; *camphor 30, veratrum 30* or *cuprum 30.* A trained homoeopath would only take a few minutes to assess each patient and prescribe the right remedy. The medicine to save the patient's life would only cost a few cents, which is the main reason why the pharmaceutical industry does not allow WHO to use it. Malaria and bilharzia (schistosoma) are the biggest killers in Africa. Both diseases can be cured with homoeopathic medicine costing less than a dollar for each individual.

Dr. Quin founded The London Homoeopathic Hospital in 1849 because he wanted to make homoeopathy available to the people. In 1854 cholera broke out in London, and 16% of the cholera patients at the homoeopathic hospital died, while in Middlesex hospital nearby, which used conventional treatments, 53% of the cholera patients died. The doctor who compiled the parliamentary report on cholera intentionally excluded the homoeopathic hospital's success from his report, but the truth was published after the chairman of the hospital board made a great fuss.[417]

TYPHOID

The germs that cause typhoid are good survivors. When they enter a human body, they can live there for years, and they shed billions of offspring which go into the sewage. They do this whether or not the human they have entered gets clinical symptoms of the disease. This means that typhoid can be caught by drinking water that is contaminated with sewage, or from food prepared by someone with faeces on their hands, or from food that has been walked on by flies with dirty feet. The typhoid germ belongs to the salmonella family. All types of salmonella are good survivors, and many of them cause serious symptoms that can lead to death. They thrive in hot weather, but they also survive in cold weather. Typhoid is caused by Salmonella Typhi, which is the worst member of the salmonella family. It does not always strike fast. Sometimes it starts by looking like a bad case of flu, and sometimes it starts with mental symptoms, or nausea and vomiting. The wide variety of symptoms that the typhoid germ can cause means that there is a bigger range of possible homoeopathic remedies for it than for a disease like cholera.

All kinds of salmonella contaminate water in countries where sewage is not properly disposed of, so always boil the water in dubious places. Gastro-enteritis from any type of salmonella is often called "food poisoning", but it is not caused by the food being rancid. Perfectly fresh food can carry salmonella, and there is no warning smell or taste. Flies can carry salmonella on their feet. Always cover food so that flies cannot land on it. Salmonella germs go through phases of increased virulence, but it is safer to practice hygiene as if they are always virulent. Outbreaks of salmonella poisoning seldom occur in modern, developed cities, but there are sometimes a few cases when the germ becomes virulent, because some people do not practice hygiene.

Franklin D. Roosevelt suffered from typhoid for five weeks when he was thirty years old, but fortunately he did not die. An Australian politician named John Gellibrand survived getting typhoid during the Boer War, being vaccinated against typhoid at the beginning of World War I, then getting typhoid again during that war. The fact that some people survive typhoid is no reason to take it lightly - it is a very serious disease.

The vaccine industry has established the myth that typhoid vaccine was effective among Allied troops in World War I, when in fact the vaccine was a spectacular failure.[418,419,420] When soldiers were exposed to typhoid they were not protected by vaccination. Ninety six percent of those with laboratory confirmed typhoid had been vaccinated against typhoid.[420] Modern typhoid vaccines are ineffective and dangerous.[421] The vaccine industry is hoping that genetic engineering will help them come up with a typhoid vaccine that works.

Penicillin was able to kill salmonella typhi until the germ mutated. New antibiotics can kill the germ, but have to be redeveloped as the germ mutates. The mutations tend to happen in regions, so the doctors have a general idea of which antibiotic will work in which area. Life support greatly reduces the death rate, but of course is not available in far flung poverty stricken areas. Aid and development agencies are stamping out typhoid in these areas by providing clean water supplies.

When a homoeopath is confronted with a patient with any kind of salmonella poisoning, he or she does not need to know the name of the germ that caused the problem. The homoeopath must take note of the symptoms that are showing in that particular patient, and after deciding on the right remedy, must move on to the next patient and start all over again.

TYPHUS

The symptoms of typhus are very different to the symptoms of typhoid, and the germ that causes typhus is completely different to the germ that causes typhoid. Typhus is caused by a tiny germ called rickettsia prowazekii, which is carried by lice. There are other types of rickettsia that are carried by fleas and ticks. Many cause illnesses that are similar to typhus, and some are almost as severe as typhus.

Typhus breaks out when people are crowded together and cannot get rid of lice because they lack washing facilities. Typhus has disappeared from most parts of the world because of better living conditions, but thousands of people still die every year from typhus in impoverished areas of the world. Typhus thrives on wars and other social upheavals. Typhus was rife in army camps when Napoleon Bonaparte was causing a disturbance in Europe, and it spread to civilians. Typhus killed millions of people during both world wars, and the Balkans were particularly badly affected. The greatest number of deaths was in Serbia, where many of the doctors who tried to help the victims died from the disease themselves. If those doctors had known how to use homoeopathy, they could have saved themselves as well as their patients. The apothecaries of the 19th century who suppressed homoeopathy so viciously are responsible for the deaths of all those Serbian doctors.

When twelve million people were kidnapped from Africa and shipped to America to be sold as slaves, about 10% of them died of typhus on the way over, and their bodies were thrown into the sea. In 1899 the Boers were in possession of the gold and diamonds of central southern Africa, and the British wanted it for themselves. As they could not beat the Boers militarily, they burned down their homes and herded the Boer women and children into concentration camps, where twenty thousand of them died of typhus and typhoid. In 1948 the Boers regained possession of the gold and diamonds, and they herded the Blacks into concentration camps called bantustans. Hundreds of thousands of Blacks died of typhus and typhoid. The exact figure is not known because accurate records were not kept.

Lice are not always infected with typhus. During World War I there were lots of armies and groups of refugees who were tormented by lice because they had no washing facilities, yet did not suffer from typhus. The ANZACS at Gallipoli suffered from "a prodigious plague of lice,"[422] but the lice were not infected with typhus. When the lice themselves are not infected with typhus they do not pass it on to humans. On the other hand, people cannot get typhus if there are no lice.

The first recorded instance of typhus being cured was when Dr. Samuel Hahnemann, the person who discovered homoeopathy, cured 178 people during an outbreak in 1813. The opportunity for him to do this was created by Napoleon Bonaparte. After Napoleon was forced to retreat from Russia in 1812, he gathered up a new army and marched against Prussia and Austria. He won a battle at Dresden, and then marched on to Leipzig. For three days a battle raged in and around Leipzig, and then Napoleon retreated back to France. Eighty thousand corpses were left in the city of Leipzig, and there were another eighty thousand wounded soldiers. A handful of doctors from the university did their best to tend the wounded.

To make matters worse, an epidemic of typhus broke out.[423]

Dr. Hahnemann happened to be in Leipzig at the time. He treated 180 people who had typhus, and only two died, one of whom was a very old man. He chose the appropriate remedy by observing the symptoms of each patient who had typhus, and giving them the homoeopathic similar. He needed only two remedies, because there was not a great variation in symptoms. This seemingly amazing feat of curing typhus made the fame of Dr. Hahnemann spread throughout Europe.[423] All the people who get typhus today could be cured cheaply and quickly if the drug companies would allow WHO and Médecins Sans Frontières to use homoeopathy.

RABIES

After a bite from an animal that is carrying rabies, the germ that causes rabies can live in the human body for up to two years, although once six months has gone by without any sign of rabies, the chance of the disease developing is very much reduced. The fact that an animal bites does not automatically mean that it has rabies. Rabies is a very rare disease, and always has been. A bite from an animal seldom results in rabies, but when it does, the consequences are dire, unless homoeopathic treatment is used. Rabies can enter a human without a bite. A young girl in South Africa got rabies from the saliva of a cow that splashed into her eye. The poor girl suffered terribly and then died, quite unnecessarily, as there are so many good homoeopaths in South Africa.

An old medical book says, "If the symptoms of rabies have begun to appear, all treatment is useless to save life..."[424] It is typical of pharmaceutical medicine to call a disease incurable because pharmaceutical medicine cannot cure it. There are modern and old-fashioned drugs that relieve spasms, and they can save a victim of rabies who would otherwise have died from the throat closing up. However, drugs cannot stop the virus from attacking and destroying the brain, whereas homoeopathy can. The primary homoeopathic cure for rabies is lachesis. This is made from the venom of a deadly snake that lives in the Amazon jungle. This is how John Henry Clarke describes the discovery,

> To the genius and heroism of Hering the world owes this remedy and many another of which this has been the forerunner. When Hering's first experiments were made he was botanising and zoologising on the Upper Amazon for the German Government. Except his wife, all those about him were natives, who told him so much about the dreaded

> Surukuku that he offered a good reward for a live specimen. At last one was brought in a bamboo box, and those who brought it immediately fled, and all his native servants with them. Hering stunned the snake with a blow on the head as the box opened, then, holding its head in a forked stick, he pressed its venom out of the poison bag upon sugar of milk.[425]

Hering made low potency dilutions with the poison, and while handling the poison he breathed in the fumes. He went into an altered state, which included fever, tossing, delirium, and mania. The next day his wife described his symptoms and how he had behaved, and Hering wrote down what she said. That was the first proving of lachesis.[425]

Another remedy for rabies is lyssin, which is made by homoeopathically potentising the saliva of a rabid dog. This remedy was thought of by Dr. Hering, made by Dr. Swann, and introduced in 1833,[426] fifty two years before Louis Pasteur injected Joseph Meister with rabbit spinal cords. Once potentised, the saliva loses all toxicity, unlike what happens in a crude vaccine. The manufacture of lyssin does not involve the infliction of pain on animals, and the use of it does not cause pain to humans.

"SMALLPOX WAS ERADICATED BY VACCINATION"

Vaccine Myth Number Nine: Edward Jenner discovered that by inoculating people with cowpox he could make them immune to smallpox. He took cowpox pus from the teat of a cow and scratched it into a human. This meant that it was no longer necessary to inoculate people with pus from a human smallpox pustule. After the introduction of cowpox vaccination, smallpox disappeared from England. In the 20th century the World Health Organisation vaccinated everyone, and the disease has now been eliminated from every country in the world.

I was taught at school that Edward Jenner observed that dairymaids who caught cowpox from cows never got smallpox afterwards. I was told that this observation led him to carry out scientific experiments, which proved that by inoculating people with cowpox, he could prevent them from getting smallpox. I was also taught that smallpox had been a terrible disease that had killed someone from every family, until Edward Jenner saved us by discovering how to prevent it. For three decades that misinformation sat in my head as part of my general knowledge. Then I was stunned to learn that the only part that was true was that smallpox had been a deadly disease in Jenner's time.

All infectious diseases come and go on a natural cycle, which human beings can neither predict nor alter. Smallpox entered Europe from the Middle East in the 6th century AD, and while it became more common in the 11th century, it remained a mild disease until the 17th century. Smallpox suddenly became a virulent disease in the 17th century.[427] The reason why smallpox became so virulent in the 17th century is not known. For that matter, the reason why any disease becomes virulent for a time, and then fades away, is unknown. Between the time that smallpox entered Europe, and the time that it became the most feared disease in Europe, a number of other diseases came and went, like bubonic plague, sweating sickness, and leprosy.

Sweating sickness was the greatest cause of death in England at one time, and yet it has completely disappeared without any action being taken against it by human beings. Its disappearance was so absolute that the germs that caused the disease were no longer available to be studied when microscopes were invented. Leprosy and bubonic plague are still present on the planet, but they have become quite rare. They waned in Europe without any help from human beings.

The history of smallpox indicates that, like other diseases, smallpox came and went of its own accord, and struck various countries at different times, with different levels of severity. The introduction of hygiene to some parts of the world has had absolutely nothing to do with the disappearance of smallpox. It is not possible to know whether the vaccine made smallpox wane faster than it would have waned without vaccination, because scientific studies were never done to see whether or not the vaccine worked. Edward Jenner's research was ridiculously unscientific, and once the vaccinators had succeeded in getting the medical establishment to accept the vaccine, there was no need to do scientific experiments to justify it. All that was needed was politicians who were prepared to pass laws making vaccination compulsory.

In the European countries that made vaccination compulsory, smallpox became more virulent and more widespread, and this led some observers to wrongly believe that vaccination was causing the increase in virulence. The vaccine did not increase the virulence of the disease.

Smallpox does not create immunity to itself,[428,429,430] so the idea that scratching the pus from a completely different disease into the flesh of a person will make that person immune to smallpox is just absurd.

From the start the vaccine industry said that it was going to eradicate smallpox, even though it was blatantly obvious that the vaccine did not work. In 1877 an anti-vaxxer wrote,

> … if it were possible to 'stamp out' smallpox by vaccination, that desirable result would long ago have been accomplished. The doctors have had it all their own way for seventy-six years.[431]

After 180 years they eventually "succeeded", coincidentally with the natural demise of smallpox. Vaccination did not put an end to smallpox, and it caused devastating illness for millions of people.

With modern vaccines they use a hypodermic syringe to neatly inject all the poisons deep into the flesh, but smallpox vaccination was not so tidy. They did it by scratching lacerations into the skin, and then pushing pus into the wound that they had made. When this resulted in a flare-up, it was said that the vaccination had "taken". If there was no flare-up, it was said that the vaccination "had not taken", and needed to be done again.

Sometimes the flare-up involved the whole limb, causing a great deal of pain and suffering. Sometimes it involved the whole body, and the person died. Sometimes the vaccination caused cancer at the site of vaccination,[432,433,434,435] and in other cases it caused systemic cancer. The start of the vaccination era was the start of the cancer era. Encephalitis and urticaria were common adverse effects of vaccination. Some people were permanently disabled, while others were hampered by poor health for the rest of their lives, unless they consulted with a homoeopath who knew how to treat vaccine damage.

Orthodox medicine treated the effects of vaccination with mercury. In those days orthodox medicine treated just about everything with mercury. Mercury was the paracetamol/tylenol of the 18th century. Before vaccination with cowpox was introduced, variolation had been practiced. Variolation was different to vaccination in that some pus was taken from a human smallpox pustule instead of from a cow, and the pus was scratched into the skin of anyone who was willing to undergo the procedure. Mercury had been used to treat the harmful effects of variolation. In 1768 the Empress of Russia swallowed mercury in an attempt to counteract the effects of variolation.[436]

The medical establishment dismissed discussion of adverse effects with the claim that severe reactions were just "one in a million". However, shortly before smallpox vaccination ceased, some countries attempted to find out the true incidence of adverse effects. The American authorities conducted a survey of adverse effects in 1968.[434] The method they used meant that they missed a lot, and they also did some pruning to make the results look better. Despite this they were left with the figure that more than one person per thousand suffered a severe reaction to his or her first smallpox vaccination. Instead of "one in a million", they found it was over a thousand in a million.

Reports of serious reactions were collected in Bavaria between 1956 and 1965.[437] The method of gathering reports failed to detect all the cases,[437] but it was a sincere attempt to assess the adverse effects. The finding was that 1 out of every 8000 children died from vaccination, and that the younger a child is when vaccinated, the higher is the risk of death.[437]

The mythical history of smallpox vaccination is lovingly nurtured by the modern vaccine industry. Children's books are a major source of brainwashing. The myths are continually repeated in the media, so that people incorporate the false history into their world view. It does not stop.

In August 2002 the British Medical Journal (BMJ) published an article on the "history" of the anti-vaccination movement.[438] The article portrays non-believers as silly people who need to be treated gently, and it portrays smallpox vaccination as safe and effective. A favourite myth of the vaccine defenders is that people objected to compulsory smallpox vaccination for intellectual reasons concerning personal liberty, rather than for health reasons. The BMJ article reinforces that idea. It also gets its facts about Edward Jenner wrong. The article states,

> Widespread vaccination began in the early 1800s following Edward Jenner's presentation of an article to the Royal Society of London in 1796 detailing his success in preventing smallpox in 13 people by inoculation with live infectious material from the pustules or scabs of people infected with cowpox. The process induced cowpox, a mild viral disease that conferred immunity to smallpox.[438]

Well, it is true that Jenner presented an article to the Royal Society in 1796, but the Royal Society was very wise and refused to publish it.[439] Two years later Jenner had a slightly different version of his article published by a vanity publisher.[440] The writers of the British Medical Journal article are not correct in saying that Jenner presented 13 cases which detailed his success in preventing smallpox. Jenner presented 23 cases, and only one case comes anywhere near to inoculating someone with cowpox to try to prevent smallpox. Most of the cases he presented were descriptions of people who had had cowpox naturally at some time in the past, and then did not catch smallpox when exposed to people with smallpox, or did not get full-blown smallpox when inoculated with pus from a person with smallpox. He presumably presented these cases because he believed that they demonstrated that the subjects were made immune by having had cowpox.

Of course they demonstrated nothing of the kind. Lots of people can be exposed to smallpox without getting it. Without a control group of people who have not previously had cowpox being included in the investigation, it is not possible to know whether or not the cowpox made any difference to the subjects' chances of catching smallpox.

Some of Jenner's cases were people who had previously had smallpox, and then did not catch cowpox when exposed, or else they only got a mild dose of cowpox. He does not explain what this is supposed to prove, but presumably it is supposed to indicate that smallpox can create immunity to cowpox. The fact that some people who had had smallpox still got cowpox does not seem to bother him. One of the cases had had natural cowpox three times, with no decrease in severity. Jenner stated that cowpox could not prevent itself, but it could prevent smallpox. In the real world smallpox did not prevent itself either.[428,429,430] A Swiss doctor showed mathematically that a person who had had smallpox once was 63% more likely to get it again in the next epidemic, than a person who had never had it.[429]

Three of Jenner's cases had had natural horsepox, not cowpox. Two of these were challenged by having pus from a smallpox pustule scratched into their skin, and they did not get very sick from it. One of the two was later exposed to smallpox and did not catch it. The third case was exposed to smallpox 20 years after having horsepox, and did get smallpox. From this Edward Jenner deduces that horsepox has to be cultivated on the nipple of a cow before it can create immunity to smallpox in a human being. That is not a logical deduction.

In all, 16 of the 23 cases were not inoculated with anything, and 6 of the cases were not challenged with anything. Some of the "cases" involved a group of people, and it is difficult to know which individual out of the group Jenner intended to be the one that proves his point.

Case number 17 was an eight-year-old boy named James Phipps. Jenner inoculated him with "matter" that was taken from the hand of a dairymaid with cowpox. James became quite sick, but he recovered. Six weeks later Jenner inoculated him with smallpox pus, and he did not react. Children's story books tell us that Jenner proved that his vaccine worked by experimenting on a boy named James Phipps. They do not mention that James was not exposed to real smallpox. The vaccine industry has latched onto this case as "proof" that vaccination works. One case, in which the patient was not exposed to wild smallpox, with no control cases, is the backbone of the propaganda machine that makes people grow up believing in vaccination.

Case number 18 was a five-year-old boy named John Baker, whom Jenner inoculated with pus from the hand of a man who had caught horsepox from a horse. Jenner reports that the boy had a reaction to the inoculation, then got better, and then he came down with a "contagious fever … soon after this experiment was made."[441] As Jenner believed that horsepox could not prevent smallpox unless it had first been grown on a cow, he wanted to see if horsepox worked when it had been grown on a human. But, says Jenner in his *Inquiry*, he could not administer the challenge dose because "the boy had been rendered unfit for inoculation."[442] The reason why the boy had become unfit for inoculation was because he had died. Jenner does not mention the fact that the boy had died in his *Inquiry*, but in other writings he mentions that this boy died after a bad reaction to the vaccination.[443,440] The name of John Baker is not mentioned in children's story books. In the long-term, the name John Baker will go down in history as the first person to be killed by Jennerian vaccination.

So out of 23 cases that were supposed to prove that inoculation with cowpox makes a person immune to the wild smallpox virus, none were inoculated with cowpox and then exposed to the wild smallpox virus, one was vaccinated with cowpox and then challenged with smallpox pus, one was vaccinated with attenuated horsepox and died before he could be challenged, and there were no controls at all.

I wrote to the authors of the article in the British Medical Journal twice and asked them which 13 of Jenner's 23 cases are the ones to which they were referring when they said that he succeeded in preventing smallpox in 13 people by inoculation with live infectious material from the pustules or scabs of people infected with cowpox. They did not reply. So I sent a referenced letter (by post) to the editor of the British Medical Journal. It said,

> Dear Editor,
>
> Wolfe and Sharp's inaccurate and patronising "history" of the anti-vaccination movement uses omission and implication to perpetuate the myths of smallpox vaccination. They mention an epidemic in Sweden which subsided after the vaccination rate was increased, but they do not mention any of the epidemics which broke out after mass vaccination. One of the epidemics that is never mentioned by vaccine promoters broke out in Italy from 1887-89 against a background vaccination rate of 98.5%. Attack rates and death rates were higher in the revaccinated than in the vaccinated, and also higher in those whose vaccinations had "taken". Wolf and Sharp mention widespread protests and riots against vaccination, including one of 100,000 people in Leicester. But they imply that people objected to compulsory vaccination because it infringed their liberty. One hundred thousand illiterate, disenfranchised people did not demonstrate in the streets of Leicester because of an intellectual concept about civil rights. They protested because vaccination maimed and killed their babies.
>
> The authors of the article state that Edward Jenner demonstrated his success at preventing smallpox in 13 people by inoculating them with cowpox. Jenner presented 23 cases in his Inquiry. I have twice asked the authors to inform me which 13 were the cases to which they were referring, but they do not reply. I contend that they have never read Jenner's Inquiry, and as

> with the rest of their article, they are just repeating popular myths which promote the concept of vaccination. If they had taken the time to read Jenner's Inquiry, they would have known that out of 23 cases which were supposed to prove that inoculation with cowpox makes a person immune to the wild smallpox virus, none were inoculated with cowpox and then exposed to the wild smallpox virus, one was vaccinated with cowpox and then challenged with smallpox pus, and there were no controls at all.
>
> Apologists for Jenner claim that his method is not important as the cowpox and vaccinia vaccines were effective. But a huge amount of data, including that presented by WHO, shows that it was not. In 1899 the president of the AMA said that doctors who do not believe in vaccination are "mad" and "misguided". Modern doctors suffer more than name-calling when they don't believe in the faith.

The British Medical Journal acknowledged receipt of my letter (by post), but, as expected, they did not publish it. They have allowed a minority group to be disparaged on their pages, and have given the group no right of reply. It is typical of the behaviour of most media outlets in regards to vaccination. In the "debate" about vaccination, the playing field is so unlevel, that the debate cannot proceed.

During the 1887-89 smallpox epidemic in Italy over forty seven thousand people died of smallpox.[278] At that time Italy had a 98.5% vaccination rate. A 95% vaccination rate is supposed to provide "herd immunity", and therefore is supposed to prevent smallpox in the unvaccinated as well as in the vaccinated. The Italian epidemic is one of many that showed that neither the vaccinated nor the unvaccinated were protected.

On the 8th May 1980 the World Health Organisation declared that they had eliminated smallpox from the planet. They published a 1400 page book about how they had done it.[445] This book gives details about the coming and going of smallpox epidemics in some European countries, but it does not mention Italy at all. I believe that this is a deliberate omission. Despite many omissions of this nature, a careful reading of this book reveals that the demise of smallpox was coincidental to the world-wide vaccination campaign. In South America the World Health Organisation missed a whole country because of a clerical error, but they still claim that they "eliminated" smallpox in that country.

At first it was claimed that one vaccination would give life-long immunity. When vaccinated people got smallpox, more doses were introduced, and it was called "revaccination". There were many epidemics which showed that revaccination did not work. The Italian epidemic mentioned above is one of them.

In his first article Jenner says,

> what renders the Cow-pox virus so extremely singular, is, that the person who has been thus affected is for ever after secure from the infection of the Small Pox.[446]

But 10 years later, when it was obvious that vaccination did not prevent smallpox, he did a complete about-face, and claimed that revaccination was necessary. He published an article in support of revaccination, in which he described cases of people who had smallpox more than once as part of his argument.[430] The authors of the World Health Organisation's 1400 page book say that Jenner never abandoned the stance that one vaccination is sufficient to create life-long immunity.[447] As with many things, they are wrong.

During the 1887-89 epidemic in Italy, the incidence of deaths from smallpox in people under the age of 20 was exactly the same in males as in females. Men were revaccinated at the age of 20 for military purposes, while women were not. Yet in people older than 20, the death rate from smallpox was much higher in men than in women.[278] In the town of Vittoria in Sicily, there was official proof that all the people had been vaccinated during their six monthly vaccination campaigns. When the epidemic of 1887-89 broke out, the number of deaths from smallpox was 2,100.[278] As the total population of the village was only 2,600, this meant that less than 20% of the population was left alive. It is no wonder that this example, and examples from other villages in Sicily, Sardinia, and Calabria, are not mentioned by anyone trying to promote the myths of vaccination. The spectacular failure of vaccination in intensively vaccinated areas like Japan and the Philippines is also not a popular topic with vaccine promoters.

When revaccination was introduced, the length of time that immunity created by vaccination was supposed to last was arbitrarily set at seven years. It then continually decreased until two years became the official length of immunity. When people caught smallpox soon after vaccination, the reason was said to be because the vaccination "had not taken". So here we have a situation where the vaccinators win no matter what happens. If the vaccinated person does not catch smallpox, then they say that he or she was protected by vaccination. If the person catches smallpox more than two years after vaccination, they say it is because he or she was remiss about being revaccinated. If the person catches smallpox within two years of vaccination, they say it is because the vaccination "did not take".

The World Health Organisation claims that revaccination was what conquered smallpox. On page 273 of their book there is a table that compares the number of smallpox deaths in Germany and Austria from 1866 to 1897. Revaccination was made compulsory in Germany in 1874. In the text they say,

> The results, when compared with the prevailing situation in Austria, in which general conditions were similar but re-vaccination had not been introduced, were dramatic (Table 6.4) and hardly require comment.[448]

But a look at Table 6.4 shows that the results very much require comment. The figures show that there was the same drop in Austria between 1874 and 1875 as there was in Germany. And between 1873 and 1874 the drop in Austria was more than double the drop in Germany. And they show that smallpox continued to rise and fall in Germany with the same disregard for revaccination as it had shown for vaccination. And they show that there was an overall decline in Austria as well as in Germany, despite the fact that Austria was doing the "wrong thing" by not revaccinating. Their own "proof" shows that they are talking nonsense.

If a terrorist were to release smallpox from a laboratory, a few people would get smallpox, but the virus would not spread into the community because it lacks the natural virulence that it had 200 years ago. The vaccine industry would vaccinate as many people as they could, and they would claim that their actions were the reason why it did not spread.

"LOUIS PASTEUR DEFEATED RABIES"

Vaccine Myth Number Ten: Louis Pasteur discovered germs, which are tiny creatures that pounce on people and cause disease. He saved the French wine industry and silk industry from ruin, and made milk safe to drink by inventing pasteurisation. He conducted public experiments with sheep, which showed that when they had been vaccinated, they were safe from anthrax. He invented a vaccine that cured and prevented rabies, thereby saving the world from mad dogs.

Louis Pasteur was a pioneer of scientific fraud. It is significant that he is the darling of the vaccine industry. The true story of Louis Pasteur's life is far more interesting than the one they teach in schools. Popular mythology holds that Pasteur was the first person to think of the germ theory, but the theory was already written down nearly 300 years before Pasteur was born. In 1546 someone called Fracastoro published a treatise on contagious disease in which he said that these diseases are caused by particles that are too small to be seen. He said that the particles move from person to person by contact, or they travel on items that an infected person has touched, or they travel through the air. He also said that the particles can reproduce themselves within the human body.[449,450] Germs were first seen through a microscope by Antonius van Leenwenhoek in 1675.[451] He called them "little animals", but he did not associate them with disease. The theory that germs cause disease was causing heated debate long before Pasteur came on the scene, and there are still people today who deny that infectious diseases are caused by germs.

The extent of Louis Pasteur's fraud is quite amazing. He plagiarised the research of other scientists, and he made pronouncements that he had experimentally proven certain "facts" when he had not done the experiments. He deliberately lied about what he had done in his experiments with both the anthrax vaccine for sheep and the rabies vaccine for humans. He put far more effort into cultivating favour with the aristocracy than he put into cultivating things in his laboratory, and his greatest affectation was that of pretending to be a humble person. He made himself into a celebrity during his life time, and the cult of hero worship that was built up during his life time still exists after more than a century. None of the adulation is justified. The products he invented have harmed millions of people, and the commercial success of his endeavours has hindered scientific inquiry into how to make people healthy.

Louis Pasteur "laid the foundations of his own legend,"[452] both through his behaviour and through his writing.[453] The myths about him are perpetuated in books, cartoons, a Hollywood movie, websites, school curricula, and by journalists who think they are referring to historical fact when they mention Louis Pasteur in the media. For almost a century nearly every child in French and English speaking countries was taught that Louis Pasteur saved the world from germs. Nowadays fewer children are exposed to the myth, because school curricula are crowded with other topics.

Right from the start there were vociferous critics of Louis Pasteur. Some of them published articles or pamphlets saying that his work was unscientific and that his vaccines were killing people and animals, while not preventing disease. In 1923 Ethel Douglas Hume published a lengthy book in which she showed that Pasteur was dishonest, and that his vaccines were harmful and ineffective.[454] In 1937 and 1938 Pasteur's nephew, Adrien Loir, published some essays about his famous uncle that exposed more of the deception.[455]

Before he died, Louis Pasteur instructed his family never to allow anyone access to his notebooks,[456,457] but his grandson donated them to a library in 1964,[457,458] and in 1971 some historians were permitted to have access to them.[456] Gerald Geison of Princeton University studied them, and at the 1993 meeting of the American Association for the Advancement of Science, he spoke about the dishonesty that he had unearthed.[456,457] Later he published a book detailing what he had discovered.[455]

One of Pasteur's co-workers was a scientist named Antoine Béchamp. Béchamp held some strange views, but he did discover that fermentation is caused by yeast, and that the disease that was killing French silkworms was caused by little parasites. Béchamp and Pasteur both published a lot of articles, and Ethel Douglas Hume took on the task of reading these articles. She documented the sequence in which Béchamp made his discoveries, and Louis Pasteur first denounced them, and then stole them.[454]

Pasteur believed in spontaneous generation.[459] This is the theory that small things appear out of nothing, spontaneously. Pasteur was in line with the thinking of the times. For instance, it was believed that maggots appeared spontaneously out of rotting meat. In Pasteur's day it had already been scientifically proven by an Italian scientist that maggots cannot appear in meat unless flies first land on the meat and lay eggs, but this finding had not yet been accepted by the scientific establishment. One of Pasteur's experiments aimed to "prove" the popular theory of spontaneous generation. He lied that he had managed to make yeast appear by spontaneous generation in a medium formed only of sugar, a salt of ammonia, and of unspecified mineral elements, when he had actually added yeast to the mixture.[460]

The misconception that Pasteur saved the French silk industry from ruin has been entrenched in medical mythology. This is not only due to Louis Pasteur's personality, but also because bureaucracies suffer from paralysis when a wrong idea needs to be put right. Silkworms had started dying en masse in 1850. The silk farmers were desperate because production dropped from 30 million kilograms per year to 8 million kilograms per year. After Pasteur had allegedly "saved" the industry, silk production dropped to 2 million kilograms per year.[461]

Béchamp investigated silkworm disease and found that a parasite that came from the air was making the silkworms sick. He experimented, and found that the parasite could be killed by the vapour of creosote, without harming the silkworms. However, Louis Pasteur had been appointed by the Minister of Health to solve the problem, so the bureaucrats ignored Béchamp.

> No one who understands anything of departmental red tape will wonder that, instead of at once accepting Béchamp's verdict, agricultural societies waited to hear the pronouncement of the official representative. Plenty of patience had to be exercised.[462]

Louis Pasteur flitted around, ingratiating himself with the Empress Eugenie and Napoleon III, and occasionally making pronouncements about silkworms. He also found time to launch attacks against Béchamp for saying that the disease was caused by a parasite.

On June 18, 1866, Béchamp sent a report to the Academy of Science on how the silkworms could be saved by making them hatch in the presence of creosote, so that the fumes of the creosote would kill the parasites.[463] His advice was ignored, and the silk industry suffered more and more from the ravages of the disease. Some entrepreneurs took advantage of Pasteur's claim that healthy eggs from healthy moths would be disease free, and sold eggs at high prices. The farmers who bought these eggs saw the caterpillars sicken and die because of the parasite. After a year of waiting for some words of wisdom from the celebrity Pasteur, the scientific world was treated to,

> I am very much inclined to believe that there is not actual disease of silk-worms. I cannot better make clear my opinion of silk-worm disease than by comparing it to the effects of pulmonary phthisis. My observations of this year have fortified me in the opinion that these little organisms are neither animalcules nor cryptogamic plants. It appears to me that it is chiefly the cellular tissue of all the organs that is transformed into corpuscles or produces them.[464]

When Pasteur finally realised that Béchamp was right about silkworm disease, he had no qualms about publicly claiming that he himself had discovered what Béchamp had discovered. It was, however, too late for the silk industry. The Academy of Science and some government officials knew the truth about what had happened, but the mythological version became regarded as historical fact.

Popular mythology says, "Pasteur proved the value of vaccination by vaccinating sheep against a disease called anthrax."[465] Fifty sheep were used in this experiment, and by the time the public came to see the results, half the sheep lay dead or were dying. The vaccine appeared to be 100% effective, yet it did not produce those results for farmers who bought it to protect their stocks from anthrax. By reading Pasteur's personal notebooks, Gerald Geison discovered that Pasteur had lied to the officials and the public about the way that the vaccine he had used had been manufactured.[456,457,466] Geison suggests that this lie was told for the purposes of personal advancement.[466] The track record of the vaccine suggests that the problem went deeper than the method of manufacture.

In March 1882, a commission that had been established by the Italian authorities to investigate whether or not Pasteur's anthrax vaccine worked, tested Pasteur's vaccine at Turin University. They injected half of a group of sheep with it, and later challenged all the sheep with an injection of blood from a sheep that had died of anthrax the day before. Every single one of the vaccinated and unvaccinated sheep died.[467] Angry letters passed backwards and forwards between Pasteur and the professors at Turin. On the 10th June, 1883, the professors of Turin published a document detailing the way Pasteur had contradicted himself in his correspondence with them. The document highlighted Pasteur's ignorance about anthrax and septicaemia, and it was published in French two months later. But the adoring public adored on.

A factory for manufacturing vaccines had been opened at Odessa in Russia. They trialled Pasteur's anthrax vaccine on a farm near Kachowka by vaccinating 4564 sheep, and 81% of the sheep died from the vaccine.[468] Pasteur ended up paying financial compensation to some of the farmers whose stock had been killed by the vaccine,[469] which is more than can be said for the British, American, and Australian governments. They will not pay compensation to the families of the soldiers who have been killed by anthrax vaccine, nor to the soldiers whose lives have been ruined by the health problems caused by the vaccine. Because of the nature of the anthrax germ, anthrax vaccines made by any method will always be the most deadly of vaccines. These vaccines kill and cause terrible infirmity in the fittest and healthiest of our young men. It is not likely that an anthrax vaccine that is able to protect a person in the case of a biological warfare attack will ever be developed.[470]

A commission set up in Hungary recommended that Pasteur's anthrax vaccine should be prohibited,[469] and in 1881 the Hungarian government said,

> The worst diseases, pneumonia, catarrhal fever, etc., have exclusively struck down the animals subjected to injection. It follows from this that the Pasteur inoculation tends to accelerate the action of certain latent diseases and to hasten the mortal issue of other grave affections.[471]

This is the same phenomenon as that which Sir Graham Wilson called "provocation disease" eighty five years later, in his book *The Hazards of Immunization*.[379] The sickness is not a direct reaction to the vaccine, but a consequence of the immune system having been compromised by the vaccine. The phenomenon has been well documented with regards to polio,[380,384,385] but it is not generally acknowledged by the medical establishment. The phenomenon is seldom mentioned in the medical literature. One exception is in a study of 3801 Swedish children who had been injected with DPT vaccine.[472] Three of the children died of a bacterial infection in the weeks following vaccination, and the study authors believed that their deaths were caused by provocation. Without doing really big studies, it is not possible to know how often vaccination causes conditions that superficially appear to be unrelated.

The story of Joseph Meister still features on many a school curriculum. This boy was bitten by a rabid dog, and his mother brought him to Pasteur because she had heard that he had a treatment for rabies. Joseph was injected each day for 11 days with stuff made in Pasteur's laboratory, and he did not develop rabies. Schoolchildren are taught that this proved that the vaccine Pasteur had invented for rabies was effective, and that since then, thousands of people have been saved from rabies by the vaccine.

Schoolchildren are not taught that for 52 years homoeopaths all over the world had already been successfully curing cases of rabies in humans.[426] Dying of rabies is a prolonged and painful experience. The victim suffers severe pain and terrible mental anguish. The pharmaceutical industry prevents people from having access to homoeopathic cures, simply because it would damage their profits.

Pasteur claimed that before he injected the vaccine into Joseph Meister, he had already tested it on a large number of dogs that had suffered bites from rabid animals. But Gerald Geison found in the notebooks that he had experimented on only a few dogs, and not in the same way as with Joseph Meister.[456,473] Pasteur had given the vaccine to 26 dogs that had been bitten by rabid animals, and 10 of them had died.[474] There were also 7 dogs which Pasteur had used as controls. They had been given no treatment after being bitten by a rabid animal, and 4 of them never developed rabies.[475] This means that out of the dogs that were vaccinated, 62% survived, while out of the ones that had no treatment, 57% survived.[476] It was a good indication of what the vaccine would do in the real world. Geison also found that some of the dogs had not been injected with the same potion as that which had been injected into Joseph Meister.[477] Some had been injected with rabbit brain, some with guinea pig brain, and the rest with rabbit spinal cords. The latter is what had been injected into Joseph Meister. When he had used rabbit spinal cords on the dogs, he had injected dried out ones first, and then moved on to fresher cords. But with Joseph he had used the fresh cords first, and then moved on to drier ones. These gruesome details are not important in the big picture, because rabies vaccine is a disgusting, harmful substance no matter how it is made. However, the details are relevant in that Louis Pasteur lied about what he had done. The vaccine industry was founded on lies, and the lies have just kept on coming.

Three months later Pasteur treated a shepherd boy who had been bitten by a rabid dog, and this boy also survived. The vaccine was greeted with enthusiastic approval by most of the medical establishment, and by most of the public. No studies were ever done to see whether it worked, nor what adverse effects it caused.

The vaccine to be injected into people who had not yet been bitten was made in different ways at different times. At first it was made by taking bits of brain from a rabid dog and "inoculating it directly onto the surface of the brain of a healthy dog through a hole drilled into its skull."[478] Later it was made by placing brain from a dog into a monkey, and through a series of monkeys.[479] Then later it was made by inoculating the spinal marrow of a rabid dog onto the brain of a rabbit through a hole bored in its skull, and then from rabbit to rabbit through holes in their skulls.[480] With the latter method, he took the spinal cord of each rabbit that had died, cut it into strips several centimetres long, suspended it in a flask for about two weeks, made a broth with it, and then injected it into dogs.[481] According to Ethel Douglas Hume, the broth contained cow matter as well.[482] The World Health Organisation defined Pasteur's vaccine as,

> …a suspension of infected tissue from the central nervous system of an animal.[483]

Lionel Dole's comment is,

> The manner in which Pasteur made rabbits "rabid" by boring holes in their skulls and inserting filth into their brains was not science but simply brutal quackery.[484]

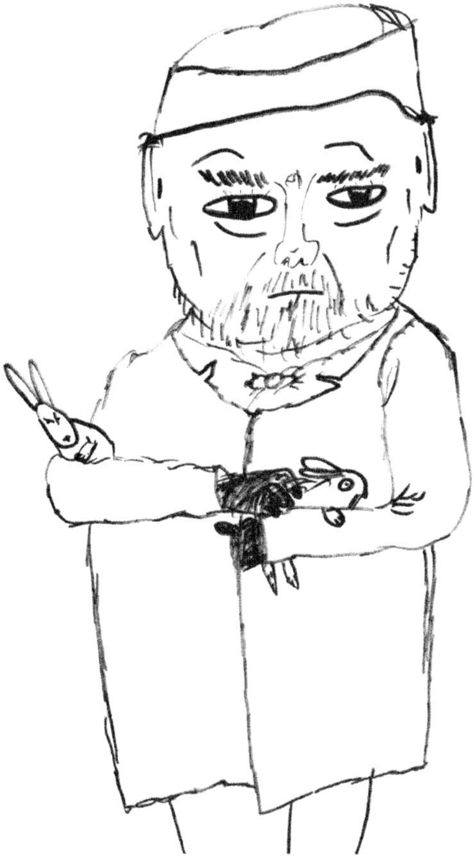

Louis Pasteur loved rabbits so much that he bored holes in their skulls and inserted rabid dogs' brains onto their brains.

One of Pasteur's co-workers thought that injecting the saliva of humans who were healthy, and the saliva of humans who had died of rabies, into rabbits, was a worthwhile pastime. He found that the two types of saliva were equally harmful to the rabbits.[485]

There are numerous written records of the failure of the rabies vaccine, and of it causing death. In 1890 a doctor published a list of people who had died after being vaccinated with Pasteur's rabies vaccine, while the dogs that had bitten them remained healthy.[285] The National Anti-Vivisection Society collected the names of 1,220 people who died from the vaccine between 1885 and 1901.[486] Just like all the people whom the vaccine industry has killed, these people do not count in the eyes of "science". They are dismissed as "anecdotal evidence". Louis Pasteur's cousin-by-marriage, Dr. Michel Peter, spoke out about deaths that were happening after the treatment, and questioned the secretiveness of Pasteur's research. He was hissed and booed when he tried to speak at the Academy of Medicine.[487]

Manufacturing vaccines became a booming commercial enterprise, with Pasteur Institutes opening up in many countries. At the International Rabies Conference held in Paris in 1927, the Director of the Pasteur Institute in Morocco reported that certain of the other Pasteur Institutes were concealing cases of rabies vaccine failure.[322]

The vaccine not only failed to prevent rabies in many people, it also caused rabies in recipients. A postman named Pierre Rascol, and another man, were attacked by a dog. The postman's clothing was sufficient to protect him from having his skin penetrated, but the other man was badly bitten. The postal authorities required Rascol to undergo a course of rabies injections, but the other man was not treated. A month after the course of injections was started, Rascol developed symptoms of rabies, and two days later he died. The other man remained well.[285]

Eleanor McBean tells the tragic and ironic story of what happened to a young English girl in staid Victorian times. She went to the "baths" with her friends, and came home with a bite. Her parents rushed her off for Pasteur treatments, and she then got ill and died. On the way home from her funeral, her friends told her parents that she had not been bitten by a dog, but by her boyfriend.[488]

In October 1920 King Alexander of Greece was washing his car when his dog and his gardener's two monkeys got into a fight. While trying to stop the fight he was bitten on the leg by one of the monkeys. It is unlikely that the monkey was infected with rabies, but the wound was infected with something, and it did not heal properly. Penicillin might have been able to save him, but it had not yet been discovered. As part of the treatment the king was given a course of rabies vaccinations. He suffered fits of delirium as his health worsened,[320] and he died four weeks after the bite. We do not know if he died from the monkey bite or from the injections, but can you imagine the fanfare there would have been if he had survived? Schoolchildren all over the world would enthusiastically be taught that Louis Pasteur saved the life of the King of Greece.

By 1982 it was admitted that Louis Pasteur's vaccine does not work. A host of new rabies vaccines are available instead. They are made with tissue from aborted babies,[489,490,491,492] goats' brains,[493] hamsters' kidneys,[494] fertilised eggs,[495] and dogs' kidneys.[496]

"VACCINES ARE SCIENTIFICALLY TESTED FOR SAFETY AND EFFECTIVENESS"

Vaccine Myth Number Eleven: Before a vaccine is licensed for use, it is tested for safety and effectiveness. The vaccine is first tested on animals, and if it proves to be safe and effective, it is then tested on a small group of humans, then on a larger group of humans. If the vaccine does not prevent the disease it is supposed to prevent, it is discarded. The exact dosage needed to produce immunity is worked out according to the weight of the person. If the vaccine causes bad side effects during the trials, it is not released for mass immunisation. If, despite all these precautions, the vaccine causes bad side effects once it is used on the general population, it is immediately recalled.

Since its historical beginnings, the testing of vaccines has been left to the people who manufacture and sell the vaccine, when it should be done by people who are financially independent of the manufacturer. The way that the vaccine industry pretends to research vaccines has become more sophisticated since the days of Jenner and Pasteur, but it has not become more scientific. Vaccines that are licensed cause a high incidence of serious adverse effects, and they often fail to prevent the target disease when the germ becomes virulent in the environment. This shows that they are not being properly tested before they are released.

Most vaccine manufacturers know that a vaccine will not be a commercial success if the serious adverse effects occur too frequently for them to be denied by the usual level of cover-up, so not every vaccine that has been invented has ended up being released for general use. Herpes vaccine was tested on orphans in Melbourne in the 1940s, and it was found to be far too harmful to release for mass vaccination. The "orphans" were mostly children who had been forcibly taken away from poor parents and put into institutions. Scarlet fever was another vaccine that was tested in Melbourne and never released. The British Ministry of Health has unpublished records of scarlet fever vaccine causing collapse and death from circulatory failure.[497]

There have also been vaccines that were introduced for mass vaccination and then withdrawn. Robert Koch invented a product called tuberculin that was intended to be used as a vaccine as well as to be used as a treatment for TB.[498] I have noticed that nowadays pharmaphiles are not keen on mentioning that it was once intended to be a vaccine; they only mention that it was useless and deadly as a treatment for TB. It was also deadly as a vaccine. When tuberculin is homoeopathically potentised it cures TB.

Quadrigen was another extremely toxic vaccine that was introduced for mass vaccination, but ended up being withdrawn because it was too dangerous for them to be able to conceal the danger. It was made of DPT vaccine (diphtheria, whooping cough, tetanus vaccine) combined with polio vaccine, and it was used on three million babies in the USA from 1959 to 1968.[499] DPT vaccine on its own was very toxic and killed and maimed numerous babies, but when it was combined with polio vaccine it became even more dangerous. Before Quadrigen was licensed it had been trialled on a small number of impoverished babies, and on a small number of institutionalised babies. One baby had died during the trialling, and a professor of paediatrics had confirmed that the death was caused by the vaccine.[500] Severe reactions were extremely common during the trialling, but that did not stop the manufacturer from announcing on the package insert that reactions were mild and no greater than with DPT.[501] DPT vaccine combined with polio vaccine was also used in Australia between 1960 and 1963. It had been trialled on 56 "orphans", one of whom died of meningitis soon after.[502]

DPT vaccine has now been withdrawn from affluent countries and replaced with the far less toxic DTaP vaccine, but DPT vaccine has not been withdrawn from non-affluent countries. During the decades that DPT vaccine was in use in affluent countries, the vaccine industry produced many white-wash "studies" aimed at denying that DPT caused a high rate of severe reactions. It also tried to damage the careers of the doctors who warned that the vaccine was dangerous and ineffective. The Emeritus Professor of Public Health at Glasgow University, Professor Gordon Stewart MD, BSc, FRCP, FRCPath., FFPHM, FRSS, DTM&H spent much of his career trying to persuade the British government to stop using DPT vaccine. He provided the relevant authorities with masses of evidence that the vaccine was dangerous and was not the reason for the decline in the natural virulence of whooping cough, but the British authorities were not going to admit that they had made a terrible mistake by introducing the vaccine. The German and Swedish governments were not so obstinate.

They listened to their doctors and stopped using DPT vaccine. Whooping cough, which had begun to decline before the introduction of the vaccine, continued to decline in Germany and Sweden after the vaccine was withdrawn.

DPT vaccine was invented in the 1920s, and was used in various countries before mass vaccination began. During this time a number of doctors reported that the vaccine caused convulsions, collapse, and death.[503] Mass vaccination with DPT was started in the US without any trials having been done. In Britain the Medical Research Council ran three clinical trials from 1946 to 1957 to see if the vaccine was effective at reducing the incidence of whooping cough,[504] but the trials were not designed to assess adverse effects. The babies in the trials were aged 6 to 18 months.[504] Children who had contraindications to vaccination were excluded from the British trials, which made the number of serious reactions in the trials lower than it is in real life. Yet the rate of convulsions in the trials was more than one per thousand.[504] The unsolicited reports from doctors about the vaccine causing death were just ignored. From the point of view of effectiveness, it was found that during the three years following vaccination, vaccinated children had a lower rate of whooping cough than unvaccinated children.[504]

Mass vaccination of babies in the USA was already underway before the results of the British trials came out. Even though the British trials were not designed to test for safety, the US medical authorities used the unfinished British trials as "proof" that the vaccine is safe for babies aged only six weeks.[505] They did not tell the American public that the babies in the British trials were aged 6 to 18 months, and that no trials had been done on 6-week-old babies. There was no suggestion that the dosage should be decreased in the USA, even though the recipients had a much smaller body weight.[506] Unlike six-month-old babies, six-week-old babies manufacture only a few antibodies, so a second dose of vaccine was introduced in the USA to compensate for the lack of antibodies created at that early age. Later on a third dose was introduced. Some countries now use four doses, and some use five.

A fraudulent study that was published in 1981[507] has frequently been used to claim that DPT vaccine is safe. In 1986 Barbara Loe Fisher and Harris Coulter exposed the fact that the study had been deviously designed to prevent most of the symptoms that occurred after vaccination from being recorded, and that then on top of that, the published version was a fraudulent misrepresentation of the raw data that had been collected.[508]

The batches of DPT vaccine being used in non-affluent countries are still tested for safety and effectiveness by means of the absurdly unscientific "mouse toxicity test" that was introduced in 1953.[509] To test each batch for effectiveness, the mice are vaccinated, then three weeks later they have a challenge dose of the bacteria that cause whooping cough in humans injected into their brains. If more than a certain number of mice survive, that is taken to mean that the vaccine will prevent whooping cough in humans.[510] To test each batch for safety, the vaccine is injected into the abdomens of young mice, and if the mice continue to gain weight, that is taken to mean that the vaccine will not cause brain damage in a human baby.[510] The breed of mouse that is used determines whether 4% or 43% die from the same batch of vaccine.[511]

These methods of testing the vaccine obviously do not work because DPT vaccine does cause death and severe as well as mild brain damage in human babies. The researchers do not ask the mice if they have a headache after vaccination, and they do not test the mice for dyslexia when they start school. The fact that the mice continue to grow bigger does not mean that they have not suffered neurological damage. Human babies who are neurologically damaged by the vaccine continue to grow bigger. They grow to adult size, but their brain remains damaged. If the motor section of the brain is damaged, they grow bigger, but they cannot look after themselves. If the intellectual segment is damaged, their bodies keep growing, but their minds do not mature. I speak with parents of children in their 30s and 40s who have the mentality and behaviour of toddlers. The vaccine industry and government agencies that coercively promote vaccination are not interested in hearing about the problems associated with caring for adult-sized toddlers. When doing the mouse toxicity test, some laboratories are careful to use a breed of mouse that has a low susceptibility to the toxic effects of the vaccine,[512] but when doing mass vaccination of humans, the industry is not careful to exclude vulnerable children.

The new genetically engineered vaccines are batch tested by counting antigens and measuring levels of toxin.[509] This new method still does not address the issue of whether or not the substance that has been manufactured is harmful to humans. That is supposed to be gauged by post marketing surveillance.[509] As post marketing surveillance is not done, the validity of this type of batch testing cannot be assessed.

In 1974 an Irish doctor wrote,

> In addition to persistent screaming and collapse, which are presumably of central rather than peripheral origin, serious brain damage occasionally follows whooping-cough vaccination. The onset of these encephalopathies usually occurs within twenty-four hours of inoculation and half of them within six hours; about one-third of the patients die, one-third appear to recover and one-third have residual and

> often severe brain damage. I knew of 2 such cases while working in Belfast and I estimated that the rate was about 1:10 000 immunized children. There are few such reports from the rest of the United Kingdom. If the rates which I have calculated for Belfast, the Midlands and Portsmouth in the 1960s (Dick 1971) are applicable for the rest of the country, there could have been 80 such cases per year. There is, in general, a considerable underreporting of all reactions following immunization by physicians.[513]

The article from which this quote was taken is immediately followed by a sophisticated denial from a doctor who was employed by a drug company that makes vaccines. It is not unethical for a doctor to be employed by a vaccine manufacturer, but this particular doctor behaved unethically because he produced and published papers that were designed to prevent vaccine-damaged children from obtaining compensation. He also misrepresented the incidence of severe neurological effects of DPT in an official reply to the department of health in Ireland.[514]

This individual's efforts at protecting his employer against accountability for the damage done by DPT vaccine emerged after the employer was forced by a court order to send all their documentation about DPT vaccine to the mother of a child who had been severely brain damaged by DPT vaccine. The child suffered the same life ruination as all the other victims of DPT, but the way that his mother persevered in fighting the system for over 20 years was so unusual that the BBC made a documentary[515] that told the story. The child was Kenneth Best, and his mother, Margaret Best, lived on a low income in Ireland. She received no state assistance to help her cope with her vaccine-damaged child. He is incontinent as well as having no intellect. Usually, coping with a brain damaged child uses up all of a family's time and resources, but Margaret somehow also found the energy to fight the giant. The measures she took to obtain compensation were extreme, but extreme hindrance requires extreme measures. One of the things that she did was to stage a sit-in with a group of her friends at a government office in order to get hold of her son's medical records. Medical records belong to the patient, so she should have been given them as soon as she asked for them, but she had to go to this extreme action to get what was rightfully hers. After 15 years of this type of battling she won a court ruling that the drug company that made the vaccine, Wellcome, had to allow her to see their documents relating to DPT. Of course drug companies do not want the public to see their internal paperwork, and for three years they succeeded in disobeying the court order.

Eventually Wellcome shipped a roomful of files to their office in

Dublin, perhaps thinking that she would be daunted by the amount of reading required. Margaret and five friends took two weeks to photocopy every page, and then she and one friend read the photocopies over the next 18 months. Among the things they discovered is that Wellcome pays doctors to write fraudulent articles for medical journals about the safety of DPT, and that Wellcome releases batches of vaccine that have failed mouse toxicity tests. Wellcome had also paid a British doctor to try to discredit a German doctor who had provided part of the evidence about DPT vaccine that had made the German government stop vaccinating against whooping cough.[516]

After 20 years Kenneth Best was finally awarded a large amount of financial compensation for what the vaccine had done to him. In talking to parents of vaccine-damaged children, I find that the thing that worries them the most is what will happen to their child after they die. Now there will be money to pay for carers after Margaret dies. Margaret spent some of the money on electric gates so that Kenneth could not wander off and come to harm. The journalist who instigated the defamation of Dr. Andrew Wakefield, the doctor who suggested there may be a connection between MMR vaccine and autism, has used the electric gates as part of his attempt to smear Margaret Best. This journalist has also written articles that try to portray Professor Gordon Stewart as having a dull intellect. The drug companies know that public opinion is far more important than science for achieving sales of their products, and the mainstream media is their vehicle for influencing public opinion. The articles that Gordon Stewart published in medical journals about DPT vaccine, and the letters that he wrote to medical officials in an effort to stop them harming British children, stand as testament to his towering intellect. However, it is not his intellect, but his courage and his tenacity that sets him apart from all the spineless doctors. In the current climate of oppression, doctors like Gordon Stewart are not allowed to publish data in mainstream medical journals, and those who are employed by health departments are treated harshly if they speak the truth about vaccination.

At one of the lectures I gave to Public Health nurses during the nineties, the nurses started barking that a big court case had "proved conclusively" that DPT vaccine never causes brain damage. They were referring to the case of case of Loveday versus Crown, which had ended before the Kenneth Best case, and in which the judge had made the finding that the plaintiff had not provided sufficient evidence that DPT vaccine causes brain damage.[517,518] This is not the same thing as proving that the vaccine does not cause brain damage, yet the vaccine bureaucracy had presented the case around the world as if it had conclusively proven that DPT does not cause brain damage. I told these Public Health nurses about Margaret

Best's great effort and her great victory, and the corruption that she had unearthed, and I showed them photos of the family. But some of those very same Public Health nurses continued to tell parents that a big court case had "proved conclusively" that DPT vaccine never causes brain damage.

The method of trialling vaccines for safety has not undergone an improvement since the 1950s. When a new vaccine is looking for a market, studies with favourable results are published to help it along. Consumer groups are trying to make it compulsory for studies with unfavourable results to be published too.

The main aim of publishing vaccine studies is to show that the vaccine works, but the authors know that these days they have to mention adverse effects. A study of a new vaccine for pneumonia that was done in a poor part of Africa[519] is an example of the typical way in which data about adverse reactions is collected. The authors of the study say, "We undertook a randomised, placebo-controlled, double-blind trial in eastern Gambia". That sounds impressive, but a careful look at the method used to collect data about reactions reveals that it is just a sham, and the authors have no right to conclude that the vaccine causes no serious adverse effects.

There are three features of the study that render it unscientific; the vaccine and the placebo were given at the same time as six other vaccines, the substance used as the placebo was not inert, and the method for collecting data about adverse reactions was ridiculous.

Half of the 16,340 children received the new vaccine as well as six other vaccines, while the other half of the children received a placebo as well as six other vaccines. Bear in mind that the other six vaccines have also not been properly tested for safety. Most placebo-controlled studies do not reveal the ingredients in the placebo,[520] but this one gives a bit of information, while not saying exactly what the placebo is. The reader is told that it is "lyophilised powders". Lyophilised powders are made from freeze dried biological matter like blood or tissue from humans or animals, and metals, drugs, and dyes are sometimes added. Freeze drying does not make biological matter become inert.[521] No studies are carried out to ensure that placebos are inert,[522] and there are no regulations about what can be included in a placebo.[522,523] It is absurd to use a substance that is not inert as a placebo, but the vaccine industry has been getting away with doing this since placebo-controlled studies replaced non-controlled studies.

Lyophilised powders come in different colours, so different ingredients are needed to achieve a particular appearance. The authors of the article say that the vaccine and the placebo "were identical in appearance", but they do not say what ingredients were added to the placebo to make it the same colour and consistency as the vaccine. It is considered very important to make sure that the people who administer the injections and those who receive the injections do not know whether placebo or vaccine is being used, but it is not considered important to ensure that the placebo is non-toxic and inert.

The study authors defined an adverse event as death or a hospital admission that occurred within seven days after the injection. An adverse event is anything bad that happens after vaccination, but is not necessarily a reaction to vaccination. The doctor on duty at the hospital when a child was admitted had to assess whether the symptoms were related to vaccination. The doctors who were tasked with making this subjective decision did not know which children had been given the new vaccine plus six vaccines, and which had been given the placebo plus six vaccines, so they could not be influenced by bias in favour of the new vaccine. They found the same number of reactions in the group that had the new vaccine plus six vaccines as they found in the group that had the placebo plus six vaccines. The study authors claim that this means that the new vaccine caused no reactions. In reality it means nothing of the kind. Children who exhibited severe reactions might have been reacting to any of the seven vaccines, or to the placebo that was not inert. The finding that there were the same number of reactions in both groups does not in any way support the conclusion that the new vaccine did not cause any reactions.

The seven day limit meant that slow reactions that do not prompt a parent to visit a hospital during the first week were missed. Parents do not take their child to a hospital right away when there is a subtle change in behaviour, or when they fall over more than usual, or when they stop making eye contact.

The vaccine industry finds this type of study satisfactory, but the dubious method does not inspire confidence in parents who want to see studies that compare the long-term health of children who have been vaccinated with the long-term health of children who have never been vaccinated. If the vaccine industry really wanted to assess the long-term consequences of vaccination they could do comparative studies, without having to spend a fortune, and without having to withhold vaccines from the children whose parents actually want them.

THE ROLE OF GOVERNMENTS IN TESTING VACCINES

The USA is the heart of the vaccine industry, even though there are independent manufacturers in other countries. Just as stock exchanges around the world react to happenings on Wall Street, so too does the vaccine industry regard the USA as its point of reference. There are many countries that permit the use of a drug or a vaccine simply because the American Food and Drug Administration (FDA) has given it approval, but they are making a mistake in trusting the FDA. The FDA was founded in 1906 when Teddy Roosevelt was president of the USA, but back then it had very little power. In 1937 a drug that was labelled as an "elixir", even though it contained diethylene glycol, killed 73 people. This motivated Franklin D. Roosevelt, who was president of the USA at the time, to tighten up the law. In 1938 the *Federal Food, Drug and Cosmetics Act* was passed. This law is supposed to ensure that manufacturers cannot sell foods, drugs, or cosmetics that are toxic or unhygienic. The FDA is supposed to enforce the law, but they approve dangerous drugs and vaccines because they get most of their funding from the pharmaceutical industry. The way the system works is that the manufacturer of a new product collects raw data on the safety and effectiveness of their product by doing a series of studies. The manufacturer then compiles a report supposedly based on this data, and the manufacturer pays the FDA to read the report. If the people at the FDA are impressed by the report, they license the substance for sale to the public. The FDA does not look at the manufacturer's raw data to see if the report is an honest representation of the information collected. "Unlike almost every other federal agency, the FDA lacks the legal clout to subpoena a company's internal records."[524]

A further problem is that the the law regarding vaccines is different to the law regarding drugs. Manufacturers of drugs have to present evidence to the FDA that their drugs are safe, pure, and effective, but the manufacturers of vaccines do not have to supply evidence that their product is pure, nor that it is effective.[525] So the FDA is not required to take an interest in how rancid the rotten monkey kidney in the vaccine has become, nor what other viruses and bacteria are in the vaccine, nor whether the vaccine is actually capable of preventing the disease.

Most health conscious people are aware that there is corruption within the drug industry, but few realise the extent of the corruption. When drugs are trialled, researchers deliberately withhold information about harmful effects that they observe, even going to the extent of forging the signatures of human participants who have died from the substance being trialled, and of replacing animals that have died with healthy animals.[526]

The story of the insomnia drug called Halcion highlights the flaws in the system. The information presented to the FDA by the makers of Halcion was fraudulent as it omitted to mention frequent side effects like insanity and violent aggression.[527] One person within the FDA was dissatisfied with the information about the drug that was presented to the FDA, but others within the FDA suppressed her concerns.[527] After the drug was licensed and was in use by the public, some doctors spoke out about side effects that they were observing, so the drug company bribed other doctors to say that the product was safe.[527] Other dangerous drugs have similar histories.

The FDA is supposed to protect the public, but historically it has been more inclined to protect money interests, and it indulges in corruption itself. For instance, when 182 reports of death caused by Hib vaccine were reported to them between 1 November 1990 and 30 September 1992, they set about trying to discredit the reports, instead of trying to determine whether or not the vaccine is safe. The FDA does get some funding from the US government, but most of its income is derived from drug company payments for its services.

In 1979 the FDA made a conscious decision to tell the public that a cluster of infant deaths soon after DPT vaccine was not related to the vaccine, even though their data showed that it was. The vaccine manufacturer was even more devious and arranged for vaccine vials with the same lot number to be spread geographically, so that overly toxic lots would be spread out, and the deaths they caused would not be detected. On 29 August 2016 a group of CDC employees sent an open letter to the Chief of Staff of the CDC, which is a branch of the FDA, pointing out that various frauds, cover-ups, and financial conflicts of interest within the CDC prevent them from doing their job of serving the public interest. The film *Vaxxed: from Cover-Up to Catastrophe* reveals how the CDC committed fraud to hide their own evidence that MMR vaccine causes autism when administered before the age of three years. The situation will not improve until the voting public demands that clinical trials be done by people other than those aiming to market the product, and that CDC activities become transparent and accountable.

In 2000 there was a Congressional committee investigation into the fact that the individuals who make US policy on vaccination are on the payroll of drug companies that manufacture vaccines. The committee found that,

> US government officials are failing to enforce conflict of interest regulations and are allowing experts with industry ties to sit on vaccine approval panels.[528]

During the hearing a congressman whose grandchild is autistic as a result of vaccination pointed out that there are 700,000 doctors in the USA, so it should be possible to find 15 doctors who do not have financial ties with the drug companies.[529] The phenomenon of financial ties between policy makers and vaccine manufacturers is not restricted to the USA. Many of the individuals who are employed by governments to decide which drugs and which vaccines will be approved for sale in their country, and which will be funded by the taxpayer, are receiving money from drug and vaccine manufacturers. Governments and bureaucracies find it acceptable that some of the people who decide what injections are going to be forced on babies have a financial interest in promoting those injections. Most people are not aware of how the system works. Professor Gordon Stewart says that the international vaccination scene is controlled by a "closed circle" of about 100 people.[530]

While some governments simply permit the use of a drug or a vaccine in their own country once it has been approved by the American FDA, other countries establish their own panel of bureaucrats to wield the stamp of approval. These panels of bureaucrats are assigned the task of ensuring that medical substances are safe and effective, but they themselves do not have to verify the safety and effectiveness of any product. All that these panels have to do is to read a report that is handed to them by the manufacturer, and approve the product if the report makes the product look good.

At the time that the measles vaccine was put on the British schedule, the two institutions that were supposed to have ensured that it did not cause serious adverse effects were named the *Committee on the Safety of Medicines* and the *National Institute for Biological Standards and Control.* I started correspondence with them in 1989, asking them questions about how the vaccine was tested for safety. The replies I received were evasive. Their inability to provide me with the information made me realise that they had not tested the vaccine for safety in a scientific manner before putting it on the schedule.

When measles cases started happening in Britain in 2012 the government escalated their vendetta against Dr. Andrew Wakefield, and their brainless lackeys in the media did not allow him to defend himself against their false allegations. So he posted a video online, and this is what he said about the trialling of MMR vaccine;

> Such was my concern about the safety of that vaccine that I went back and reviewed every safety study, every pre-licensing study of the MMR vaccine and other measles containing vaccines before they were put into children and after. And I was appalled with the quality of that science. It really was totally below par and that has been reiterated by other authoritative sources since.

In Australia the panel that has the task of protecting the public from unsafe substances is called the Therapeutic Goods Administration (TGA), and it works out of a building in Canberra. Canberra is the seat of government in Australia. When the people who work for the TGA write a letter, they use letterhead paper that has the Australian coat of arms at the top. The emu and the kangaroo stand proudly next to the shield containing the badges of the six Australian states. This letterhead gives the impression that the TGA is a government body, yet the TGA gets absolutely no funding from the government. The TGA's entire income comes from the companies that want their products licensed. This arrangement has a profound effect on the attitude that the TGA adopts towards their clients, and towards the products for which their clients seek approval.

Their attitude towards their clients came to light when some investigative journalists produced a documentary about a drug that suppresses the symptoms of arthritis, but also causes heart attacks. The TGA licensed the drug although the manufacturer did not even pretend that they had conducted a proper comparative study on it. Then once the TGA learned that the drug causes heart attacks, they failed to warn doctors not to prescribe it. When a journalist questioned a member of the TGA about this behaviour, the bloke being interviewed made it quite clear that the TGA is accountable to the drug company and not to the consumer, and that the TGA has reason to be afraid of the drug companies.[531] With this system in place it is no wonder that the TGA approves vaccines that kill and maim babies.

Australia has a Freedom of Information Act which means that one is supposed to be able to obtain information about how vaccines are tested for safety. When DPT was due to be replaced with DTaP in Australia, an Australian vaccine manufacturer made their own brand of the new vaccine. In 2001 I applied under the Freedom of Information Act for a copy of the pre-licensure documentation that the company had submitted to the TGA when applying to have their vaccine included on the Australian Register of Therapeutic Goods. My request caused a flurry, and it took a whole year before they complied with the law and sent me the documents. Some parts of the text were blacked out, and so were all of the reference numbers in the text. The latter made me suspicious that they did not want me to be able to check whether they had used the references honestly. Previously I had encountered promotional material and articles in medical journals that provided references that did not support the statements to which they were linked, and I presume it is done because the writers know that it is unlikely that any reader will bother to check. However, the TGA knew that it *was* likely that I would check, so they made it impossible for me to check the honesty of the references.

Nothing that I read in the documents that they sent me would have convinced me that the vaccine was safe and effective, had I been the person making the decision. It was a lot of waffle that never came to the point. There were five pages of references at the end, and one of the references was to a study of DPT vaccine that had been published in 1981, and exposed as fraudulent in 1986.[508] Because I am familiar with this fraudulent study I could see that there was no explanation in the text as to what it was supposed to prove about the new DTaP vaccine. This increased my suspicion that the reason why they blacked out all the reference numbers in the text was that they did not want me to be able to look them up and see that they had no relevance to their submission.

At the time that I read this report I was unaware that the TGA received no funding from the government, and that the manufacturer of the vaccine was paying the TGA to read this stuff, so I was mystified as to why the TGA had accepted such drivel. Now I know why, but the public is not aware of what is going on as this blatant conflict of interest is kept out of the public eye. Australians naturally assume that the TGA is funded by the government, and neither the government nor the mainstream media inform the public of the true situation. I go around telling people how the TGA is funded, and they are astonished. If the Australian government cannot afford to pay for the testing of medicinal products, then they should inform the public that this area of their responsibility has been privatised.

A VACCINE TRIAL IN NEW ZEALAND

Modern vaccines are tested on human beings to see whether they produce antibodies. If they do, it is declared that the vaccine is able to produce immunity. There is no requirement to prove that antibodies reflect immunity. The manufacturer of the vaccine has total control over which adverse effects are going to be acknowledged during the trials, and which are going to be ignored.

In September 1990, while I was living in New Zealand, I received a phone call from someone whose sister had been asked by her doctor to allow her baby to take part in an experiment with a new vaccine. The caller wanted IAS to get the trial halted. We knew that that would be impossible, but we decided to investigate the details of the experiment, and then ask the Minister of Health to appoint an independent, unbiased individual to monitor the results of the experiment.

The vaccine was intended to prevent a disease called haemophilus influenza type b, which is called Hib for short. It is a rare disease, but it does cause serious damage or death in some babies. Babies are unable to make antibodies to the germ that causes Hib, even when they have the full-blown disease. This poses a problem for the vaccine industry, because they can only justify the use of a vaccine if it makes antibodies. To add to their commercial troubles, adults of European extraction had been shown to produce antibodies in response to the vaccine, but adults of other genetic types had failed to make antibodies when injected.

The aim of the New Zealand experiment was to find out whether attaching the outer shell of the Hib germ to diphtheria toxoid could cause babies under 18 months of age to produce antibodies to Hib. The drug company was particularly interested in finding out what the antibody response would be in Maori and Pacific Islander babies.

Two doctors who were in full time employment with the New Zealand Health Department were being paid by a multinational drug company to do the trial. We asked two people who worked for the Health Department to go and interview them on our behalf. The trial doctors fell into the trap of assuming that the interviewers were devotees of vaccination, and they enthusiastically answered the questions. The only question they would not answer was how much they were being paid by the drug company.

The study was not designed to assess adverse effects, but passive reporting by parents was permitted. It was then up to the two doctors to decide which of the parents' reports to include in the data. Our two moles who interviewed the two doctors asked about adverse reactions, and the response was most enlightening. The doctors said that the reactions would be at the injection site, like redness, swelling, or heat, and where it did occur, it would go away pretty quickly. They said that some children might experience a mild fever as in DPT, but the fever would be much lower with Hib. They said that there are no serious long-term effects of the vaccine, because it had already been safely administered to thousands and thousands of children. They said they would encourage the mothers to monitor temperatures, and they would be providing a follow up service. One of them could be paged at all times. They did not give a cut-off point for the follow up, but they were quite adamant that anything relating to the vaccine would be happening close to the time of the shot.

This confirmed all our fears about the likelihood of getting a true report on any adverse reactions that may occur. The doctors had decided, before they even started, which symptoms they were going to acknowledge as adverse reactions. They had also made up their minds that all adverse effects would show up soon after vaccination, and there would be no damage of a permanent nature. We know that when a mother rushes to get medical help during the acute stage of a baby's vaccine reaction, the doctors and nurses prescribe a painkiller, and deny that the baby is having a vaccine reaction. We had no reason to believe that if a mother in a panic paged one of these doctors, she would be treated any differently.

As the researchers already "knew" before they started the study that all adverse effects would show up soon after vaccination, any reactions that took two or three weeks to emerge would be discounted. As the germ itself is capable of causing permanent brain damage, it is absurd to suggest that the surface antigen of the germ that has been attached to a foreign protein cannot do the same. If any babies suffered severe reactions to the vaccine, the study doctors could simply choose to believe that it was a coincidence, and then fail to mention it in the report. It is especially easy to ignore subtle symptoms that are a precursor to a long-term handicap.

My greatest concern was that if a baby died from the vaccine, it could be replaced by another baby in the final report, because the two doctors who were being paid by the drug company were the only people who knew the names of all the babies who started into the experiment. So we asked the Minister of Health to appoint an independent ombudsman to monitor all the babies who started in to the experiment, and we recommended that the ombudsman should be a person who has credibility with both the medical establishment and with consumer groups.

We expected to be fobbed off, and we were fobbed off. Perhaps this was partly because the Ministry of Health was very busy at the time fobbing off all the people who were trying to warn them that the Factor 9 blood product being used in New Zealand at that time was contaminated with hepatitis C. So the study went ahead without an independent observer being able to note any cases of encephalitis, seizure, or death that might have occurred.

When our moles had interviewed the study doctors during the recruitment for the trial, they had queried whether the number of babies in the study was big enough to be valid. Our moles wrote in their report, "The intention is to have 2 groups with 50 in each. However they may go for 60 in each group to allow for dropouts along the way. They have had approval from the Ethics Committee & the FDA that the numbers in their study will be statistically significant."

As the Maori SIDS rate at that time was 8 per 1000, there was a strong possibility of a death occurring within the trial group. That would of course not necessarily have meant that the vaccine was responsible for the death, but it would have been good if an unbiased observer had had viewing rights. It is common practice in medical trials to treat deaths as "dropouts along the way", instead of investigating the cause of death. Statistically they are treated as if they had moved to another city.

We tried to find out from the Ethics Committee what protocols had been accepted before they gave permission for the trial to go ahead, but the committee lost the file for a few years, and then when they found it again, they said that the contents were none of our business. In any case, even if they did give approval for a good method of recording adverse events, that does not mean that the events would have been honestly recorded.

The only indication we had that the study was over was a newspaper report in September 1992, which said that the vaccine had not proven effective in Maoris and Pacific Islanders.[532] A spokesperson for the Health Department was quoted as saying that a Hib vaccine for babies of six months would not be introduced unless it were "proven effective" in Maoris and Pacific Islanders, because that would be "poor public health practice".

Shortly afterwards, a different brand of Hib vaccine, made in exactly the same way as the one in the trial (conjugated polysaccharide), was included in the New Zealand schedule. The vaccine was started at six weeks, not at six months. I wrote to the Ministry of Health and asked if this brand of vaccine had been tested to see whether it made antibodies in Maoris and Pacific Islanders, and the reply I received said that it had not.

Soon after VAERS was established the FDA received 182 reports of death caused by the vaccine. They conducted a complicated whitewash, and proclaimed the vaccine to be free of responsibility. One of the contortions they used for the whitewash was to say that the rate of adverse events was not known, because none of the trials had been big enough to detect them.

"THE EFFECTIVENESS AND SIDE EFFECTS OF VACCINES ARE MONITORED AFTER THEY ARE INTRODUCED"

Vaccine Myth Number Twelve: Once a vaccine has been introduced, the medical authorities keep a record of the side effects. They also keep a record of the vaccination status of people who catch the disease, so that they can assess how effective the vaccine is. They compile data about side effects by getting doctors and nurses to report any side effects that occur. Every vaccine reaction is then recorded in a central data collecting system.

The biggest factor that prevents an accurate appraisal of adverse effects is the pathological denial into which most doctors and nurses retreat when they see a case of vaccine damage. Pathological denial is a term used to describe the reaction of a person who does not want to face up to the reality of the consequences of his or her actions. Medical people even resort to pathological denial when a large group of children have the same violent reaction to a vaccine at the same time in the same place.

A friend of mine's cousin had a violent reaction to BCG vaccine at the age of 13, and died after 3 days. The doctors and nurses who were involved with the case went to absurd lengths to deny that the vaccine was the cause. One of them even said that her death was more likely to have been caused by some seagull poo landing on her sandwich at playtime than by the vaccine. The girl's mother managed to establish that other children in New Zealand had died from that vaccination campaign, but she never got official acknowledgment.

Because of the media blackout on the topic, people who are not personally affected by a vaccine reaction are blissfully unaware that vaccination is causing so much death, disablement, and distress. In the old days families who were victims of vaccine damage were isolated from other affected families, and they tended to think that their child was just a rare unlucky exception. Now they can post their stories on the internet, but all the stories of life-spoiling reactions that are being posted on the internet do not rattle the consciences of the vaccine zealots. They still say that any parent who thinks that they have observed a bad reaction is mistaken and ignorant, and that the timing of the symptoms is just a coincidence. They believe that parents are not intelligent enough to make accurate observations about their own children, because the parents have not spent seven years at medical school being trained to treat measles with paracetamol/tylenol.

I get a steady stream of requests for help from parents of vaccine-damaged children who have received no help from the authorities whose job it is to help them, and so do other vaccination activists. In the 1990s Hilary Butler noticed that two of the families that she was helping lived in the same suburb in Wellington. She put them in touch with each other, and they discovered that they lived in the same block, around the corner from one another, yet they had never met. Both families had boys who had had violent reactions within hours of the measles vaccine, and have ongoing behavioural problems, as well as recurrent immune system troubles. The boys are both intellectually damaged in specific areas, and in both of them the immune system damage flares up periodically with the same dramatic symptoms. They were both being seen by the same paediatrician, who was telling both the mothers that the fact that the brain damage occurred at the time of vaccination was just a coincidence. One of the mothers had said to the doctor, "You say that my child can't have been affected by the vaccine because it only happens to one in a million. Well how do you know that he's not that one in a million. Someone has to be the one in a million. How do you know that it's not my child?" But the doctor still would not admit it. One day the two mothers confronted him together, and he almost admitted that the vaccine was the cause. Afterwards they talked to his receptionist, and she told them that four other mothers who brought their children to him regularly had told her that their child's condition was caused by vaccination.

Each vial of vaccine comes with a piece of paper called the package insert, that among other things lists ingredients and possible adverse reactions. Most doctors do not read package inserts. In fact some do not even know that the package insert exists. The latter becomes apparent when a parent who is being pressurised to vaccinate asks to see the package insert, and the doctor rummages around and finds a glossy pamphlet that has been left behind by a drug rep. When mothers point out to their doctors that the very symptoms that their child has experienced are mentioned on the package insert, the doctors still insist that it must have been "something else" that caused the symptoms, because it definitely could not have been the vaccine.

When there is a convulsion after vaccination they say it is a coincidence. When there is another convulsion after the next vaccination, they say that too is a coincidence. Convulsions are not uncommon in the first year of life, so it is possible for a convulsion to occur after vaccination without it being caused by the vaccination. However, when it happens a second time, the likelihood of it being a coincidence is greatly diminished. The chance of a convulsion that is not caused by vaccination happening in the three days after vaccination is one in four thousand, and the chance of it happening a second time after a subsequent vaccination without being caused by the vaccination is one in five million.[533] Yet many parents are told that the second one is also a coincidence.

Ultimately the responsibility for monitoring the effect of a vaccine does not lie with the drug company nor with the doctor. It lies with the government agents who bought the vaccine from the manufacturer and foisted it on the population. They are the ones who should be on the lookout for an upsurge of any kind of disease or disorder after a new vaccine is introduced, and they should withdraw the vaccine as soon as there is doubt about its safety. Unfortunately bureaucracies do not work like that. A culture of denial prevails, and doctors who do not partake of the denial are viewed as traitors. Professor Gordon Stewart hit the nail on the head when he said in 1984,

> The crux of the matter is the risk benefit equation. Assumption that this favours vaccination creates the danger, not only of accepting a hypothesis which is untested but also, because the assumption is already adopted as policy, of creating conditions whereby it can never be tested.[259]

Vaccines are introduced on the assumption that they will be safe, and once they are part of the schedule, any evidence that they are not safe is ignored because they are already a part of the schedule.

A CASE OF MASS PATHOLOGICAL DENIAL

A startling example of mass pathological denial occurred during a meningitis vaccination campaign held in New Zealand schools in 1987. A polysaccharide vaccine was used, and it was designed to give immunity to one strain of bacterial meningitis for two or three years. The way that the information was presented to parents led many to believe that it would make their child immune to all types of meningitis for life.

When this vaccine was used at a primary school in a town called Drury, which is just 10 miles south of Auckland, two mothers who had brought their pre-schoolers to school to be vaccinated saw children reacting violently to the injection. They decided to stay at school to see what was going to happen. Some of the children vomited or collapsed within minutes of being injected with the vaccine, while others took a few hours to become ill. These two mothers saw scores of children seriously affected by the vaccine. One of them described it to me later as, "It was like one of those old Florence Nightingale movies. The war-wounded were lying all around."

The children did not all have the same reaction. Interestingly the trend was for the older children to react immediately, while the younger ones took longer to become affected. Some of the children got severe headaches, some got dizzy, some got fevers, some fainted, some got tingling sensations in their arms and hands, some vomited, some lost control over their legs, some got numb feet, some could not concentrate on the person who was speaking to them, some got sore necks, some got glassy eyes, some lost eye/hand coordination, some slowly became floppy and slowly fell off their chairs while trying to do schoolwork. Some children were only beginning to react when it was time to go home. Some of them went home by bus and had to be carried off the busses. Some of the children slept abnormally that afternoon.

Most of the children suffered more than one of these symptoms, and they had all been perfectly fit and healthy before being injected with the vaccine. All of these symptoms, including the vomiting, can be caused by neurological disturbance.

The two mothers who witnessed these reactions went to the press, and two newspapers decided not to withhold the information from the public. A journalist contacted the medical officer of health for comment, and was told that only 14 children had shown any symptoms, and the symptoms had no physical cause, they were just caused by mass hysteria. The reason he gave for the hysteria was that the vaccine had been delayed for an hour, and "all sorts of nasty rumours developed, and the youngsters got themselves worked up into quite a state." It is true that the vaccine had been delayed for an hour, but the children were not aware that it had been delayed. They were just working in their classrooms until they were called out to be jabbed.

Another person in the Health Department said that the neurological effects were not caused by the vaccine, they were caused by an unrelated meningitis virus that was "rippling through the community" at the time. It is of course absurd to suggest that a large group of children suddenly got very sick from a virus in the air, just minutes after they are injected with a bacteria that causes the same symptoms, and that the injection of the bacteria had absolutely nothing to do with the symptoms. But it worked as a public relations exercise.

The Health Department did not have it all their own way. After ten days the medical officer of health admitted that the reactions were not psychological, and said that they were now treating all complaints with concern. Despite this quiet admission, much of the New Zealand public is still left with the impression that there was an incident of mass hysteria after vaccination at a school. The medical officer also said that adverse effects like this had not been heard of before, and were apparently not known to the makers of the vaccine. He said, "It is potentially of world-wide importance."[534]

Eventually it emerged that the same thing had happened at another school at the start of the campaign, but the director-general of health had decided to suppress the information, because he thought it might jeopardise the rest of the campaign. It had then happened at other schools as well, and they had managed to keep it out of the press, until the incident at Drury Primary School. The thing that I find most shocking about all of this is that so many teachers kept quiet about what they saw. One expects the doctors and nurses who are promoting the campaign to be callous and dishonest, and only concerned with preserving the status of modern medicine, but teachers are supposed to care about the welfare of children, and in New Zealand they will not lose their jobs if they speak out about a pharmaceutical product.

Once the cat was out of the bag, the Health Department decided to improve its image. When the publicity first started, various medicrats made statements that contradicted one another, so to avoid further embarrassment the chief bigwig issued a decree that only he and one other bigwig were allowed to make statements to the press. They also advertised a phone number for parents to call if they were concerned about their child's reaction. The phone number was only available for a short time, and some parents who tried to use it received no answer. I was not living in New Zealand when all this happened, but I have since spoken to a number of parents whose children were affected by the vaccine. Two of them told me that they contacted the phone company to see if there was something wrong with the phone line because they could not get through.

Two paediatric neurologists were appointed to examine the 546 victims who had managed to make contact. One of the neurologists is an individual who has been appointed to assess other cases with which IAS has been involved in compensation claims. His behaviour towards the parents of these cases suggests that he has made up his mind that there is no such thing as vaccine damage. I believe that this prejudice very strongly clouds his judgment.

Six weeks after the reactions had first reached the media, the official report came out saying that there was no evidence to suggest that the reactions were associated with permanent harm, but that children under the age of two who had reacted badly should not have the booster shot. Two weeks later a group of medicrats declared that there was no evidence of long-term damage in any of the children, and there was no clear link between neurological problems experienced by some children and the vaccine. This was going beyond the findings of the official report. They had no new data on which to base this declaration, they just made it up.

They said that the same vaccine was used in a major campaign in Finland in the 1970s, and no neurological reactions were reported there. I can think of a number of possible reasons why no neurological reactions were reported in Finland. Perhaps it is because the medicrats in Finland are also pathological liars and were more successful at keeping the truth hidden. Perhaps there were much fewer reactions in Finland, and it was easier to keep it out of the press. Or perhaps Finnish children are made of stronger stuff, and none of them experienced bad reactions to the vaccine. But even if all the children in Finland were strong enough to cope with this injection, that still does not alter the fact that thousands of New Zealand children were not strong enough to cope with it.

This episode in history was not a case of mass hysteria by "youngsters" who got themselves worked up about a needle. It was a case of adults in a position of responsibility and power resorting to mass pathological denial in order to protect their own status. When children lose the use of their legs for three hours after an injection, what has actually happened to them? What did the vaccine do that made that possible? What are the long-term implications of such a symptom? The Health Department should be researching the biological reality of this symptom, instead of pretending that they know the symptoms are not important. No attempt was ever made to find out what the immediate reactions indicated about the long-term adverse effects of the vaccine.

Hilary Butler documented the story of one girl who was damaged by the vaccine, and was still in pain and could not play sport five years after the injection.[535] I have received phone calls from many people whose children were damaged by that campaign, and were still suffering effects of the vaccine years later. Most of them were suffering from mild uncoordination, which affected their movements, and made them unsuccessful at sports they had previously enjoyed. All of these people telephoned me because they were being pressurised to accept yet another vaccine for the damaged child, or for one of its siblings, and they wanted IAS to help them avoid it. Some have told me that they did not know about the hotline at the time that it was available, while others made contact with the Health Department, but were successfully told to get lost. Two have told me that their children were examined by the paediatric neurologists and given a clean bill of health when they were still affected by the vaccine.

Two doctors reviewed the official report that was presented by the paediatric neurologists, and published an article in the *New Zealand Medical Journal*.[536] This article keeps on harping about the possibility that other things may have caused the severe symptoms, and they will not let go of that psychological bit. "The initial explanation seemed to be related to a delay in the arrival of the vaccine, and therefore an anxious waiting period for the children at the school." They make this claim despite the fact that it had been admitted in the press that there had not been an anxious waiting period.

Although it is regrettable that the true figures were well pruned and trimmed, at least there is something in a medical journal to say that something happened. They said that there were 63 reports of headache, stiff neck, and myalgia within 48 hours of vaccination, although, "other causes, particularly viral illness, cannot be excluded." They also mentioned 152 cases of fever, and 85 of fever, rash, and local reaction.

> There were 92 reports suggesting peripheral nerve involvement. Motor symptoms consisted of 80 reports of unexplained weakness and subjective "heaviness" unrelated to injection site, and there were 57 reports of sensory symptoms suggesting paraesthesia or dysaesthesia. Both categories occurred in some children, and in younger children, reluctance to use a limb may have been due to either. The majority of cases, both sensory and motor, were transient and had gone within 48 hours of immunisation although symptoms persisted for up to three weeks in some cases. These symptoms could have been vaccine related as they are less likely to be related to intercurrent illness, and many episodes occurred within a plausible time interval. On the other hand it is clear that absolute causality cannot be ascribed on the basis of the data.

So they are not quite admitting that the vaccine was responsible, and they are certainly not admitting that some children were permanently damaged.

> All reported cases of fainting, nausea and dizziness occurred within 24 hours and can probably be ascribed to psychological

> effects of the procedure.

They show their contempt for the victims by accusing them of being emotional and scared of the needle.

> Other symptoms which were reported only occasionally were considered too subject to confounding to warrant further consideration.

In other words, "Some children suffered unusual symptoms from the vaccine, but as there were not a large group of each of these symptoms, we will choose to ignore them." Although this report is mildly infuriating, it at least makes it official that there were some neurological adverse effects. This is important because one of the features of medical denial is that it is often claimed that something cannot be happening here if it has not been reported as having happened somewhere else. So although the incidence of reactions is greatly reduced in this report, and although the children who are still suffering bad effects years afterwards are not acknowledged, the fact that the report was published in a medical journal means that medicrats in other countries will not be justified in brushing aside similar events in their own country on the grounds that "there has never before been a report of serious reactions to this vaccine anywhere in the world."

It would be interesting to know what percentage of medicrats actually take cognisance of things that are printed in medical journals. Two and a half years after this report was published, a journalist interviewed a highly placed New Zealand medicrat about vaccination. When discussing the Drury incident, the medicrat told her that a specialist had been called in to check the reactions, and had concluded that it was a case of mass hysteria, and there were no problems with the vaccine.

Five years after the event, members of the IAS had discussions with a number of school principals about an MMR vaccination campaign that was planned in schools. Many of these principals were still under the impression that the Drury incident had been a case of mass hysteria. A lie once told is very powerful.

The person who was the Medical Assessor for New Zealand at the time reported to the World Health Assembly in Geneva that there had been problems with the vaccine. The World Health Organisation had two excuses for not acting on his report. The first was that he had no controls.[537] According to them, he should have selected some children who were not injected with the vaccine, and investigated whether they were vomiting and collapsing at 11 am on vaccination day. Their second excuse was that no other country had reported any adverse effects.[538] The first excuse is almost valid because all data should have controls. Even though it is quite obvious to anyone with common sense that those children were vomiting and collapsing because of the vaccine, to be scientifically correct, the Medical Assessor should have sent evidence that children of the same age who had not been vaccinated, were not vomiting and collapsing at the same time on the same day. If the World Health Organisation actually cared about the welfare of children, they would have investigated the matter for themselves. They could easily do it, seeing as they have billions of dollars to work with. Their second excuse for ignoring his report has no validity, because most countries that bought the vaccine make no effort to record the adverse effects of any vaccine. Later the Medical Assessor spoke on radio about adverse effects of vaccination, and was verbally rebuked for doing this. When his contract with the New Zealand Health Department was due for renewal, which normally happens automatically every year, it was not renewed. Basically he got fired for talking about vaccine reactions.

In 1987 Hilary Butler published a paper that documented the events of this mass vaccination campaign.[539] In it she discusses the immunological reasons why those particular reactions occurred. She mentions that some doctors recognised the syndrome and diagnosed correctly, while

> … the hospitals, paediatric neurologists and Health Department chose to ignore such blatantly obvious facts. As one doctor put it: "Well, we'll never really know, until in maybe five years time in some other country, the same syndrome is reported in the literature." Such statements are somewhat of an oxymoron, since in the hypothetical five years time, said doctors would probably look at the literature and say "Can't be - never happened before!" and it wouldn't get within an arm's length of a medical journal. This is the way that information which should be classified as *fact* and reported, is continually ridiculed and put-down as *anecdotal*.[540]

Those were prophetic words. In 1991 there was a minor controversy in South Africa about the death of a child after a meningitis vaccination campaign in schools. My friend Arlene in Cape Town wrote to a member of parliament who was in parliament on an anti-apartheid ticket and expressed her concern about the child's death. The child who had died had a black skin, so there would have been no point in contacting a pro-apartheid parliamentarian about the death. The member of parliament replied that he knew that the death was not caused by the vaccine, because no other country had reported adverse effects.

I wrote to the World Health Organisation and asked how they monitor the adverse effects of vaccines in South Africa. They replied that they do not, and they gave me the address of the Medicines Control Council in Cape Town, and suggested I should ask them how the South Africans monitor adverse effects.

I knew very well that the South African medical authorities did not monitor adverse effects of vaccines, but I wanted them to put it in writing. So I wrote to the Medicines Control Council and asked them how they monitor adverse effects. They replied that they have a system for the voluntary reporting of adverse drug reactions by medical doctors, dentists, pharmacists, and the pharmaceutical industry, but they do not have a system that specifically solicits adverse reactions to vaccines. Their letter ended, "Because the system is a voluntary reporting system it does not allow for monitoring the incidence of adverse reports."

It was a very tidy arrangement for the drug companies. The World Health Organisation promoted vaccination around the world, but made no effort to find out what adverse effects occur. The governments that accepted the vaccines did not monitor adverse effects. Yet the World Health Organisation could reject a report from an official in New Zealand because there were no similar reports from other countries. In 2019 South Africa still relies on voluntary reporting of vaccine reactions, and makes no effort to determine the adverse effects of mass vaccination campaigns in schools.

RELIANCE ON PASSIVE REPORTING

The United States government was the first to set up an institution to collect reports of adverse effects, but the reason they set it up was not because they suddenly developed a conscience. They did it because of the effort of a group of parents whose children had been killed or severely damaged by DPT vaccine.[541] The *National Childhood Vaccine Injury Compensation Act* was passed after a tremendous struggle on the part of a group that called itself Dissatisfied Parents Together (DPT).

> Like David against Goliath, DPT represented essentially powerless vaccine injured victims pitted against three of the most powerful and wealthy segments of our society: the pharmaceutical industry, organised medicine, and the federal government.[541]

The group DPT worked hard for four and a half years to compile and submit legislation that would allow reports of reactions to be recorded, and allow families to be paid compensation for severe damage. The powerful drug companies blocked the legislation every year, but finally they said that they would allow the law to be passed as long as it went through at the same time as a law that they wanted introduced. The law that they wanted to introduce made it possible for them to sell new drugs to countries outside of the USA without having to wait for the drug to be passed by the FDA.[541] This is not as bad as it sounds for those of us who live outside of the USA, because the FDA is a corrupt organisation that passes unsafe drugs anyway. Both laws were passed at the same time, and the Vaccine Adverse Events Reporting System (VAERS) was established to collect reports of vaccine reactions.

VAERS is a branch of the FDA. The Act states that a doctor must report a side effect of a vaccine to the FDA if they "judge the event warrants reporting."[542] If a doctor decides to retreat into pathological denial the event will not be reported, but at least when a doctor is prepared to face up to the reality of what he or she is seeing, there is now a central register to which the observation can be reported. A list of symptoms that were considered acceptable to be recognized as adverse effects of each vaccine was drawn up, and an arbitrary time frame was established in which these events had to occur if they were to be accepted as related to the vaccine.[542] A large sum of taxpayers' money was set aside for paying compensation each calendar year, but in the first year that the system went into operation, they ran out of money in March.[543] Despite the fact that only symptoms that were on their list could be reported, and that not all cases get reported, they were still getting far more cases than they had expected. When it was seen that paying for some of the damage done by vaccines was going to cost far too much money, they decided to decrease the length of time after vaccination in which the reactions have to occur in order for compensation to be paid.[544]

The parents consumer group called Dissatisfied Parents Together has changed its name to National Vaccination Information Center (NVIC). When a doctor refuses to report a reaction, NVIC can submit the report on behalf of the parent, that is, if the parent is fortunate enough to know that NVIC exists. VAERS claims that when it receives reports, "All reports received are entered into the database."[545] NVIC used the Freedom of Information Act to obtain a copy of the data about vaccine reactions that the FDA had in their computer. Despite the court order, the FDA tried to avoid complying. When NVIC finally obtained the data, they discovered that it was not accurate. Some of the cases they had assisted in getting reported were not even there, and others had the details wrong.[546]

The medicrats have built in an escape chute so that they do not have to take too much notice of the reports that do end up being typed into the computer. "Submission of a report does not necessarily denote that the vaccine caused the adverse event."[542] Any reports they do not like can simply be quashed by saying that the doctor's judgment was wrong.

Since VAERS was created many countries have set up similar institutions so that they can claim that they are acknowledging all serious reactions to vaccination. It is a world-wide problem that most doctors refuse to report vaccine reactions, and in the countries that allow parents to make the reports themselves, parents do not know that they have the right to do so.

The vaccine industry does not like the term "vaccine reactions". They are conducting a worldwide push to substitute it with "adverse events". New Zealand has the Adverse Event Reporting Committee that is based in Dunedin. Doctors can report reactions to them if they feel so inclined, but the bureaucrats in Dunedin are not obliged to enter the report into their computer. The IAS does not know what percentage of reports is simply thrown away instead of being entered into the database, but we do know of some that were not entered. Any member of the public who wants to know how many reports are entered for each vaccine for each year has to pay a lot of money for the information. So we at the IAS started our own collection of reports of adverse effects, so that at least some would be documented for posterity. One of the questions we ask on the form is whether the doctor or nurse to whom the parent reported the reaction reported it to the committee in Dunedin.

The Australian consumer group the Australian Vaccination Network (AVN) also started their own database for Australian vaccine reactions. The official body to which reports of vaccine reactions can be made in Australia was called ADRAC, and is now called ACSOM. The official policy is, "Any serious or unexpected adverse event should be reported."[547] No limits have been put on the type of reactions that can be reported, and the cut-off time within which reactions have to occur has been lifted, "as some adverse events related to vaccination could occur many years later."[547] Serious reports are supposed to be followed up, and the victim is supposed to be helped if possible, but victims are neither followed up, nor helped. In 1999 three AVN members met with ADRAC representatives in Canberra. The ADRAC representatives admitted that less than 10% of reactions are ever reported in Australia, and of those that are, almost none are followed up to see if there have been any long-term complications, or, in fact, if the person involved has survived the reaction.[548,549] By 2009 the AVN had more than 700 cases of severe reactions on its own adverse reactions database. None of them had been reported to ADRAC by the vaccinator, nor by any health professional who has been consulted about the vaccine damage.

In 1997, when there were only 200 cases on the AVN database, the AVN sent the reports, with names and addresses, stating which of them had already died from the reaction, to the Minister of Health, and asked him to investigate them all and add them to the official statistics. After six months of evasive action, the Minister finally said that he would neither investigate the reactions, nor add them to the statistics, as they had not been reported by doctors. Since then, hundreds of deaths caused by vaccination have been reported to ADRAC by doctors, but the Australian politicians are only interested in persecuting parents who do not vaccinate.

In 1996 the World Health Organisation founded the Global Training Network (GTN) "to improve the quality of vaccines and their use."[550] As part of this initiative they commissioned the Department of Pharmacology at the University of Cape Town, South Africa, to design a system that each country can use for monitoring and responding to adverse reactions, and to train people to put the system into practice.[550] The system they developed relies on passive reporting for the collection of data, and makes no attempt at assessing long-term adverse effects. Countries that use this system do not get an accurate picture of what vaccination is doing to the health of the nation, but politicians use it to claim that they are monitoring adverse effects. In an article that describes the system the authors say,

> The limitations of the system and training programme described in this paper are such that long-term effects are not detected. The passive surveillance methods need to be supplemented with a variety of other epidemiological methods, including long-term follow up using registries of patients and dedicated studies of individual problems and concerns.[550]

So who is going to do these dedicated studies and follow ups of registries of patients? They should have been done seventy years ago, but they are not likely to be done while the drug companies control the World Health Organisation.

Some of the processes recommended by the people in Cape Town are that;

* each country should establish a body for receiving reports,

* all vaccine reactions should be reported,

* people in supervisory positions should encourage those who

interact with patients to report reactions,

* all data should be kept in a permanent record,

* the data collected should be made available for research purposes, "to provide a stronger scientific basis for causality assessment"[550]

* top government officials and the public should be provided with information about adverse effects, and

* governments should consider terminating contracts with companies that manufacture unsafe vaccines.

If human beings were honest creatures, this system would result in the collection of accurate data on short-term adverse effects, truthful communications to the public, and all companies that produce unsafe vaccines going out of business. However, human beings are not honest creatures, and there is too much pride, prestige, and money at stake for honesty to prevail. Even though there are a minority of individual doctors and nurses who want to do the right thing, they know that they would put their jobs and careers in jeopardy if they told the truth.

As the authors themselves admit, this system would not result in the collection of data about long-term adverse effects. Long-term adverse effects ruin the lives of millions, yet they are completely ignored.

One of the recommendations made by the people in Cape Town is that when patients go to a medical outlet to report a reaction, "the supervisor and the health care worker concerned [should] … comfort the patients and their parents."[550] Wouldn't that be nice.

In the background waffle of the article the authors adopt the stance that vaccination is known to be safe and beneficial. It does not seem to occur to them that the reason why they are establishing a method for recording adverse effects is that the adverse effects of vaccination have not been properly assessed in the past, and therefore vaccination is not known to be safe and beneficial. They say that vaccines "have a favourable risk-benefit profile," and an "impressive performance record."[550] They have no right to claim that vaccination has a good record when no records have been kept. Vaccination has a good reputation, but it does not have a good record. And they have no basis on which to believe that vaccines have a favourable risk-benefit profile, because no country has ever kept an accurate record of short-term or long-term adverse effects, nor a record of the effectiveness of vaccines.

One of the things they teach people in the courses that are being run at Cape Town University is how to handle the media when the public complains about a cluster of bad reactions. "Trainees are required to develop and present action plans and communication reports such as press statements. Mock television interviews with journalists are included."[550] I would like to be a fly on the wall to watch what goes on during these training sessions. I am not optimistic that the culture of denial that pervades the field of vaccination is about to disappear.

Early in 1988 I had an encounter that highlights the typical attitude of keen vaccinators. It was with a high-ranking doctor from Groote Schuur Hospital in Cape Town. My second child, Kenny, was born at home in a small town south of Cape Town on the Cape Peninsula. When he was two months old, the local public health nurse telephoned me, and I told her that he was not going to be vaccinated. A few weeks later two women unexpectedly turned up on my doorstep. One was the public health nurse, the other was the doctor from Groote Schuur Hospital. Ever since Chris Barnard did the world's first heart transplant at Groote Schuur Hospital, anyone associated with the hospital has bathed in reflected glory. The public health nurse thought that this doctor would be able to intimidate me. I invited them to sit down, and a lively discussion ensued between myself and the doctor. I had a number of people living with me at the time, and they gathered around to watch. The public health nurse switched off her ears and got that same glazed look in her eyes that white South Africans used to get when you told them that apartheid should be abolished. I was quite taken aback by the doctor's ignorance about the immune system. One of her clangers was, "Natural measles does not cause IgA antibodies." I was amused by the expression on her face when she found out that I knew that the polio vaccine was no longer compulsory. No member of the public was supposed to know that.

I gave a number of reasons for not vaccinating Kenny. She told me that she knew that measles vaccine has no adverse effects because they had just done a mass vaccination campaign against measles in Khayelitsha, and, "They would be turning up in droves at the hospital if there was any problem."

I replied, "They'll be turning up in droves in ten years' time, and you won't know that it's because of the vaccine." Khayelitsha was a slum on the eastern side of Cape Town that attracted people who faced starvation in the Ciskei and Transkei "bantustans". This doctor knew what conditions were like in Khayelitsha. She had been there and she knew that the people lived in tents or self-built shacks, that there was no public transport and there were no telephones, that the people had no money, and that while the ambulance drivers did their best to get every dangerously ill person to hospital, the ambulance service was hopelessly under-funded and over-stretched. According to her method of assessing adverse effects, a child who suffered a severe immediate reaction was supposed to make it to hospital 30 miles away despite these difficulties. I tried to impress on this doctor that a reaction might only show up some time after the vaccination, in the form of chronic disease or ill-health, but her mind was absolutely closed to the idea. In any case, even if a child who had suffered a severe immediate reaction had made it to the hospital alive, there would have been little chance of the case being recorded as a vaccine reaction.

When it was time for the two ladies to leave, the public health nurse snapped back into consciousness and said to me, "When you bring him down to the clinic I will leave out the whooping cough part of the vaccine." She had not heard a word I had said. With all the sickness and misery that prevailed in Cape Town, it is amazing that a doctor from Groote Schuur had nothing better to do with five hours than travel to the home of an affluent person in order to try to achieve compliance. At least she was friendly and non-aggressive. Some doctors do not attempt to discuss vaccination, choosing instead to launch an attack on the non-believer's character.

An "evaluation" of the mass vaccination campaign in Khayelitsha was later published in the South African Medical Journal.[551] The article evaluates how successful they were at reaching the target population, and does not even mention adverse effects. Did it not occur to them that adverse effects might happen, or did they just not care? I am not optimistic that the culture of not acknowledging adverse effects can be changed by the World Health Organisation's training course in Cape Town. There needs to be a fundamental change in attitude towards the suppression of information about the adverse effects of vaccines, but this is not likely to occur while most doctors and nurses see their self-worth as being tied up in the prestige of pharmaceutical medicine.

Any country that does make a serious effort to evaluate adverse effects is in for a shock. When the measles vaccine was introduced, East Germany was under communist rule. The government made measles vaccine compulsory, and passed a law that every person who suffered vaccine damage must be compensated.[282] Once the claims for compensation started rolling in, the government was shocked to discover how very common severe long-term adverse effects were.[146]

The three most serious problems in regard to the recording of adverse effects are those of pathological denial at the patient/provider interface, pernicious dishonesty among medical bureaucrats, and financial relationships between vaccine manufacturers and some of the highest-ranking officials.

An American mother whose child was killed by DPT vaccine failed to get acknowledgment of the cause of death despite going to a lot of effort to get it. During a telephone conversation with a CDC official, she was told by the official that he knew that DPT was the cause of her son's death, but he did not dare say so to anyone else.[552] Dr. Paul Offit, in his first pro-vaccine propaganda book for parents, makes the outrageous statement, "No child has died from the 'old' pertussis vaccine (DPT vaccine)."[553]

In 1967 a Swedish scientist published his finding that whooping cough vaccine encouraged the growth of cancer cells.[554] In 1983 Dr. Richard Moskowitz related how a doctor confided in him that a five-year-old boy patient had developed cancer after DPT vaccine, been treated, and been on the road to recovery until another dose of DPT caused a full relapse.[555] Dr. Moskowitz says,

> The idea that vaccination might also be implicated in some cases of childhood leukemia was shocking enough in itself, but … perhaps even more shocking to me is the fact that the boy's own physician dared not communicate his suspicion of vaccine-related illness to the parents, let alone to the general public. It was this case that convinced me, once and for all, of the need for serious, public discussion of our collected experiences with vaccine-related illness, precisely because rigorous experimental proof will require years of investigation and a firm public commitment that has not even been made yet.[555]

More than three decades later those studies have still not been started, and the vaccine industry has absolutely no intention of starting them.

The vaccine defenders scorn the anecdotal evidence that MMR vaccine causes autism in some children, saying that anecdotal evidence is "not scientific". If they truly believed in science, they would want the anecdotal evidence to be followed up with methodologically sound scientific studies. Anecdotal evidence is not enough to draw scientific conclusions, but it is an indicator that proper scientific research needs to be done. While the industry is refusing to do proper studies on the possible relationship between MMR and autism, they have no right to dismiss the anecdotal evidence. No study that compares the rate of autism in the vaccinated and the unvaccinated has been published. So while the vaccine pushers scorn the anecdotal evidence that MMR vaccine causes autism in some children, they have no scientific evidence to support their claim that MMR vaccine does not cause autism.

An example of anecdotal evidence is the Irish toddler who was using some words at 18 months, and was "chatting" in the morning before his

MMR vaccination. He suffered a violent reaction to the vaccination and lost the use of words. At ten years old he still has no language, and just like the millions of other cases where it is obvious that the vaccine was the cause, the doctors and government are denying that his lack of language and all of the other problems that started with the injection were caused by the injection. They say that it is all just a coincidence, and that anecdotal evidence is worthless. What these vaccine defenders are saying is that if that child had not been injected with MMR that morning, he still would have screamed while clutching his head all afternoon, banged his head and jerked his limbs all night, lain on his bed and stared at the ceiling the whole of the next day, never made eye contact again, and never spoken again. They are saying that all of these things would have happened if he had not had the injection. It is a ridiculous claim for them to make, but for them there is more than just billions of dollars at stake, there is also the terrible fear that they would lose prestige if they admitted the truth.

The vaccinators are also saying that it is a complete coincidence that similar reactions with similar long term outcomes have presented in millions of other toddlers soon after injection with MMR. They defend themselves from facing up to reality by claiming that they believe in "science", not in anecdotal reports. But the "science" to which they are referring is a raft of shonky studies that do not compare the rate of autism in the vaccinated and the unvaccinated. The existing studies use absurd methods like looking at the age at which autism is diagnosed, or comparing autistic children who have older siblings that are autistic with autistic children whose older siblings are not autistic. Dr. Paul Offit, the dude who says that aluminium is a nutrient, not a neurotoxin, did not serve his masters well when he made the admission that the lack of studies that compare vaccinated with unvaccinated means that there is, "limited ability to assess associations between vaccination and adverse events with delayed or insidious onset (eg, autism)."[556]

The vaccine industry has a variety of excuses for not doing studies that compare the incidence of chronic disease in the vaccinated and the unvaccinated, the most ridiculous of which is that it would be unethical to do these studies. The makers of this excuse range from hysterical bloggers to the sedate pharmashills at the Institute of Medicine. In its 2013 report, the Institute of Medicine admits that comparing vaccinated children with unvaccinated children would be the best kind of study, and it admits that the existing research about vaccine safety is not adequate, but it then goes on to say that it would be unethical and too expensive to do comparative studies.[557] Another reason given by the Institute of Medicine for not doing comparative studies is that, "there are very low observed rates of adverse events with vaccination".[558] Wrong. Very high rates of adverse events have been observed, but most adverse events are not recorded as such, and are dismissed as "just a coincidence". So high rates of adverse events are observed, but very low rates of adverse events *are acknowledged.* Ironically, by talking about "observed rates of adverse events with vaccination", the Institute of Medicine is basing its stance on anecdotal evidence. They are saying that there is not the anecdotal evidence to warrant scientific studies. Wrong again. Even the tiny fraction of adverse reactions that are reported to official channels are enough to warrant proper scientific studies that compare the rate of autism in the vaccinated with the rate in the unvaccinated.

The vaccine defenders repeatedly claim that a study[559] done in Denmark compared the rate of autism in the vaccinated and the unvaccinated, and that this study proves that MMR vaccine does not cause autism. Vaccine defenders call it "the Madsen study," or "the Danish study", and they love it. The abstract says that the study compared the rate of autism in the vaccinated and the unvaccinated, but if you read the text, you see that it did not. Many well-written critiques of this ridiculously unscientific study can be read on the net, but the point I want to make is that if the researchers had actually wanted to compare vaccinated children with unvaccinated children, they could have done so. Every citizen and every resident in Denmark has a civil-registry number, which enables researchers to obtain information about the vaccination status of individuals. The Madsen study could easily have compared vaccinated children with unvaccinated children if they had wanted to do so.

Whenever a new autism/MMR study appears in the armoury of the vaccinators, journalists around the world report that another study comparing the vaccinated with the unvaccinated has been done, proving yet again that MMR vaccine does not cause autism. Journalists do not read the studies before reporting on them, they only read a press release about the study, and repeat what it says. An investigative journalist would read the actual study instead of just assuming that the study has been done properly, and that the press release is truthful.

Anecdotal reports do not tell us how often each side effect happens. Neither do case reports written by doctors. Hepatitis B vaccine is documented in medical journals as causing Guillain-Barre syndrome (a type of paralysis), optic neuritis, transverse myelitis, demyelinating lesions in the brain, and progressive demyelination.[560,561,562] These case reports, however, do not indicate what the actual risk of damage from this vaccine is for an individual.

The human immune system does not restrict itself to making antibodies to the germ that is contained in the vaccine. The immune system also makes antibodies to all the other ingredients in the vaccine, like mercury, formaldehyde, antibiotics, animal tissue, human tissue, vegetable matter, and aluminium. Some people who suffered paralysis from a rabies vaccine that was made of brain were found to have developed anti-brain antibodies.[563] When brain is injected into someone's blood, his or her immune system automatically manufactures anti-brain antibodies. While these antibodies float around in the bloodstream they have the potential to attack the person's brain. If someone were to offer to inject me with brain, I would say, "No thank you. I don't want to have anti-brain antibodies circulating in my blood stream." Recipients of vaccines that contain brain are not told that the vaccine contains brain.

It is the responsibility of governments to ensure that vaccines are safe before they are introduced into government schedules, instead of just believing the manufacturers that the vaccines are safe. Each government that provides vaccination should set up an extensive database to discover all the adverse effects that have a delayed appearance. Some countries are setting up databases to record who is vaccinated and who is not. Their intention in recording this information is to make it easier for them to persecute the families who do not vaccinate. They have no intention of using the data to evaluate adverse effects and effectiveness of vaccines, but it is possible that in the future these databasesmight be used, by people who care about the welfare of children, to assess the facts and figures which up until now government agencies have so assiduously avoided collecting.

IGNORING CONTRAINDICATIONS

In 1953, a Swiss paediatrician published an article that related his personal experience of the factors that make a baby vulnerable to suffering brain damage from whooping cough vaccine, and what he had found on the topic in the medical literature.[564] He listed five factors that greatly increase the risk of a baby suffering brain damage from the vaccine; a family history of neurological disease, a history of convulsions in the child, allergies, poor general condition, and evidence of an acute infectious disease.[564] The medical establishment as a whole acknowledged that the presence of these and some other factors meant that a child should not be vaccinated. Every English speaking country adopted the official policy that vaccination should be withheld from children with contraindications to vaccination. A British study published in 1974 confirmed that a child is more vulnerable to neurological damage from vaccination if he or she has a history of fits, or a family history of fits in first degree relatives, if he or she has had a reaction to a previous jab, has had a recent infection, or has neurodevelopmental defects.[565]

The vaccine industry did not allow this trend to continue because they lose money every time someone is not vaccinated. In 1989 the American Immunization Practices Advisory Committee announced that some contraindications were not really contraindications to vaccination.[566] I wrote to this committee and asked for evidence to support their stance, and they sent me 18 references. Some of these references were to articles that did not exist, and none of the articles that did exist supported the claim that known contraindications are not contraindications. However, it was interesting that one of the references said that a hypotonic hyporesponsive episode (limpness, paleness or blueness, and reduced responsiveness or unresponsiveness) after vaccination *is* a contraindication to further doses,[567] as many countries adopt the stance that hypotonic hyporesponsive episodes are not a contraindication to further doses of vaccine. The American bureaucrats have persuaded health departments around the world to ignore contraindications, and to vaccinate babies who are known to be at risk of suffering serious adverse effects.

An example of the callous irresponsibility of modern medical officials is that they recommend that premature babies should be vaccinated according to their date of birth, not according to their gestational age. A proper study was eventually done in 2001, and it found that premature babies are very susceptible to suffering from serious vaccine reactions.[568] The authors of the study point out that the research on which the modern British policy of vaccinating premature babies is based is inadequate, and they call on the British Department of Health to change their policy.[568]

When I lived in New Zealand I got a phone call at about 8 pm one night from a woman who wanted me to give her the name of a homoeopath who would be prepared to go to Auckland hospital and treat her niece. She said the girl had reacted violently to MMR vaccination at school that day, and was "getting worse by the hour." She told me that the doctors at the hospital were saying that it had happened because the girl had been vaccinated when she had a cold, and there was nothing wrong with the vaccine. When they want to peddle the vaccine they say that it is perfectly safe to vaccinate someone who has a cold. However, when they want to protect the reputation of a vaccine, they turn around and say it is wrong to vaccinate someone who has a cold.

In New Zealand, the medical bureaucrats use a variety of aggressive methods to try to increase the uptake of vaccines. Parents of vaccine-damaged children are repeatedly telephoned and harassed to accept another dose. The government has instructed doctors to make their receptionists do this. Hospital staff have been instructed to ask about the vaccination status of all children who come into hospital, and to persuade the parents to "get the shots up to date." The questions are asked when the child is admitted to hospital, but the jabbing is not done until the child is discharged. Because of government cutbacks, patients are usually discharged before they are fully recovered. So children are being jabbed when they are in poor health, and then sent away instead of being observed. If the parents later have a story to relate about an adverse reaction, the medical staff do not believe them because no medically trained staff saw the reaction.

Most cases of vaccine damage result in symptoms that are there all the time. For instance, the child cannot walk, or has inflamed ears, or is continually violent. A strange thing is that some children get symptoms that come and go at regular intervals. It could be once a month, or every six weeks. The child has a health crisis for a few days, and then appears normal until the health crisis returns. Sometimes the crisis is so intense and frightening that the parents rush the child to hospital. Upon entry they are aggressively asked if the child's vaccinations are up to date. When the parents aggressively reply that it is vaccination that has caused the problem in the first place, the hospital staff usually look shocked and shut up. But you get some hard cases who still carry on badgering the parents to have another dose of vaccine, while telling them that they are quite wrong in thinking that vaccination can cause such drastic and peculiar symptoms.

Parents are often told to give a drug to suppress fever after vaccination. One drug company even goes so far as to say on a vaccine package insert that if the baby is given "salicyles, barbiturates or antihistamines" in association with the vaccine, that will help the reaction to be "benign and transient," and reduce the risk of convulsions, brain inflammation, and brain damage. I wrote to the drug company and asked them how they know that giving these drugs soon after vaccination will prevent brain damage. They did not reply. They cannot have any evidence to support the claim, because giving these drugs on the same day as vaccination does not prevent brain damage. It is outrageous that a drug company can make a claim like that on a package insert. What is worse is that these drugs actually make a baby more vulnerable to damage from the vaccine.

A study was done looking at the effect of paracetamol/tylenol during the first 24 hours after vaccination.[569] With paracetamol/tylenol there was less fever, less pain at the injection site, and less fussiness. Paracetamol/tylenol was voted a huge success by the authors of the study, some of whom have been publicly exposed as being on the payroll of drug companies. Another study looked at the effect of paracetamol/tylenol in the first 48 hours after vaccination.[570] Babies with contraindications to vaccination were excluded from this study. This really infuriates me, because it shows that they know that contraindications increase the risk of a severe adverse reaction, and they do not want to have that affecting the results of their study. But they do not exclude babies with contraindications from vaccination in the real world outside of their study, because they would lose dollars for each child who is not vaccinated. This study found that paracetamol/tylenol reduced fever and pain at the site of injection, but it also looked at the symptom of drowsiness, and it found that the drug made no difference to drowsiness. We have seen earlier how fever protects the body. Fever-suppressing drugs make the baby's brain more vulnerable to attack by the germs, as well as to the proteins and the toxins that are in the vaccine. At the same time they mask any acute reaction that might show up during the period shortly after vaccination, so that parents are less likely to be successful at suing the drug company for long-term damage. It is significant that the drug did not mask the symptom of drowsiness. Drowsiness after vaccination has sinister long-term implications regarding brain damage.

Prescribing paracetamol/tylenol to prevent brain damage from vaccination is as unscientific as the claim of 200 years ago that swallowing mercury would protect people from a bad reaction to smallpox vaccination. Science is not the issue. Compliance is the issue. The latter study concluded with the statement,

> Use of acetaminophen [paracetamol/tylenol] may thereby relieve parental anxiety and improve compliance with recommended vaccination programs.[570]

Achieving compliance, not preventing adverse effects, is what the pharmaceutical industry wants. The finding of this study was reported in a magazine for doctors with the title in large print, "*Paracetamol Increases Immunisation Compliance.*"[571]

Sometimes a vaccine damages the brain without the person's body having been able to muster up a fever in order to defend itself, even in the absence of fever-suppressing drugs. The child's initial reaction is something else, like staring episodes, or somnolence, without fever. A Swedish study from the 1960s found that there was no fever in 35% of cerebral reactions, and no fever in 55% of cases of shock from whooping cough vaccine.[572]

Teething at the time of vaccination also increases the risk of vaccine damage, but that contraindication was never officially acknowledged, so it has not been discarded. Since vaccination started it has been an observable fact that a child is more vulnerable to reacting badly if the vaccination is done while the child is teething, and it is now known that during teething the blood brain barrier is more open than at other times. For some reason there has been a subsection of medical dogma that denies that teething is a time of vulnerability to any kind of onslaught. There are many articles in medical journals that angrily deny that teething causes any symptoms in a baby. The authors need psychotherapy. Their rationale is that babies can also get sick when they are not teething, so it is always a coincidence if it happens when they are teething. One doctor even goes so far as to say, "relief of symptoms by the use of an antihistamine can be attributed to its sedative and antiallergic properties, for the drug has no effect on the tooth, the gum, or the eruption of the tooth."[573] This is ironic because it has since been discovered that "the eruption of the tooth" makes the body produce histamine,[574] so obviously an antihistamine would make a teething baby feel better. (*Chamomilla 30* is a better, non-toxic option). The increase in histamine is significant because histamine opens the blood brain barrier.[575,576,577] This is one way that babies become more vulnerable to vaccine damage while teething, but there are probably also other ways that are yet to be discovered. No amount of ranting by medical dinosaurs is going to alter the fact that teething at the time of vaccination makes a baby more vulnerable to brain damage from the vaccine.

Separating jabs by 7 days, 14 days, or 21 days also increases the risk. Tell that to a keen vaccinator, and observe the scorn spread over their face. People who want to separate MMR into M, M, and R are making a terrible mistake.

Thankfully there are still doctors who have enough common sense to observe contraindications, and therefore they do not jab children who are obviously at high risk. Unfortunately, while contraindications increase the risk, the absence of contraindications does not mean there is no risk. A baby who is perfectly healthy and belongs to a family of sturdy individuals can tragically suffer serious damage from vaccination. The British Medical Journal documents the case of a boy who came from a family with no history of anything, and who was perfectly healthy until his first dose of whooping cough vaccine at eight months caused profound brain damage.[578]

VACCINE INGREDIENTS

One of the extraordinary features of vaccination is that the vast majority of doctors and nurses who inject vaccines into babies, children, and adults have absolutely no idea what they are injecting. The ingredients, over and above the antigen that is supposed to make the antibodies that are supposed to create immunity to the disease, include formaldehyde, aluminium, mercury (yes, there is still mercury in vaccines), gelatin, glycerin, castor oil, ammonium sulfate, chick embryo, chicken, chicken egg, duck egg, dog brain, monkey kidney, mouse blood, sheep blood, caterpillar ovaries (the manufacturer is really proud of this one), lung cells from aborted babies, pork, beef broth, polysorbate 80, borax, yeast, antibiotics, silicone, sucrose, lactose, casein, bicarb, monosodium glutamate (MSG), glutaraldehyde, β-propiolactone, detergents, solvents, chelating agents, polydimethylsiloxane, hydrolyzed gelatin, sodium chloride, sodium phosphate dibasic, potassium phosphate monobasic, potassium chloride, EDTA (to help the body get rid of the mercury and aluminium), neomycin, fetal bovine serum, monosodium phosphate, phenol, sorbitol, sodium borate, soy peptone, and acetone. These bizarre ingredients should not distract us from the danger posed by the antigen itself.

Angry vaccine defenders say that the amount of aluminium that is injected into infants who are vaccinated according to the schedule is lower than the amount they obtain from other sources, but the amount is actually higher.[579] The amount of aluminium that is "safe" to inject into an infant has never been scientifically determined. The claim is made that aluminium has been added to vaccines for a long time, so therefore it must be safe. That is illogical, and is further proof that vaccination is not based on science. The regulators keep on increasing the amount of aluminium that is allowed to be added, without doing any studies.[580]

There are no studies on the effects of injecting MSG into humans, and the same applies to most of the stabilizers, adjuvants, residuals, buffers, and preservatives that are in vaccines. There are plenty of studies that show that injecting rats with MSG causes brain damage, and one of them shows that injecting the rats with Calendula officinalis an hour after injecting the

MSG greatly reduces the amount of brain damage done by the MSG.[581]

Allergy to gelatin or yeast is an official contraindication to vaccines that contain those ingredients,[580] but vaccinators don't tell parents that these ingredients are about to be injected into their baby, so even if the parents know that the baby is allergic to gelatin or yeast, the official contraindication is useless.

Some vaccines have officially had the mercury removed, while other vaccines still officially contain mercury. In the US the law requires all ingredients to be listed on the package insert, unless the ingredient is a trade secret, or is DNA, or an endotoxin.[580] Two brands of vaccine that claimed to be free of mercury were tested in the USA and found to contain mercury.[582] A brand of vaccine that claimed to be free of mercury was tested in Australia and found to contain mercury.[583]

During the 60s and 70s experimental vaccines contained peanut oil, but those vaccines were not licensed for use in the USA. Peanut oil is not listed as an ingredient in modern vaccines, but there is suspicion that some do contain it.

The protein base on which vaccine germs are grown is called the substrate. Originally the substrate was obtained from animals, but in the 1960s the vaccine industry started using tissue from aborted babies and from malignant human tumours as substrates. None of the vaccines for children are made from malignant human tumours. Decades passed before the consumer became aware of the use of human cells, and now that awareness has erupted, the vaccine industry and their sycophants are working on damage control. There is heated discussion on the internet about the health implications and the ethical implications.

People who are anti-abortion but pro-vaccines have a range of excuses for supporting vaccines that contain aborted baby. "The babies were not aborted with the intention of using their bodies to make a vaccine." True. "Only two babies have been used to make vaccines." Not true. "The babies died a long time ago, and as the baby is dead anyway its body might as well be used to help mankind." "The cells have been dividing since they were removed from the fetus, so they are not the original cells." "The Vatican officially approves." True. "No religious leaders have condemned the use of aborted babies." Which only goes to show how spineless and unethical most religious leaders are. The religious leaders who are supposed to object to their flock being injected with pork, beef, and monkey are also spineless.

About the health implications, amateur vaccine defenders say that all the human cells are completely removed before the vaccine is injected, professional vaccine defenders say that the amount of residual DNA is too small to do any damage, and package inserts say that there are whole cells in the vaccine. Naturally the vaccine industry has not conducted any studies on the effects of injecting human cells or bits of human cells into babies. The claim for safety is based on the argument that human cells and fragments of human cells have already been injected into millions of people, and they are all fine. The flaw in that argument is that they are not all fine. Some are not even alive. When writers make the statement that the use of human tissue in vaccine manufacture is considered safe because it has been used for a long time on a lot of people, they usually give a reference, but that reference just refers to someone else making the same statement, without any research to back it up. Conferences have been held and reviews have been published, but no studies have been done. In 2005 the World Health Organisation stated, "The potential risk of this cellular DNA has been debated for over 40 years, without resolution".[584] The discussion has been about whether these cells might cause cancer, while the possibility that they might cause autism or autoimmune disease has not been discussed.

Dr. Paul Offit is a high profile vaccine defender, and he is one of the authors of the vaccine industry's 1513 page book called *Vaccines*.[585] The topic of vaccine ingredients is covered in the two chapters called, *Evolution of adjuvants across the centuries*, and *Vaccine additives and manufacturing residuals in the United States.* These two chapters confirm that neither adjuvants, additives, nor residual cells have been tested for safety. Another chapter, entitled *Vaccine Safety*, authored by Dr. Paul Offit and Dr. Frank DeStephano, does not mention the issue of safety of human cells. In this chapter there is a sub heading called *Vaccines contain DNA from aborted human fetuses.* There are two paragraphs in this sub section. The first paragraph chats about the two cell lines that are used in the US, and the second waffles about Vatican approval of the procedure. There is no mention of safety. Someone should tell them that Vatican approval is not the same thing as scientific studies.

Vaccine defenders say that the human DNA in vaccines is probably broken into small strands, and probably would not be able to integrate with host DNA. However, short strands of DNA can change the host DNA by integrating with it.[586,587]

The human cells need nourishment to grow, so they are fed with beef broth, which also ends up in the vaccines. In the laboratory, mitosis keeps on happening, as long as the cells are fed. A commonly used cell line is called WI-38 because it is taken from the 38th baby experimented on at the Wistar Institute. MRC-5 is taken from the fifth baby used by the Medical Research Council. WI-38 was female and aborted in Sweden, while MRC-5 was male and aborted in Britain.

After replicating in laboratories for six decades these human cells are now getting old, and are beginning to grow tumours. So a new human cell line has been developed in China. The baby was "aborted because of the presence of a uterine scar from a previous caesarean birth",[588] and the water bag method was used so that the baby would still be alive when the lungs were removed.[588] These cells are called Walvax-2, and they culture viruses better, and they replicate faster, than the sixty year old cells.[588]

"SCIENTIFIC RESEARCH HAS PROVEN THAT VACCINATION DOES NOT INCREASE THE RISK OF SIDS"

Vaccine Myth Number Thirteen: Some parents believe that their child died from vaccination just because he or she died after vaccination, but a temporal association does not mean that the vaccine was the cause. Scientific studies have shown that vaccination does not cause SIDS.

Around the world, medical authorities tell parents that it has been scientifically proven that vaccination does not cause SIDS, and sometimes they even tell parents that vaccination prevents SIDS. However, the studies that are used to justify these claims are scientifically flawed, and use research methods that do not adequately investigate the possibility that vaccination may actually increase the risk of SIDS in susceptible babies.

SIDS stands for Sudden Infant Death Syndrome, a phenomenon that claims the lives of thousands of apparently healthy babies every year. In a true case of SIDS there is no warning that death is about to occur, and an autopsy is done which finds no explanation for the death. It is called "crib death" in the Americas and "cot death" in other English speaking regions.

It is mysterious why a baby who seems to be perfectly alright can suddenly stop being alive. Some of these babies die because they stop breathing, others stop breathing because they die. These unexplained deaths have been happening since long before vaccination was invented,[589] and as records of its incidence were not kept until relatively recently, it is not possible to know whether the rate of SIDS in modern times is different to what it was in the distant past. Until such time as the natural causes of SIDS can be understood, it is important to find out which external factors increase the risk of it occurring. Some studies have been done, and it has emerged that smoking during pregnancy, a lack of breast-feeding, wrapping up the baby too warmly, and making the baby sleep on its tummy increases the risk. Characteristics and behaviour patterns of the parents, like the age and marital status of the mother, have been studied, but medical researchers steer away from looking at whether practices and customs of the medical establishment contribute to SIDS. When I pointed this out to a doctor at Auckland university who studies SIDS, he panicked and said it can *definitely* only be parental behaviour that affects SIDS. Unpopular topics for research include the use of prescription drugs during pregnancy, the habit of pulling on the baby's head during birth (which causes cervical subluxations), and the injection of vaccines into the baby. A study that compares the rate of SIDS in babies who have been vaccinated with the rate in those who have not been vaccinated has never been done.

The practice of placing babies on their tummies was actually introduced by doctors, but the medical establishment suffers corporate amnesia about that. It did not become a parental behaviour pattern until doctors told parents to do it. In the middle of the 20th century doctors started telling mothers to put *all* babies down on their tummies, because it had been observed that *premature* babies fared better that way.[590,591] Until then all cultures in the world had put babies down on their sides or on their backs, or carried them upright in a carry pack. Chiropractors warned that being face down impedes the functioning of a baby's autonomic nervous system, but they were ignored. The medics finally got around to doing some research on the matter, and the practice is now discouraged.

DISHONEST DIAGNOSIS

One of the scandalous features of SIDS is that many infant deaths that are quite obviously vaccine related end up being described as SIDS on the death certificate. Doctors do this deliberately to hide the fact that a vaccine caused the death. When dramatic symptoms have been present before the baby dies, the death cannot accurately be labelled as SIDS. Symptoms like a weird and nasty rash, prolonged high fever, blueness or lack of colour in the face, inability to move properly, violent black diarrhoea, inability to open the mouth, convulsions, and high-pitched screaming are all indications that something is wrong. SIDS is a death that happens when there has been no indication that anything is wrong.

When a doctor decides to write "SIDS" on the death certificate, and does not mention serious symptoms that were present before the baby's death on the report to the coroner, the coroner can only come to the conclusion that it was a case of SIDS. Parents I have spoken with had begged their doctors to tell the coroners about serious symptoms that were present before the baby died, but their doctors refused. Coroners cannot make a correct judgment when information is being withheld from them by the doctors. A death has also not been a case of SIDS when the baby has been exhibiting the quiet symptoms of vaccine damage before dying, like excessive sleeping, drowsiness, unresponsiveness, refusing food, petit mal epilepsy, or waving the arms in a strange way.

These cover ups of vaccine deaths are obviously not restricted to those I was involved with in New Zealand. When Barbara Loe Fisher looked into the FDA records, she found, among other scandalous things, that deaths of babies who screamed and shrieked uncontrollably for hours and hours every day from the day of vaccination to the day of death were labelled as "SIDS."[592]

SHAM STUDIES

While many deaths labelled as SIDS are not really cases of SIDS, we are still left with those which really are mysterious and inexplicable, and it would be ideal to know all the factors that increase the risk of SIDS happening. Vaccination has of course been suspected of being a factor that increases the risk of SIDS, and the vaccine establishment has produced a number of studies to try to persuade parents to believe that vaccination does not carry that risk.

One type of study that is often quoted as proving that vaccination does not cause SIDS is the temporal study. Central to these studies is the assumption that if vaccination were to cause a sudden unexplained death, it would do so within 12 hours, or 24 hours, or 48 hours, or 7 days, or 14 days.[593,594,595,596] No one knows what vaccines do once they get inside the body, so no one knows what the time frame is for a negative effect. Implying that they do know is fraudulent. Antibodies only start appearing two weeks after vaccination, and the production of antibodies continues for a few more weeks. The researchers, who are sometimes being paid to do the study by a vaccine manufacturer, have no basis for assuming that any negative effects of the ingredients in vaccines would take less time to develop than it takes for antibodies to develop.

One of the studies[596] that used assumptions about timing was done in the American state of Tennessee. The study was supported by the FDA and the CDC, partially funded by the NCHSR, and two of the four doctors in the study were Burroughs Wellcome Scholars in pharmacoepidemiology.[596] Burroughs Wellcome is a drug company that made DPT vaccine. The intention was to prove that DPT vaccine does not cause SIDS, but, ironically, it ended up proving the opposite. A typical statement about this study is,

> An American study of 129,834 babies looked at the possible risk factor between sudden infant death syndrome and immunisation against diphtheria, tetanus and pertussis. A total of 109 deaths in the ten-year period were classified as due to SIDS. The study published in 1988, concluded that there was no increase in the risk of SIDS after immunisation with the DTP vaccine.[597]

This sounds very impressive, but when you read the study, you find that it is not at all impressive. For a start, it is not a study of 129,834 babies; it is a study of 109 babies. All the other babies are discarded from the study, for one reason or another. The authors make no comparison between vaccinated and unvaccinated babies, and they use a dubious method to try to prove their point. Ironically, the method they used ends up showing that vaccination does increase the risk of SIDS.

The researchers had access to the records of all the babies born in four counties in the state of Tennessee. In those days polio vaccine and DPT vaccine (sometimes called DTP vaccine) were the only vaccines given to babies.

At the onset of the study the authors excluded the 1.9% of babies who had been vaccinated too early according to the schedule, and the 9% for whom there was no vaccination record, and the 14% who were known to be unvaccinated. That 14% should have been used as controls to be compared with the vaccinated babies, and the 1.9% who had been vaccinated too early should not have been ignored, because in the real world babies are often vaccinated earlier than the schedule recommends, and this might be a factor that contributes to SIDS.

The researchers then went on to exclude all the babies who had not died of SIDS, and they were left with 109 babies. They then measured the amount of time that had passed between the date of last vaccination and the date of death. They should instead have compared the incidence of deaths in the vaccinated group with the incidence of deaths in the 14% who were not vaccinated.

The study found that there was no increase in deaths in the seven days following vaccination, so the authors conclude that DPT vaccine does not cause SIDS. Pseudo-scientists who merely want to promote a particular point of view make baseless assumptions all the time. In this study they made the assumption that if DPT can cause SIDS, it will do so within seven days. There is no scientific reason to assume that the adverse effects of DPT vaccine, or any other vaccine, will occur only during the first seven days after vaccination. The length of time it takes for DPT to depress the immune system has not been researched, but studies of provocation disease suggest that immune suppression becomes more pronounced during the second week after vaccination. Earlier I mentioned that when there is a virulent polio virus in the environment, vaccination against other diseases suppresses the immune system, so that people who would otherwise not have caught polio, do catch it. I also mentioned a study of polio in Britain in 1949 which found that most cases of polio that are provoked by vaccination, start 8 to 17 days after vaccination.[380] Another study, covering 1951 to 1953, and done by the Medical Research Council in Britain, found that the greatest number of provocation cases started from 8 to 14 days after vaccination, with the next highest number of cases starting 15 to 21 days after.[598] In Bavaria, bad reactions to smallpox vaccination peaked 8 to 13 days after.[437]

These and other studies indicate that there is no basis for assuming that if DPT causes death, it will do so within seven days. In fact they indicate that death is more likely to occur from the eighth day onwards. In accordance with this pattern, the data from the Tennessee study showed that in the 8 to 15 days and 16 to 30 days periods there was a higher rate of SIDS than the national average. This suggests that DPT vaccine does cause SIDS. As I have mentioned, it is ironic that by attempting to prove that DPT vaccine does not cause SIDS, the Tennessee study authors ended up with data that supports the hypothesis that DPT vaccine does cause SIDS.

In an effort to increase the vaccination rate in New Zealand, a high-ranking medical bigwig issued a printed handout to be given to parents to persuade them that vaccination does not cause SIDS. On it he listed some studies, and next to the Tennessee study he wrote that it showed that "there was no increase in SIDS deaths among vaccinated vs unvaccinated children." This is a peculiar thing to say when the study did not compare vaccinated and unvaccinated children. It makes one wonder if medical bigwigs read anything while they are being paid large salaries by the taxpayer.

The Tennessee study was carried out in an attempt to convince parents that DPT vaccine does not cause SIDS, because there had been public disquiet about a cluster of deaths that had occurred soon after the administration of DPT in a part of Tennessee. Eleven babies had died, and nine of them had been injected with vials of vaccine from the same lot. Vaccine authorities had felt a need to convince the public that the deaths had been a coincidental cluster, and had not been caused by a "hot lot." The manufacturer of the vaccine, however, had its own strategy for maintaining public confidence in the vaccine. They circulated an in-house memo instructing employees that from then on, vials of vaccine from the same lot must be distributed widely, instead of each lot going to just one outlet. The purpose of this was to geographically spread any lots that were far more toxic than the officially acceptable level of toxicity. Being separated geographically would mean that if the lot did cause a high number of deaths, the deaths would not be clustered in one area, and would not attract public attention. The memo is dated 27 August 1979, and the first sentence states, "After the reporting of the SID cases in Tennessee, we discussed the merits of limiting distribution of a large number of vials from a single lot to a single state, county or city health department and obtained agreement from the senior management staff to proceed with such a plan." The last sentence ends with the phrase, "... make arrangements for split delivery."

One would expect Dr. Paul Offit, the world's most notorious vaccine defender, to actually read studies before he comments on them, yet in 1999 he made the shameless statement, "Several studies performed over the past 10 years comparing children who received the DTP vaccine with those who did not receive it proved that the DTP vaccine did not cause SIDS."[599] No such studies had been done during the previous 10 years, nor have they been done at any other time.

Another type of study used by researchers who are looking at the relationship between vaccination and SIDS is the case-control method. Case-control studies compare babies who died with babies who did not die. The researchers select a group of babies who died of SIDS within a particular geographical area, and these babies are called the cases. Each case is matched with two or three live babies who are called the controls. The vaccination history of the baby who has died is then compared with the vaccination histories of the two or three babies who have not died. Babies who have not received any vaccinations are excluded from the study.

In the case-control studies that have been published, researchers have found that when the live babies were at the age at which the case baby died, they had received more vaccine doses than those who had died. This leads the authors to conclude that vaccination does not cause SIDS, a happy conclusion for those who want to promote vaccination, but far from scientifically sound.

One problem with the case-control method is that it could be comparing fragile babies who are susceptible to dying from an immunological onslaught with tougher babies who can survive being injected with animal tissue, human tissue, attenuated germs, toxic metals, toxic chemicals, and genetically engineered yeast. Case-control studies can be useful for investigating something that is static at the time of death; for example,

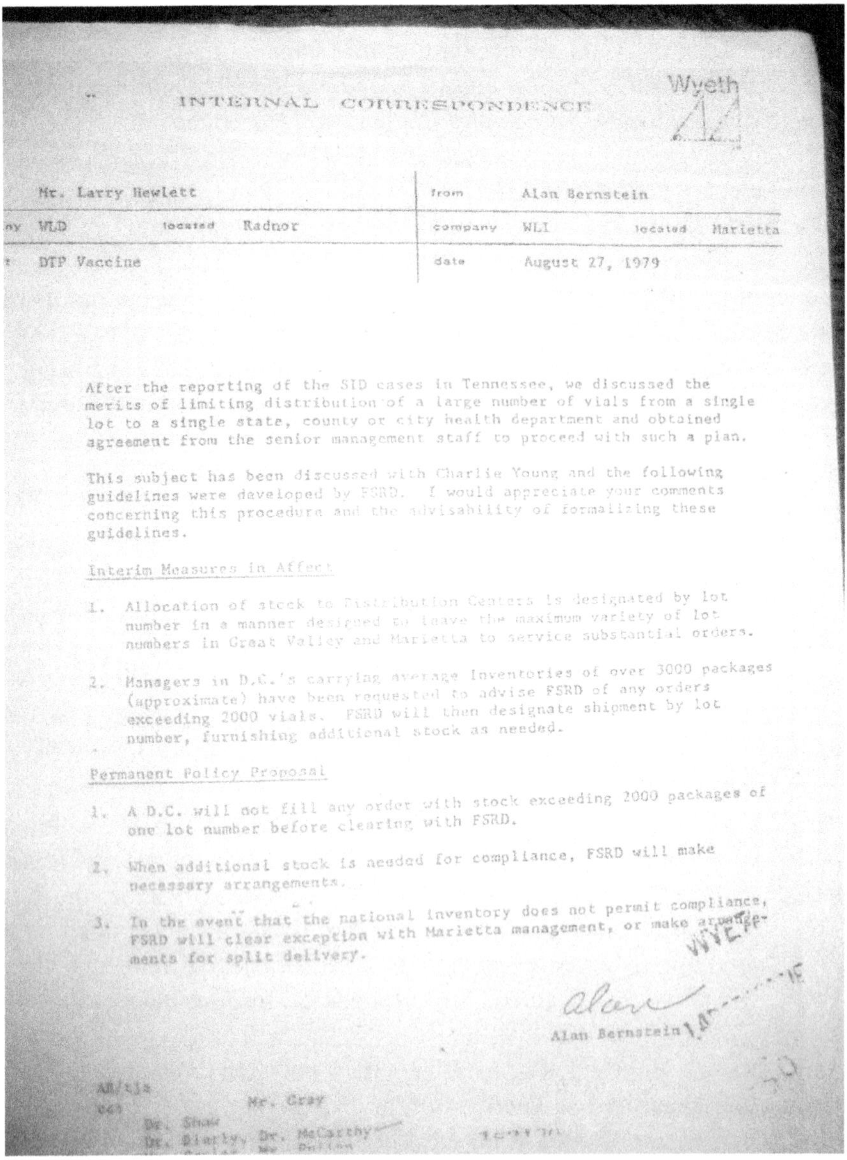

INTERNAL CORRESPONDENCE

Wyeth

Mr. Larry Hewlett		from	Alan Bernstein
WLD	located Radnor	company	WLI located Marietta
DTP Vaccine		date	August 27, 1979

After the reporting of the SID cases in Tennessee, we discussed the merits of limiting distribution of a large number of vials from a single lot to a single state, county or city health department and obtained agreement from the senior management staff to proceed with such a plan.

This subject has been discussed with Charlie Young and the following guidelines were developed by FSRD. I would appreciate your comments concerning this procedure and the advisability of formalizing these guidelines.

Interim Measures in Affect

1. Allocation of stock to Distribution Centers is designated by lot number in a manner designed to leave the maximum variety of lot numbers in Great Valley and Marietta to service substantial orders.

2. Managers in D.C.'s carrying average Inventories of over 3000 packages (approximate) have been requested to advise FSRD of any orders exceeding 2000 vials. FSRD will then designate shipment by lot number, furnishing additional stock as needed.

Permanent Policy Proposal

1. A D.C. will not fill any order with stock exceeding 2000 packages of one lot number before clearing with FSRD.

2. When additional stock is needed for compliance, FSRD will make necessary arrangements.

3. In the event that the national inventory does not permit compliance, FSRD will clear exception with Marietta management, or make arrangements for split delivery.

Alan

Alan Bernstein

AB/tjs

Mr. Gray

Dr. Shaw

Dr. Biarly, Dr. McCarthy

The 1979 memo.

whether the baby was sucking a pacifier, or lying face down, but the effects of vaccination are not static; they are ongoing, and they are unknown.

Case-control studies can also be useful if you take all the confounding factors into account, but in the case of vaccine susceptibility, no one yet knows what the confounding factors are. Controlling for factors that are known to increase the risk of SIDS does not mean that you are controlling for factors that increase the risk of SIDS from vaccination.

In the most recent case-control study, which was done in Germany, researchers found that the babies who died had had fewer vaccinations than the ones who were still alive, and that their vaccinations had been done later.[600] The latter finding may be significant. Parents can be reluctant to turn up on time for vaccinations when they feel that their baby is unusually fragile, or when they know that vaccine reactions run in the family. Some parents who are not keen on vaccination eventually comply because of the extreme pressure that is put on them, but they do it later than at the prescribed time.

Interestingly, the researchers did find a statistically significantly higher rate of developmental problems, hospital admissions, and special investigations, like x-rays or electrocardiograms, in the SIDS babies compared to the live babies.[601] This discovery might mean that the babies with these problems, who were only 22% of the SIDS babies, were more susceptible to dying unexpectedly, and that vaccination played no role in their deaths. Alternatively, it might mean that these babies were susceptible to an unknown effect of vaccination, and that vaccination killed them. The fact that these babies had had fewer doses of vaccine than the live babies with whom they were compared does not mean that they were not pushed over the edge by the vaccines that entered their bodies. It is illogical to say, "Baby A had 6 vaccines and is dead, while Baby B had 11 vaccines and is still alive, so that proves that vaccines had nothing to do with the death of Baby A."

Tobacco science compares smokers who died with smokers who did not die, instead of comparing smokers with non-smokers. Vaccine case-control studies are tobacco science.

Another problem with case-control studies is that they often begin with the data concerning all of the babies who are said to have died of SIDS in a selected geographical area, and then discard all the babies whose deaths were not really cases of SIDS. Back in the real world the babies' death certificates still say "SIDS", and the parents are still left with the impression that their child died of SIDS. One such study excluded 5% of the babies who had officially been declared to have died from SIDS.[594]

Low blood sugar might be a significant factor in SIDS. During a three-year period in New Zealand the blood sugar level of 84 babies who had died inexplicably was measured at autopsy, and in 81 of them, the level was found to be below the normal range.[602] Other studies have shown that low blood sugar is strongly associated with SIDS.[603,604,605,606] The whole cell whooping cough vaccine causes low blood sugar by stimulating insulin production.[301,607] The drop starts at about 8 days after injection, reaches its lowest point at about 12 days after injection, and becomes normal at about 24 days after injection.[608] When a person dies from low blood sugar they just lie there and quietly die. It is not obvious to an onlooker why the person has died. When a baby dies from low blood sugar, the symptoms fit the criteria of SIDS. Every vaccine that is recommended for infants should be tested to find out whether it causes blood sugar levels to drop at any time after vaccination. There is anecdotal evidence that the adult whooping cough vaccine causes a drop in blood sugar in pregnant women. An adult is able to rectify the situation, while an infant is not.

In 2010 a group of Canadian doctors published an article in which they considered the possibility that some children who were born with metabolic disorders may have died from the whole-cell whooping cough vaccine.[609] There are many types of metabolic disorders, but each one occurs in only a few children. The Canadian doctors paid special attention to a metabolic disorder called medium-chain acyl-CoA dehydrogenase deficiency. After considering the biological pathways in children with this disorder, the doctors concluded that one third of the babies who were born with it, and who were also injected with the whole-cell whooping cough vaccine, could have died from resultant low blood sugar.[609] Because medium-chain acyl-CoA dehydrogenase deficiency is very rare, this amounted to only 39 babies per year in the USA. The consideration of medium-chain acyl-CoA dehydrogenase deficiency was only done seven decades after the whole-cell whooping cough vaccine was introduced. There are more than four hundred metabolic disorders that need to be considered and studied. There may be other types of vulnerability apart from metabolic disorders that make babies susceptible to dying quietly from vaccination. Case-control studies are unable to detect deaths that occur because of individual susceptibility.

I once mentioned to a pediatrician who publishes articles about SIDS that I considered case-control studies to be an inadequate way of testing whether vaccination increases the risk of SIDS. He replied, "That's the way it has always been done." Valentina A. Soldatenkova is a mathematician and physicist who has also expressed the opinion that case-control studies are inadequate for assessing the relationship between vaccination and SIDS. In her published critique of the existing case-control studies, she criticises the study designs employed and the statistical methods used.610 The Institute of Medicine in the USA has the job of publishing complicated whitewashes about vaccine adverse effects, and they, of course, have done exactly that in regard to the question of whether vaccination may cause some cases of SIDS. Their lengthy report on the existing studies concludes that "the evidence does not support a causal link" between vaccination and SIDS. Soldatenkova says that their report should have stated that "the evidence is inadequate to accept or reject a causal relation between SIDS and vaccines."[610]

In recent years many countries have passed legislation that an autopsy must be done after every SIDS death, and they have introduced protocols that have to be followed. This is a great step forward. Previously autopsies were only done if someone felt like doing one, and they could decide what to investigate and what to ignore. One of the benefits of the introduction of autopsy protocols is that explanations are found for some of the otherwise mysterious deaths. In Germany, for example, a non-SIDS explanation for 11.2% of the SIDS deaths was found because of the autopsies.[611] In the future, the protocols will help to identify ways to reduce the incidence of SIDS. In the mean time they help to detect infant abuse, and they help to prevent parents from being falsely accused of abuse. The protocols also mean that doctors can no longer write off blatantly obvious reactions to vaccination as SIDS. The usefulness of the autopsies would be enhanced if they were to include an assessment of the blood sugar level at the time of death, which can be done even though blood glucose continues to be broken down for a short while after death.[603,612]

There are some absurd studies that have been done to "prove" that vaccination does not cause SIDS. One of them[613] compared the number of SIDS deaths that occurred in a geographical region during the time that a certain batch of DPT vaccine was in use with the number of deaths that had occurred in the same region when the previous batch of DPT had been in use. There were a similar number of deaths in the two time periods, so the conclusion was made that DPT does not cause SIDS. The fact that one batch of DPT is not shown to cause more deaths than another batch does not prove that DPT vaccine cannot cause death. Another absurd study surveyed the breathing patterns of "at risk" babies for twelve hours after injection with DPT vaccine.[593] They found that there was no increase in abnormal breathing during this time frame, and they concluded that this proves that vaccination does not cause SIDS. The twelve hour cut-off time is ridiculous, and periodic breathing is not an indicator of SIDS. Most babies who die of SIDS do not have a history of apnoea,[614,615] and in most cases asphyxiation is not the primary cause of death. Out of 629 autopsy reports on SIDS cases in New Zealand, only 4.9% showed evidence of oxygen deprivation.[602]

The studies that already exist range from seriously flawed to absurd, and the vaccine industry is assiduously avoiding carrying out studies that compare the incidence of SIDS in vaccinated and unvaccinated babies.

In 1988 New Zealand had the highest SIDS rate in the world. DPT vaccine was given at the tender age of six weeks, together with hepatitis B vaccine, and Maori and Pacific Islander babies were also given BCG vaccine at birth. At that time the SIDS rate in New Zealand was ten times higher than in Sweden. The vaccine schedules of the two countries had significant differences. Sweden omitted the whooping cough component of DPT, so that it became DT vaccine. They did not use hepatitis B vaccine at all, and they started the first dose of DT at 3 months.

At that same time, the SIDS rate in New Zealand was four times higher than in Britain. In Britain they did include the P component of DPT, but they started vaccinating at three and a half months and did not use hepatitis B.

The difference in vaccine schedules was not only reflected in the number of babies who died, it also affected the age at which they died. In Britain when DPT was started at 3.5 months, SIDS peaked during the fourth month. In New Zealand when DPT was started at 6 weeks, SIDS peaked during the second month. The medical establishment claims that SIDS happens at the age when vaccinations are being done because that is the "natural age" for SIDS. If there were such a thing as a "typical pattern for SIDS", the age at which SIDS deaths peaked would have been the same in New Zealand as it was in Britain.

MEDICAL MALICE

Some doctors take revenge on parents who say that their child is vaccine-damaged by accusing them of having caused the child's symptoms. In some countries the false accusation against a parent makes it possible for the vaccine-damaged child and its siblings to be taken away and put into foster care. Sometimes vaccination causes a haemorrhage in the brain, and in most cases when this happens the doctor says that the haemorrhage had no cause, and the fact that it happened soon after vaccination is just a coincidence. However, sometimes the doctor feels irate with the parent for believing that the vaccine is the cause, and decides to punish the parent by saying that the haemorrhage must have been caused by the baby being assaulted. This can result in a huge problem for the parent.

Another situation that can result from complaining about vaccine damage is that a mother can be accused of having the mental illness that goes by the large name of *Munchausen's syndrome by proxy*. Mothers who actually suffer from this mental illness deliberately make their children sick because they crave attention from the medical establishment. *Munchausen's syndrome by proxy* really does exist, but unfortunately the existence of the condition is sometimes used as a device by doctors who want to persecute an innocent mother.

In Wellington, New Zealand, a young mother took her vaccine-damaged child to hospital in the belief that the staff would be willing and able to help her. Instead of helping her they wrote "unfit parent" on the baby's record. This put the mother in a vulnerable position because when a comment like that is included on a medical record, it can be used to justify taking the child away from her. She asked Hilary Butler to help her get the words removed from the medical record. Eventually Hilary succeeded in getting the words removed, but the child never got compensation for the damage done by the vaccine.

Hilary says that it is common for a mother to be sent for mental evaluation when she reports that her child is vaccine-damaged, because the medics assume that someone who does not believe in vaccination must be mentally unstable. Having a properly conducted mental evaluation can be beneficial because it provides evidence that the mother has a sound mind, and there is less opportunity for her to be punished for her beliefs later on. The doctors who will not face up to reality about vaccine damage are the ones who have the psychological problem, not the parents. I propose the label *Denialus medicalus arrogantus* for their condition.

Many parents and baby minders have been wrongly accused and some even convicted of assaulting a baby after vaccination caused physical trauma or death. Some wrongful convictions have been overturned on appeal, while other victims are still waiting for justice. Alan Yurko is a parent who was wrongly convicted of harming his baby son after the baby was killed by vaccination. Vaccine zealots have created a number of websites that defame Alan Yurko, so let's take a look at what actually happened. The baby had been born prematurely, and had suffered from pneumonia and respiratory distress syndrome. Despite these contraindications he was injected with five vaccines at the age of eight weeks. The next day he developed a fever and started to fuss. Ten days later he elicited a high-pitched scream, but the parents were told not to worry. A couple of days later the baby stopped breathing, and Alan rushed him to hospital, where he was subjected to harmful interventions. The baby died, and Alan was blamed for his death because he had been alone with the baby when he stopped breathing. Alan was charged with murder, and rapidly, without proper legal representation, sentenced to life without parole. This all happened in the US state of Florida in 1997.

After six years of being incarcerated Alan was given the right to appeal the conviction. One hundred and fifty doctors from fifteen countries either did travel to Florida, or were prepared to travel to Florida, to testify that the baby had been killed by the vaccine. However, most of the doctors never appeared in court because the judge ended the case early and ordered that Alan be released. At this point Alan should have been able to walk free, but the prosecution immediately launched a new charge against him. They called it "manslaughter by negligence". Prosecutors like to have a track record of successful convictions, so their motivation for doing this was to enhance their careers, not to protect the reputation of vaccines. Alan's lawyers advised him to register "no contest" because that would mean he would be released immediately due to time already served, whereas if he did not register "no contest" he would be in jail forever, as the manslaughter case would never come to trial because the autopsy had been botched. "No contest" is not the same thing as pleading guilty, but Alan felt that he actually was guilty of negligence because he had allowed his son to be vaccinated, and he had not stopped the doctors from doing bad things to the baby in the hospital. This is how Alan expressed his belief that he was partly to blame for the death of his baby,

> I do take responsibility for the fact that as a parent I could have and should have taken a stronger role in his health care. I could have stopped his vaccinations, I could have been more inquiring and demanding about his care in the hospital, and I could have researched the health and science issues thoroughly. I did not do any of these things, and therefore I cannot escape the fact that I have some culpable negligence in his death.[616]

I do not agree. He was brought up to believe that doctors know what they are doing, and he believed it. That is not a crime.

Australia's own Archie Kalokerinos was one of the doctors who travelled to Florida to help release this innocent man. Archie was disappointed that he missed out on the opportunity of presenting to the court all his evidence that vaccines can cause brain haemorrhages. Alan's supporters and the doctors who were planning to testify on his behalf are now directing their energy towards helping other parents who are imprisoned because a vaccine killed their baby. Some of these parents face the death penalty.

CONTAMINATION AND THE ORIGIN OF AIDS

When vaccine cultures are grown on animal tissue they can accidentally pick up bacteria and viruses that are not supposed to be included in the vaccine. In 2010 bits of a pig virus were found in both brands of rotavirus vaccine, but the FDA said that the virus was not harmful to humans. In 1993 the virus that causes hog cholera in pigs, and diarrhoea and sterility in cows, was found in MMR vaccine,[617] and the researchers pointed out that the virus is associated with microcephaly and gastroenteritis in humans.[618,619]

Vaccines that contain ingredients like blood or pus from humans are also sometimes unintentionally contaminated. In 1942 twenty eight thousand five hundred and eighty five (28,585) American men who were waiting to be transported across the Atlantic in preparation for D-Day got hepatitis B from a contaminated yellow fever vaccine, and sixty two of them died.[620,621] The ingredients of that particular vaccine were chick embryos (with the head and spinal cord removed), mouse brains, and "normal human serum".[622]

Smallpox vaccine was said to be made from cowpox, but manufactures sometimes added pus from humans to make the reaction look more impressive, with the result that it was sometimes contaminated with germs of human diseases, like syphilis[623] or leprosy.[624,625,626] In 1884 one thousand seven hundred and seventy three (1,773) babies died because the smallpox vaccine with which they had been scratched contained human syphilis germs.[627]

There is a virus called the stealth virus that is associated with chronic fatigue syndrome in humans. A geneticist who is investigating this virus has found that it is more closely related to a monkey virus than to a human virus.[628,629] This finding implies that polio vaccine may have caused the current epidemic of chronic fatigue syndrome, so it has thrown the vaccine industry into damage control/research suppression mode.

Asian monkeys carry a type of virus called SV40. In the late 1950s it was discovered that American polio vaccine contained the SV40 virus,[630] and that this virus causes cancer in laboratory animals.[631,632] This is how *Time* magazine told the story of the capture and transportation of the Asian monkeys in 1954;

> In northern India's state of Uttar Pradesh last week, Moslem trappers working in teams of four set out their nets before dawn. While three hid, one man walked to a clump of trees. Loudly he called "Ao! ao! ao!" (Come! come! come!), and began to scatter grain. Rhesus monkeys scrambled down and followed his grain trail. When the monkeys got to the grain in the trap, a hidden operator pulled a cord and meshed them in the netting, an average dozen at a time.
>
> The Moslems (no Hindu will do this work because of religious scruples) stuffed the monkeys into bamboo cages and carried them on shoulder poles into Lucknow. The train hauled them 260 miles to New Delhi. There, 1,000 specimens carefully chosen for health and size (4 to 8 lbs. apiece) were collected. Then a four-engine transport flew them, with a full-time attendant to feed and water them three times a day, the 4,000 miles to London. Next, another plane and another attendant took them 3,000 miles to New York's Idlewild Airport and trucks carried them 700 miles to Okatie Farms in South Carolina. There the rhesus monkeys from India were caged with other hordes of "Java" (Cynomolgus) monkeys from the Philippines, to be used as ammunition in a great battle now being fought by medical science. The enemy: polio.
>
> Though Okatie Farms may receive 5,000 or more monkeys a month, the supply never catches up with the demand.[633]

In order to avoid the virus, the manufacturers started getting their monkeys from Africa instead of from Asia, because the virus does not exist in African monkeys. They sold all remaining stocks of contaminated vaccine to other countries. Despite knowing that it was contaminated, New Zealand and Australia bought stocks of this vaccine, because it was going cheap. Many studies have found the SV40 virus in malignant tumours in humans and in other types of cancer, but that is not proof that the virus caused those tumours to appear. However, recent advances in technology have enabled researchers to establish that the SV40 does cause cancer in human tissue.[634] It may never be possible to calculate how many cases of cancer were caused by contamination of polio vaccine with SV40.[635]

The contamination that has had the most far reaching consequences occurred in Central Africa in 1957, when the HIV virus, which causes AIDS, was transferred into humans through the use of an experimental polio vaccine.[636] HIV is not a monkey virus, it is a chimpanzee virus. In 1957 some American and European vaccine manufacturers built a compound in the African jungle, and their servants caught chimpanzees in the forest and brought them to the compound, where they were kept in cages until they were killed. The kidneys of these chimpanzees were then used to manufacture the experimental polio vaccine, which the manufacturers were hoping would be accepted by the FDA for use on Americans. It was not yet known that the HIV virus existed, and the manufacturers were unaware that some of the chimp kidneys that they were using contained the HIV virus. More than one million people in Central Africa were vaccinated with the experimental vaccine, but not all of them were vaccinated with the contaminated batch. A map of the region that was covered by the experimental vaccine was published in the British Medical Journal in 1958.[637] The earliest evidence of HIV in a human being was found in a blood sample that was taken in the Belgian Congo in 1959.[638,639,640] A retrospective search for cases of AIDS occurring before 1957 has not unearthed even one.

The polio vaccination campaign created a pool of HIV infected Africans, and the virus was spread further when the World Health Organisation vaccinated 96 million people against smallpox in the same region. When the World Health Organisation started their smallpox vaccination campaign they used jet injectors. Jet injectors do not need to be sterilised after each vaccination because they can shoot smallpox pus through the skin, without making contact with the skin. Only the pus goes through the skin, and the jet injector does not become contaminated with the recipient's blood. However, the jet injectors kept on breaking down, so in 1968 they changed to using the bifurcated needle. A bifurcated needle has two prongs at the tip, with a U shaped gap between them. A clump of pus hangs in the gap, clinging to the prongs. When the prongs are stabbed into the flesh of a recipient, some of the pus goes through the person's skin, and some of the person's blood in turn clings to the prongs. The bifurcated needle takes 20 minutes to sterilise, so they did not sterilise it between vaccinations.

> The bifurcated needle was developed by Wyeth Laboratories, Philadelphia, which allowed the eradication program to use it without patent costs. It became a basic tool in the program, and enabled a vaccinator to give up to 1,500 vaccinations a day.[641]

This is how small amounts of blood from people who already carried the HIV virus got into other people who were standing behind them in the same queue, and a million cases of AIDS suddenly appeared in Central Africa. Ed Hooper, the author of *The River: A journey to the source of HIV and AIDS*, interviewed a doctor who had "personally witnessed smallpox vaccinations being conducted in the Ruzizi Valley with no attempt being made to sterilize the needles between jabs."[642] At a party in Johannesburg in 1982 I overheard a group of doctors talking about the unhygienic way in which the smallpox vaccinations had been done in Central Africa.

In 1986 the World Health Organisation employed an outside consultant to go to Central Africa and find out what had caused AIDS to appear there. This researcher realised that the explosion of AIDS cases had followed the intensive smallpox vaccination campaign that the World Health Organisation had conducted in Zaire, Uganda, Tanzania, Zambia, Malawi, Rwanda, and Burundi. The World Health Organisation's brag book about the vaccination campaign says,

> In the African Region, Zaire strategically had the highest priority for the allocation of WHO resources.[643]

The outside consultant concluded that the vaccination campaign had sparked AIDS. When he reported his findings to the World Health Organisation, they fired him. So he went to the London Times with his story. On the 11th May 1987 the London Times carried a front page article entitled *Smallpox vaccine 'triggered Aids virus'*. It told how the countries in which smallpox vaccination was done were the countries in which AIDS had suddenly appeared, and how the researcher had been fired by the World Health Organisation for making that discovery.

At this point the plot thickens. It is normal procedure for any news item that appears in the British press to be networked to the USA on the same day, so that when the sun comes up in the Americas, the morning papers have already printed the story. But this story was intercepted. American readers were not going to be allowed to be exposed to this piece of information. Jon Rappaport investigated the blackout, and found that the news had been cut off in London, so that it never reached the news distributors at Associated Press, Reuters, nor United Press International.[644]

One of the reasons that the vaccine industry is increasingly moving towards manufacturing vaccines on aborted babies is that human tissue is not likely to be contaminated with unwanted microbes. However, the main reason is that it is much cheaper to buy the bodies of aborted babies than it is to breed animals or to obtain animals from the wild. Organs that have been stolen from babies who have died of SIDS are not suitable for manufacturing vaccines, because when babies have lived out in the world for a while, they have germs and antibodies in their tissue. Polio vaccine made on aborted babies was already being used in 1962.[645] Naturally the vaccine industry does not want its customer base to know that they and their children are being fed with or injected with cells from aborted babies, which is why the matter is not discussed in the mainstream media.

COPING WITH DISAPPROVAL

If you decide to keep your child vaccine free, or to decline some of the vaccines on the schedule, you not only have to contend with irate officials, you also have to deal with relatives and friends who voice their disapproval and try to make you conform. This can cause emotional stress and drain the energy of new parents. Before you decide how to handle your critics, consider their reasons for condemning you. Be careful to differentiate between people who want to persuade you to "immunise" because they are genuinely concerned about the welfare of your baby, and those who are just angry with you because you threaten their belief in modern medicine. For some people vaccination is a religion, and they get very upset when they meet a non-believer.

When someone is genuinely concerned that you are exposing your baby to dangerous diseases by not vaccinating, you owe them an explanation for your decision. That does not mean that they will necessarily listen, but give them a chance. They should be willing to discuss the matter with you in a civilized manner. It is not easy for people to come to terms with the facts when their own children have been vaccinated, but some do. You will find that elderly people who had their children before the vaccine industry went rampant are less likely to feel threatened by your decision, and therefore are less likely to condemn you. I have found that elderly people who were nurses during the era of smallpox vaccination tend to have severe doubts about the practice of vaccination.

There is no point in trying to defend your decision to a vaccine zealot who is angry with you and is not actually interested in knowing your reasons for not vaccinating. This kind of person just wants to make you conform so that they can feel comfortable about their beliefs. They are likely to stop bothering you sooner than the ones who are genuinely concerned about your baby, but they will be more stressful to cope with while they are still harassing you. It is no fun having accusations flung at you, and then not being given a chance to explain. With this kind of person it is best to try to distance yourself from the emotional baggage that is being thrown at you, and to try to work out what is making them behave so badly. It might be because they love modern medicine and cannot accept that one part of it is not perfect, or because they don't want to think about what they have done to their children, or perhaps they are afraid that you are going to start an epidemic. Defending yourself is not going to work because they are not interested in your reasons.

The people who condemn you the most are the ones who are the least likely to be willing to look at scientific information about vaccination. If you offer them literature and documentation to read, and they refuse, then you have grounds for telling them that they are not to mention the subject again until they have read what you are offering. No matter what evidence you present to some people, they will continue to cling to the myths of vaccination. If you have photocopies of articles from medical journals they will refuse to look at them. If you tell them about someone you know who suffered a severe injury from vaccination they will scoff at it. If you try to talk about the history of diseases or the failure of vaccines, they won't want to know.

Some people get angry with you for "endangering" their children. Many vaccine believing parents think that vaccine free children are spewing out germs and will make their vaccinated children get sick with diseases that they have been vaccinated against. This is of course irrational if they believe that vaccination works, but although you know that they are being irrational, their attacks on you can still cause a lot of stress. Raising a child is stressful enough without having to cope with a barrage of criticism. If you are being harassed by people telling you that you are bad parents because you are not "protecting" your child with vaccination, you would find it helpful to make contact with other vaccine free families. They are also being accused and abused, so they will have a good understanding of your situation.

One of the vicious tactics of the vaccine industry is to make new parents fearful of people of any age who have not recently been jabbed with whooping cough vaccine. This is succeeding in causing great hurt in family members who are not allowed to get to know the new arrival.

Some people do not want to take responsibility for their children's health, so they prefer to let a bureaucracy make the decisions. My husband offered a business colleague some information about vaccination, and the latter displayed unusual honesty when refusing to read it. He said, "If I don't immunise my children and they get sick, it would be my fault. If I do immunise them and they get sick, then the doctor is to blame. So it's better to have it done."

TREATING VACCINE DAMAGE

Homoeopaths have been treating vaccine damage ever since Edward Jenner started creating vaccine damage, but nowadays there are many approaches to helping those who have been harmed by vaccines. I am going to discuss the three approaches that I have seen to be effective; homoeopathy, conductive education, and cranial osteopathy, while not claiming that they are the only methods for treating vaccine damage.

Homoeopathic treatment of vaccine damage is usually done with a potentised version of the vaccine that did the damage, but some homoeopaths prefer to prescribe a constitutional remedy first. A potentised vaccine usually brings about some degree of improvement in the victim's condition. Sometimes the improvement is dramatic and total, but usually it does not go that far. The potentised form of DPT vaccine, for example, is often effective at curing chronic ear problems and asthma in vaccinated children, but it does not reverse severe brain damage. Likewise, potentised BCG vaccine usually helps the lymph system recover from BCG.

It is sensible to homoeopathically antidote vaccines one at a time, in the reverse order to which they were administered. Enough time should be allowed to lapse between each antidote, so that all the symptoms associated with that vaccine can work their way out of the body. Sometimes when a homoeopathically potentised vaccine is used to treat the symptoms that are known to have arisen as a result of that particular vaccine, other symptoms unexpectedly clear up too. With hindsight, this makes the victim or the victim's parents realise that those symptoms arose soon after vaccination, and that they must have also been caused by the vaccine.

It is ideal for the potentised vaccine to be made from the same brand as the vaccine that did the harm. This is because different manufacturers put different ingredients into their vaccines, along with the antigens that are there to create antibodies to the target diseases. Ingredients like aluminium, formaldehyde, mercury, animal tissue, animal blood, human tissue, human blood, and emulsifiers may have contributed to the harm. It is even more ideal for the remedy to be made from the same batch as the vaccine that did the damage, as vaccines differ from batch to batch, and, more importantly, if there is a contaminating microbe in a particular batch, it would be useful to have the contaminant potentised as well. For instance, if a person has a condition like chronic fatigue syndrome that was caused by measles vaccine, the extra viruses in the vaccine mixture could be contributing to the slow but relentless attack on the muscles. Antidoting the measles vaccine with homoeopathically potentised measles vaccine from another batch that does not contain the contaminating virus might only solve part of the problem.

When I was living in New Zealand I saw potentised MMR vaccine work very well on a little boy whose reaction started two days after vaccination. From the time he woke up he was hyperactive. "Off his head," was the phrase his mother used. He also had a weird rash. That night he had difficulty sleeping, and the next day he had changed to being listless and floppy, rubbing his head as if it hurt, and sometimes seeming semiconscious. A fever developed and in the afternoon he had a major convulsion. An ambulance took him to hospital, where they gave him paracetamol/tylenol. One of the doctors told the parents that vaccine reactions do not start until 3 or 4 days after vaccination, so his symptoms could not have been caused by the vaccine. (When the reaction does start 3 or 4 days after, they tell parents that it is not a vaccine reaction, because it did not start straight after the injection.) Blood tests and X rays found nothing, and the toddler was much improved the next day, so he was discharged. There were no more convulsions, and the mother thought that he was better because the weird rash had gone, and he was neither wreaking havoc in the house, nor flopping into an immobile state.

The doctor who had administered the vaccine refused to report the incident to the Adverse Reactions Committee. The mother contacted me to express her fury about what had happened to her boy, and she was especially angry that she had not been warned of the possibility of a convulsion before she agreed to vaccination. "If I had known that this could happen, I wouldn't have had him vaccinated," she said.

"That's why they didn't tell you," I replied.

She wanted to warn other parents through the media. Television New Zealand had a programme after the news on Channel One called *The Holmes Show,* which presented itself as a programme that fearlessly exposed the wrongs of the world. The mother thought that this would be a suitable platform for her to warn other mothers. A junior journalist from the programme team was keen to do the story, and she was optimistic that it would be permitted. I warned them that Paul Holmes, the programme director, was an ardent supporter of vaccination. They persevered in their attempts to get the story aired, but it was not permitted.

During my first conversation with the mother, I asked tactful but pointed questions about the child's condition. Her feeling at that time was one of great relief that it was all over, but I knew that there was no certainty that it really was all over. As is often the case, the subtle early symptoms of long-term brain damage were present, but she had not recognised them. The toddler was clumsy and uncoordinated, and he was not alert. He was troubled and listless, and unable to settle. I was placed in the position of having to recommend homoeopathic treatment for those symptoms, without wanting to scare her. She was an intelligent lady, and my guarded questions did scare her.

I gave her the phone number of her nearest homoeopathic chemist, and she ordered six doses of *MMR 30*. After only one dose he reverted back to being the same little boy he had been before the vaccination. His clumsy lack of coordination just evaporated, he went back to sleeping through the night, and he began to play again. It was only when she saw the dramatic change brought about by the remedy that she fully realised how changed he had been by the vaccine reaction. I spoke to her again three days after he had had the potentised MMR.

"He's pottering and playing again. I hadn't noticed that he had stopped playing. The difference is quite remarkable. It's lovely having him play again. I can do things." Whew. The mother had learned enough during her crash course on vaccine damage to realise that the change brought about by the remedy meant that the insidious progress of brain damage had been halted, and that their family had had a narrow escape. Perhaps one of the reasons why the antidote was so effective in this case was that it was made from the same brand of vaccine as had been injected into the boy, which meant that it contained the same type of egg yolk, the same toxic metals, and so on, as had been in the vaccine. I knew that it was made from the same batch of vaccine because I knew the person who had obtained a vial of the vaccine from a doctor and taken it to the homoeopathic chemist to potentise. Another factor would be the timing. The vibration of the remedy cut off the deterioration of the central nervous system before it had gone too far.

When I was twenty-six years old and had been under homoeopathic treatment for six months, my practitioner decided that it was time to antidote the ten smallpox vaccinations that I had had between the ages of twelve and twenty four. Nine of the vaccinations had been done with the vaccine gunk that was manufactured in Johannesburg. The other one was done at Heathrow Airport, so I do not know in which country the vaccine was manufactured. I know that it was not manufactured in Britain as the British government banned the manufacture of smallpox vaccine in 1932 because the means of production was so cruel to cows. Smallpox vaccine was made by slicing long slits along the flanks of cows and rubbing pus into the wounds. The cows' heads were braced so that they could not lick the wounds. The pus then foamed and grew in volume, and was harvested off the flanks of the cows and stored in vials. It was kept in the vials until it was scratched into the skin of humans. Although this procedure had been banned in Britain, the British government was not concerned about cruelty to foreign cows, so they purchased the vaccine from other countries.

The remedy that the homoeopath gave me had been made by potentising the brand of smallpox vaccine that had been produced in Johannesburg. I only had one dose, I do not know in what potency, and it caused a radical improvement in my state of health. I was already on the upward path to good health because of having been under homoeopathic treatment for six months, but the effect of that potentised smallpox vaccine was like jumping up a cliff on the path.

A Dutch medical doctor who is also a homoeopathic practitioner has discovered that the benefits of antidoting vaccines using potentised versions of the vaccine can be enhanced by also antidoting the other toxic insults to which a person has been subjected during his or her early years.[646] He is Dr. Tinus Smits, and he and the people who use his method have had spectacular success at curing conditions like vaccine-induced autism and ADHD. Dr. Smits says that real brain damage is not curable, but "most autistic children are curable because their brains are not damaged, but blocked".[646] Orthomolecular medicine and diet restrictions are used in combination with the homoeopathic treatment. The aim of the orthomolecular treatment is to support the healing process, not to compensate for deficiencies, because the conditions being treated are not deficiency diseases.

Occupational therapists in New Zealand have used a Hungarian method of brain training to bring about great improvements in children who are brain damaged by vaccination. The method was developed during the 1940s by Professor András Pető, who called it "conductive education". He was taking advantage of the neuroplasticity of the human brain long before the medical establishment caught up with the fact that the brain has neuroplasticity. The Hungarian government established a dedicated institute named the *Peto Institute* in Budapest in 1950. The aim of the treatment is to train the damaged nervous system to form new neural connections. The most common cause of central nervous system damage in young children is stroke, which sometimes occurs before birth. However, the central nervous system can also be damaged by a bad reaction to vaccination. Children from all over the world are treated at the Peto Institute, and there is also a network of satellite clinics in other countries.

The Peto Institute does not accept cases that cannot be helped by conductive education. Conditions that fall under the umbrella of "cerebral palsy" are ones that they will consider, but they cannot help children with Rhett's Syndrome, autism, myopathy, progressive neurological disease, or serious intelligence deficits. Professionals who can incorporate conductive education into their work, like teachers, nurses, and physiotherapists, can undergo training in Budapest or at one of the satellite clinics.

Some children who have developed neurological problems from vaccination can be helped by cranial osteopathy. Some osteopaths take on extra training in order to specialise as cranial osteopaths, and they are trained to gently move the bones of the skull into the correct position. The treatment is painless; it feels like the osteopath is just lightly touching the head and neck, but the results are profound. Pharmaceutical medicine adheres to the medieval belief that the bones of the cranium are fused to one another, forming a solid plate. However, the bones are not fused together, and they can move out of their correct position. The movement may be less than a millimetre, but that is enough to have a negative impact on the rest of the body. Sometimes a baby's skull bones do not get back into the right position after moulding for birth, and this can affect things like the immune system or the endocrine system. A mild blow on the head of an adult can move a bone out of position, and a variety of health problems, including migraines, can result. It makes sense that moving the bones of the skull back into their correct position would fix certain problems, but why it helps with neurological problems from vaccination will remain a matter for speculation until research provides the answer.

Some babies who react to DPT vaccine suffer from persistent high-pitched screaming while they are in the acute phase of the reaction. I know of a case where a two-year-old girl who had reacted to DPT vaccine as a baby let out a long, high-pitched scream when a cranial osteopath released a particular band of tension through her head. Her mother was shaken because it sounded just like that terrible scream she had heard in the days after DPT. After the treatment the child was able to coordinate in ways that she had not been able to do before the treatment.

THE MYTH THAT *THUJA* PREVENTS VACCINE DAMAGE.

A myth has arisen that the homoeopathic remedy called *thuja* antidotes all vaccines. It is such a compelling myth that some parents think that if they give their child *thuja 30* a few minutes after the child has been vaccinated, adverse reactions will not be possible. *Thuja* is often, but not always, the correct remedy to treat the adverse effects of smallpox vaccination, but it does not match the symptoms of vaccine damage from modern vaccines.

The possible origin of the myth is a little book from the 1880s, called *Vaccinosis*, by J. Comptom Burnett MD.[647] This little book describes how the author cured many people who had been suffering from serious long-term effects of smallpox vaccination. The case histories are fascinating, but nowhere does the author suggest that a century later, parents will be able to protect their babies from the concoction of DPTHibIPVHepB by giving them a dose of *thuja* as they walk out of the clinic.

In his book Compton Burnett describes the case of a little girl with ringworm that was complicated by residual immune system disturbance from smallpox vaccine. The ringworm did not respond to *bacillinum 30,* which is the usual remedy for ringworm, but when *thuja* was given, the scabby nature of the ringworm changed, and *bacillinum 30* was then able to cure the ringworm. This principle still applies today - get the vaccine damage out of the way, and the door opens for other remedies to be effective.

Another of Compton Burnett's patients was a 19-year-old girl who had been vaccinated against smallpox as a baby, vaccinated again at the age of seven years, caught smallpox at the age of nine years, and was vaccinated again at the age of 14 years. She was suffering from severe headaches twice a week, an enlarged liver, occasional boils, and from what is now called chronic fatigue syndrome. He used a constitutional remedy, and a month later she was a little better. He then gave her low potency *thuja* every day for a month, and she had only one headache during that time. Her energy level also improved. Then he gave her a higher potency of *thuja,* and she developed nausea and fever, and broke out in smallpox pustules. Her mother said that the pustules looked exactly like the ones that were on her skin when she had smallpox. They lasted five days before turning yellow and then fading away. After that she was completely cured. This course of events strongly suggests that she had been suffering residual problems from the smallpox disease as well as from the vaccinations.

Compton Burnett also tells of a baby who became very ill from drinking the milk of a wet nurse who had been vaccinated for smallpox. The wet nurse only had a sore arm and an eruption of pus at the site of vaccination, but the baby was in dire straits. The baby and the wet nurse were treated with *thuja*, and both recovered rapidly.

THE MYTH THAT VACCINES CAN BE ANTIDOTED BY "DETOXIFICATION"

Growing awareness about the many poisons that are contained in vaccines has led some people to believe that toxins are the *only* problem in vaccines, and that the harm done by vaccination can be undone solely by a process of detoxification. Of course one does not improve a person's health by injecting him or her with toxic substances like mercury, aluminium, and formaldehyde, but the toxins are only a part of the problem. Every ingredient in a vaccine is an antigen that causes an immune response, and the ramifications of that response can be quite complicated. Vaccine damage is not simply a matter of an overload of toxins.

Some of the ingredients in vaccines are not toxic when eaten, but are clearly unsuitable for injecting into a baby. For instance, gelatine is not toxic when eaten, but it has the potential to be harmful when it is injected. The amount that is injected is tiny, but if it generates an insidious immune response that changes something in the body, simply removing the gelatine from the body is not going to make the body revert back to how it was before the injection. Substances that are added to vaccines to make them create more antibodies are called adjuvants, and even when they are injected on their own they can cause immune-mediated or autoimmune reactions.[648,649,650] The role of adjuvants in causing vaccine reactions is being researched, and preliminary studies suggest that the adjuvants can cause serious autoimmune and inflammatory conditions, as well as brain injury.[651,652] Merely removing the adjuvant from the body, if such a thing can be done by detoxification, would not stop an autoimmune process that has been set in motion.

No one has researched the effect of injecting human cells into babies. It obviously does not have a dire effect on the majority of children, but for those who are affected, detoxification is not the solution. While detoxification has its place in our polluted world, it is not the answer to vaccine damage.

"HOMOEOPATHIC VACCINATION CAN BE USED AS A SUBSTITUTE FOR BIOLOGICAL VACCINATION"

Vaccine Myth Number Fourteen: By giving a baby the homoeopathic remedy that would be used to cure an infectious disease, we can ensure that the child will never catch the disease.

Society has been seduced by the concept of artificial immunisation, so some people fall into the trap of believing that a "homoeopathic vaccine" will protect their child from infectious disease. Homoeopaths have become polarised about the issue of "homoeopathic immunisation". I have seen heated arguments break out at seminars between individuals who oppose the practice and those who support it. I do not support "homoeopathic vaccination" because I believe that it does not stimulate immunity to the scary diseases that we need to avoid, and that it can cause insidious long-term adverse effects. It also concerns me that proponents of "homoeopathic immunisation" want to prevent the beneficial, self-resolving diseases, and that they base their schedule on the local vaccination schedule. Vaccination schedules are not based on scientific reasoning, so homoeopaths who mimic the schedules demonstrate a lack of understanding about vaccination and immunity.

The people who promote homoeopathic vaccination say that if a baby is given a remedy that would normally be used to treat a particular disease, it will make the baby immune to that disease for life. However, no properly controlled studies have been done to assess effectiveness over time. Combining common sense with knowledge of how homoeopathic remedies work leads me to the conclusion that treating a disease in advance is both unsafe and ineffective. I believe that homoeopathic remedies should not be given to a person who has no symptoms in the hope that it will prevent an infection in the future.

The claim that "homoeopathic immunisation" is an effective procedure rests mainly on anecdotal reports of people not contracting a disease after being administered with a remedy. An absurd but oft quoted claim for effectiveness is that the potentised remedy *diphtherium* was able to make people immune to diphtheria, because it made them react positively to the Schick test. The Schick test is an unscientific, inaccurate skin test that has been discarded by the medical establishment. It tried to assess immunity to diphtheria by scratching disease matter into the skin, and then seeing if there was a reaction. If a potentised remedy could make a person "Schick positive", it would be of no consequence anyway. Perhaps the people who are selling this remedy to try to prevent diphtheria are not aware that diphtheria naturally ceased to be a threat in the environment more than fifty years ago.

Can a medicine that contains nothing more than a vibration alter the state of a person's vital energy in a way that would make the person unable to contract a specific disease for the rest of his or her life? That question will finally be answered when the technology to measure the vital energy in the body is invented, but in the meantime the evidence suggests that it cannot. Earlier I described how arnica keeps working in the body for a while after it is administered. The same thing happens with other remedies. At present we can judge how long a remedy keeps working by the fact that the improvement in the patient's condition stops when the remedy stops working. Most remedies stop having an effect within a month. This suggests that a remedy given to a healthy person would only alter the vital energy for a month at the most, if it alters it at all. It is probable that the vibration is a type of wave, and when a wave is set in motion it gradually loses energy and peters out. If you throw a stone into a still pool of water, rings of waves will move out from where the stone hits the surface, until they lose their energy and the surface of the pond becomes still again. Even if the energy from a homoeopathic remedy were able to keep going in the human body for five decades, the owner of the body would have to avoid any contact with the substances that antidote homoeopathic remedies for that whole time, or the wave would stop immediately.

It could be argued that although the vibration does not last, what it alters in the body does last. If the remedy is altering something in a healthy body, what is it altering? When homoeopathy is used as an intervention, the vibration alters something that is wrong in the body, and makes it right. But when it is used as prevention, the vibration is supposed to change something that is right into something that is right. It is a bad principle to try to fix something that is not broken. It seems far more sensible to stay healthy by not consuming toxic or refined food, and by getting enough sleep and exercise.

With "homoeopathic immunisation" there is also the problem that a remedy is being chosen for a person who has no symptoms. When a polio epidemic breaks out, a homoeopath has to take a look at each patient who is suffering from polio, before being able to choose the right remedy to cure that individual patient. Each polio epidemic is caused by a slightly different virus, and presents slightly different symptoms, and each victim reacts slightly differently to each virus. So how can you be sure you are choosing the right remedy 10 years before the epidemic breaks out? To give a baby three doses of one of the remedies for polio, and then tell the parents that no polio virus will ever be able to harm the child, is outrageously irresponsible. If a child has *sativa 30* as a baby, and 10 years later is exposed to a polio virus that causes symptoms that need treatment by *gelsemium 30*, or *phytolacca 30*, or *eupatorium 30*, or *aethusa 30,* or *physostigma 30*, what happens then? The homoeopaths who are using "homoeopathic immunisation" to prevent polio at present are getting away with it because there is no virulent polio virus in the environment. If the polio virus becomes virulent again, parental complacency about the danger could have tragic results.

If a potentised version of the polio vaccine were used, it would contain the vibration of the three main strains of polio virus. This is one of the remedies to consider when treating a patient with polio, or with paralysis caused by polio vaccine. But to give it to a baby and claim it will alter the vital force for the rest of the baby's life is absurd. Even if an introduced vibration could last that long in the body, it would only do so if the person never brushes their teeth with ordinary toothpaste, never picks the leaf of a eucalyptus tree and crushes it in their fingers, never catches a whiff of mosquito repellent, never has an X ray, is never on the same bus as someone chewing mint-flavoured gum, and never uses one of a thousand other homoeopathic remedies that can de-activate the polio vibration. Even if the introduced vibration could last for decades in the body, it would be totally impractical in the real world.

Some homoeopaths who support the practice do not go so far as to claim that a potentised remedy can make a person immune for life. They say that it can make a difference for a few weeks, and therefore should be used during epidemics. They do not restrict this advice to trying to prevent undesirable infectious diseases, but also recommend that parents attempt to prevent the developmental childhood diseases.

If an epidemic of polio broke out in the region where I live, I would know that my children were being exposed to a virulent polio virus, because the polio virus floats in the air. I would not give them a potentised remedy to try to protect them. I would become very vigilant about what they were eating, and what activities they were doing. Nutrition is of prime importance in preventing polio, and sufficient rest comes second. Providing children with wholesome substances to eat requires far more effort than making them suck a sweet tasting little homoeopathic pill, but no effort should be spared in trying to prevent polio. Caring for a child who has been crippled by the polio virus would require far more effort. Of course if my efforts failed and one of them did actually contract polio, I would not hesitate to use homoeopathy to cure the disease. Hundreds of studies which confirm that homoeopathy is an effective method of curing disease have been done. A few of them have even made it into medical journals. If ever any large-scale, long-term, properly controlled studies are done, and they show that "homoeopathic immunisation" is effective, I would reconsider my standpoint on effectiveness. However, I would still want solid scientific evidence that giving a potentised remedy to someone with no symptoms does not cause adverse effects.

Homoeopathic remedies that are made by potentising disease matter are called nosodes. Morbillinum, which is made from measles virus, is an example of a nosode. Classical homoeopaths say that giving a non-indicated nosode to a healthy person can cause profound negative changes in the body. When a nosode like morbillinum is given in the hope of preventing measles at some time in the future, that is an example of giving a non-indicated nosode. Giving a non-indicated nosode to a baby is particularly risky, because babies are very sensitive to waves and vibrations. It is possible that introducing the vibration of potentised viruses or bacteria could disrupt a baby's electromagnetic field, without the effects of the disruption being immediately obvious. It is easy to overlook the subtle long-term adverse effects of crude vaccines if you are not watching out for them. How much easier it would be to miss any subtle, insidious, long-term adverse effects of a potentised virus. When a homoeopath gave me potentised smallpox vaccine in 1980 I was showing symptoms of chronic illness from the ten vaccinations to which I had been subjected between 1965 and 1978. She was a classical homoeopath who would never have used that remedy to try to prevent smallpox.

Some babies and toddlers do not exhibit any symptoms after they are given a nosode, while others show what may be considered "trivial" symptoms, like becoming mucusy, or grumpy, or listless. Symptoms like these are not trivial, because they indicate that the baby's vital force has been disturbed. Some children whoop after having the whooping cough nosode. What does this mean about what has happened in their bodies? Some children who are given the measles nosode show behavioural symptoms of measles about a month afterwards, and then they break out in an atypical measles rash. This makes me shudder. Some children who have the measles nosode in infancy do get measles during childhood, but they do not get proper measles. They get one of a variety of forms of atypical measles. That is not a sign of good health.

Some people believe that the symptoms provoked by "homoeopathic immunisation" are merely the expulsion of a miasm, and are good for the child. A miasm is an inherited weakness. For example, there is the miasm of syphilis, which is medically recognised as coming down 14 generations, but is recognised by homoeopaths as having an effect for much longer than that. When you treat a miasm, you should base the choice of remedy on the presence of symptoms, not on a vaccination schedule developed by the local pharmaphiles. Proponents of "homoeopathic immunisation" recommend giving the same number of doses of their remedy as the vaccinators recommend giving their vaccine. This would amuse me if it were not so scary. If a homoeopath wants to treat a miasm, he or she should treat the miasm, not prescribe a "homoeopathic immunisation" and then claim to be treating a miasm.

To find out if trying to prevent measles with nosodes is beneficial, recipients should be followed up for at least thirty years, and their chronic disease rates should be compared with people who have had no interventions to try to prevent measles. For instance, the incidence of cancer should be compared in;

* those who had the nosode,
* those who had measles,
* those who had neither,
* and those who had both.

Only then will we be able to make concrete judgments about whether "homoeopathic immunisation" is safe.

I am particularly unhappy that the potentised Epstein Barr virus is sometimes given to babies with the promise that it will prevent glandular fever (infectious mononucleosis). This is a very nasty virus which can cause diverse things like chronic fatigue syndrome and cancer. I believe that introducing the vibration of the Epstein Barr virus into the bodies of very young babies will harm those who do not have a strong vital force. Dr. Dorothy Shepherd argues eloquently against the injection of cells and chemicals into the human body on the grounds that they can cause physical disease by changing the vibration of the body's cells.[653] But her arguments can be used equally strongly against the introduction of non-indicated homoeopathic vibrations. All living cells have a vibration.[654] Germs are living cells, and if a species of germ vibrates at a frequency that is incompatible with the natural frequency of human cells, then potentising the germ and giving it to a person with no symptoms makes no sense, unless you are trying the make the person sick for research purposes. Each type of cell has a set of metabolic oscillations that are characteristic of its type.[654] When healthy tissue becomes malignant, the oscillation of the cells changes.[655] It does not strike me as wise to introduce a homoeopathically potentised virus into the body of a tiny baby, even if the baby is perfectly healthy at the time. Too little is known about oscillations and electromagnetic fields in a baby's body to start introducing unnecessary waves and frequencies.

CONCLUSION

At the time that our first child was born we were living in a police state in which vaccination was compulsory. I was aware that some vaccines cause serious adverse effects that are not acknowledged by the medical establishment, and as I intended refusing some of the vaccines that were on the schedule, I thought I had better look up some statistics in case I found myself appearing in court. My investigations led me to discover that the vaccine industry has never bothered to collect accurate data about adverse effects, that vaccination is not the reason why diseases like diphtheria and whooping cough have declined, and that vaccination is responsible for causing a wide range of chronic diseases. I also discovered that it is not a good idea to try to prevent the self-resolving childhood infectious diseases, and that the infectious diseases that need intervention can be prevented by methods that are far more reliable than vaccination. I had heard it said by health practitioners that it is wrong to suppress fever, and I was surprised to discover that there is solid scientific evidence to support that view. Later I learned that suppressing fever is one of the most dangerous things that modern medicine does. By delving into the history of vaccination, I discovered that it is a procedure based on falsehood, cruelty, and supposition. I felt motivated to share what I had learned with other parents.

For my husband and me, protecting our children from the wiles of the vaccine industry involved more than making health related choices on their behalf. As they grew we ensured that they were equipped with sufficient knowledge to understand why we made the choices that we made for them. We also made sure that they understood why our choices were at odds with the aggressively presented ideas of the world around them. It was no different to helping them understand, as they reached the appropriate age for specific pieces of information, why we were at odds with the prevailing ideology of apartheid into which all four of us had been born. Now that they are adults they are responsible for deciding what goes into their own bodies.

There have been critics of vaccination ever since the vaccine industry started trying to scratch cowpox pus into every available arm, but it is only in recent decades that the industry has become globally organised in its efforts to silence opposition. Doctors who speak up about a problem with vaccination are regarded as traitors, and they risk persecution. Even if a doctor suggests that children should be vaccinated against thirteen diseases instead of fourteen, the industry reacts with hysteria against that doctor. The mainstream media refuses to report negative information about vaccination, but has no qualms about stirring up irrational fear of infectious diseases. Journalists who attempt to do balanced reporting are threatened with dismissal by their bosses, even in sections of the media that do not have financial ties to the pharmaceutical industry.

In more and more countries draconian laws that prevent non-vaccinating parents from accessing childcare and education for their children are being introduced. Countries that have no history or a short history of democracy find it easy to make vaccination compulsory. However, in Turkey and Lithuania, the supreme courts have ruled that compulsory vaccination laws are illegal and must be abolished. The vaccine bullies are scornful of things like constitutions, and it always takes a huge amount of effort and money for parents to assert their rights. In 1982 the province of Ontario in Canada made vaccination compulsory for school attendance. This law was unconstitutional, but it took a group of parents two years, a huge amount of work, and lots of money, to get it abolished. Now the vaccine loving politicians in Ontario are at it again, and a new generation of parents have to fight vicious laws to assert their right to keep their children healthy. Italy, Argentina, Australia, California and New York State have introduced fascist laws, and the vaccine industry is motivating other governments to do the same.

The vaccine industry establishes "non-profit" organisations that campaign for vaccines to be made mandatory for people who work in the health field, and mandatory for children to be enrolled at school.[656] These organisations are actually funded by vaccine manufacturers,[656] and they spread unsubstantiated claims about the effectiveness of vaccines.[656] Vaccine manufacturers also fund non-profit organisations that campaign for governments to spend more money on buying vaccines,[656] and they fund fake blogs that present themselves as having been written by caring mothers.[656]

There is also a vast army of unpaid vigilantes who patrol the internet and vilify non-believers on social media. They label people who believe that vaccines should be scientifically studied as "anti-science". One of their favourite chants is that it is better for a child to have a lifetime of autism than a week of measles. Bloggers write articles that defame anti-vaccination doctors and activists. There are a number of blog posts about me, full of lies and fabricated quotes. Some of the false quotes are fabricated by journalists, and then the bloggers attack me for saying things I have not said. Trolls who pretend that they are anti-vaxxers write false negative reviews about this book on Amazon. Their comments make it obvious that they have not read the book.

In the USA there are laws ensuring that the vaccine industry has no accountability, but in every other country the vaccine industry has no accountability anyway. The University of Connecticut and London University have set up well-funded spy agencies to monitor everything that is said about vaccination on the internet, with the long-term goal of controlling community sentiment. Vaccine fanatics have asked Amazon to stop selling vaccine-truth books and films, and have asked social networks to deletee vaccine-truth groups and people. The aim of the vaccine fanatics is to stop all discussion about vaccine damage, and to stop discussion about corruption in the vaccine industry. The present climate of oppression is causing difficulties for a lot of parents, but it will not succeed in silencing criticism of vaccination. As long as vaccines continue to harm children, parents will continue to talk about it.

REFERENCES

1. Miller, D.L., Frequency of Complications of Measles, 1963 - Report on a National Inquiry by the Public Health Laboratory Service in Collaboration with the Society of Medical Officers of Health. *Brit Med J.* 1964 July 11;2(5401):75-8.
2. Australian Government Department of Health and Ageing, *Understanding Childhood Immunisation*, Department of Health and Ageing Publications, Approval number 3744, Revised October 2005.
3. Therapeutic Goods Administration, Medicine Summary, Haemophilus Influenzae Type B Vaccine, 17 August 2004.
4. Cockburn, A., Ridgeway J., Scientist J. Anthony Morris - He fought the flu shots and the US fired him. *Washington Post.* 13 March 1977.
5. Researcher Denied Funds to Study DPT. *NVIC News.* October1991;1(3):3.
6. Thompson, N.P., Montgomery, S.M., et al., Is measles vaccination a risk factor for inflammatory bowel disease? *Lancet.* 1995 April 29;345:1071-4.
7. Wakefield, A.J., Pittilo, R.M., et al., Evidence of Persistent Measles Virus Infection in Crohn's Disease. *J Med Virol.* 1993 Apr;39(4):345-53.
8. Lewin, J., Dhillon, A.P., et al., Persistent measles virus infection of the intestine: confirmation by immunogold electron microscopy. *Gut.* 1995 Apr;36940:564-9.
9. Barton, J.R., Gillon, S., Ferguson, A., Incidence of inflammatory bowel disease in Scottish children between 1968 and 1983: marginal fall in ulcerative colitis, three fold rise in Crohn's disease. *Gut.* 1989 May;30(5):618-22.
10. Measles Vaccines Committee. Vaccination against measles: a clinical trial of live measles vaccine given alone and live vaccine preceded by killed vaccine. A report to the Medical Research Council. *Brit Med J.* 1966 Feb 19;1(5485):441-6.
11. Patriarca, P.A., Beeler, J.A., Measles vaccination and inflammatory bowel disease. *Lancet.* 1995 Apr 29;345(8957):1062-3.
12. Farrington, P., Miller, E., Measles vaccination as a risk factor for inflammatory bowel disease. *Lancet.* 1995 May 27;345(8961):1362

13. Calman, K.C., Measles vaccination as a risk factor for inflammatory bowel disease. *Lancet.* 1995 May 27;345(8961):1362.
14. Minor, P.D., Measles vaccination as a risk factor for inflammatory bowel disease. *Lancet.* 1995 May 27;345(8961):1362-3.
15. MacDonald, T.T., Measles vaccination as a risk factor for inflammatory bowel disease. *Lancet.* 1995 May 27;345(8961):1363.
16. Miller, D., Renton, A., Measles vaccination as a risk factor for inflammatory bowel disease. *Lancet.* 1995 May 27;345(8961):1363.
17. Baxter, T., Radford, J., Measles vaccination as a risk factor for inflammatory bowel disease. *Lancet.* 1995 May 27;345(8961):1363.
18. Thompson, N.P., Montgomery, S.M., et al., Authors' Reply. *Lancet.* 1995 May 27;345(8961):1364.
19. Sienkiewicz, D., Kułak, W., et al., Neurologic adverse events following vaccination. *Prog Health Sci.* 2012;2:129-41.
20. Dyer, C., Families win support for vaccine compensation claim. *BMJ.* 1994 Sep 24;309(6957):759.
21. Benjamin, C.M., Chew, G.C., Silman, A.J., Joint and limb symptoms in children after immunisation with measles, mumps, and rubella vaccine. *BMJ.* 1992 Apr 25;304(6834):1075-8.
22. Weibel, R.E., Benor, D.E., Chronic arthropathy and musculoskeletal symptoms associated with rubella vaccines. A review of 124 claims submitted to the National Vaccine Injury Compensation Program. *Arthritis Rheum.* 1996 Sep;39(9):1529-34.
23. Cooper, L.Z., Ziring, P.R., et al., Transient Arthritis After Rubella Vaccination. *Amer J Dis Child.* 1969 Aug;118(2):218-25.
24. Hedrich, A.W., Monthly estimates of the child population "susceptible" to measles, 1900-1931, Baltimore, MD. *Amer J Hyg.* 1933;17:613-36.
25. Kids don't spread hepatitis B. *Australian Doctor Weekly.* 6 November1992.
26. Burgess, M.A., McIntosh, E.D.G., et al., Hepatitis B in urban Australian school children - No evidence of horizontal transmission between high-risk and low-risk groups. *Med J Aust.*1993 Sep 6;159(5):315-9.
27. Hoefs, J., Sapico, F.L., et al., The Relationship of White Blood Cell (WBC) and Pyrogenic Response to Survival in Spontaneous Bacterial Peritonitis (SBP). *Gastroenterology.* 1980;78(5)Part 2:1308.
28. Weinstein, M.P., Iannini, P.B., et al., Spontaneous bacterial peritonitis. A review of 28 cases with emphasis on improved survival and factors influencing prognosis. *Am J Med.* 1978 Apr;64(4):592-8. "The presence of fever with temperatures greater than 38° was associated with significantly diminished mortality (P=0.0240)."
29. Bryant, R.E., Hood, A.F., et al., Factors Affecting Mortality of Gram-Negative Rod Bacteremia. *Arch Intern Med.* 1971 Jan;127(1):120-8. In this study 71% of humans without fever died, while 27% of those with fever died.
30. Mackowiak, P.A., Browne, R.H., et al., Polymicrobial Sepsis: An Analysis of 184 Cases Using Log Linear Models. *Am J Med Sci.* 1980 Sep-

Oct;280(2):73-80. In this study the association of fever with survival was stronger when the patient did not have an underlying terminal illness.

31. Swenson, B.R., Hedrick, T.L., et al., Is fever protective in surgical patients with bloodstream infection? J Am Coll Surg. 2007 May;204(5):815-21
32. Arons, M.M., Wheeler, A.P., et al., Effects of ibuprofen on the physiology and survival of hypothermic sepsis. Ibuprofen in Sepsis Study Group. *Crit Care Med.* 1999 Apr;27(4):699-707.
33. Sugimura, T., Fujimoto, T., et al., Risks of antipyretics in young children with fever due to infectious disease. *Acta Paediatr Jpn.* 1994 Aug;36(4):375-8.
34. Kluger, M.J., Fever. *Pediatrics.* 1980 Nov;66(5):720-4.
35. Mackowiak, P.A., Boulant, J.A., Fever's glass ceiling. *Clin Infect Dis.* 1996 Mar;22(3):525-36.
36. Nahas, G.G., Tannieres, M.L., Lennon, J.F., Direct measurement of leukocyte motility: effects of pH and temperature. *Proc Soc Exp Biol Med.* 1971 Oct;138(1):350-2.
37. Bernheim, H.A., Bodel, P.T., et al., Effects of Fever on Host Defence Mechanisms after Infection in the Lizard Diposaurus Dorsalis. *Br J Exp Pathol.* 1978 Feb;59(1):76-84.
38. Ellingson, H.V., Clark, P.F., The Influence of Artificial Fever on Mechanisms of Resistance. *J Immunol.* 1942;43:65-83.
39. Bodel, P., Atkins, E., Release of Endogenous Pyrogen by Human Monocytes. *New Engl J Med.* 1967 May 4;276(18):1002-8.
40. Cranston, W.I., Goodale, F., et al., The Role of Leukocytes in the Initial Action of Bacterial Pyrogens in Man. *Clin Sci (Lond).* 1956 May;15(2):219-26.
41. Weinberg, E.D., Iron and Infection. *Microbiol Rev.* 1978 Mar;42(1):45-66.
42. Bullen, J.J., The Significance of Iron in Infection. *Rev Infect Dis.* 1981 Nov-Dec;3(6):1127-38.
43. Kluger, M.J., Rothenburg, B.A., Fever and Reduced Iron: Their Interaction as a Host Defense Response to Bacterial Infection. *Science.* 1979 Jan 26;203(4378):374-6.
44. Ballantyne, G.H., Rapid Drop in Serum Iron Concentration as a Host Defense Mechanism. *Am Surg.* 1984 Aug;50(8):405-11.
45. Kluger, M.J., Fever: Role of Pyrogens and Cryogens. *Physiol Rev.* 1991 Jan;71(1):93-127.
46. Rager-Zisman, B., Bloom, B.R., Interferons and Natural Killer Cells. *Brit Med Bull.* 1985 Jan;41(1):22-7.
47. Heron, I., Berg, K., The actions of interferon are potentiated at elevated temperature. *Nature.* 1978 Aug 3;274(5670):508-10.
48. Roberts, N.J., Temperature and Host Defense. *Microbiol Rev.* 1979 Jun;43(2):241-59.
49. Manzella, J.P., Roberts, N.J., Human Macrophage and Lymphocyte Responses to Mitogen Stimulation after exposure to influenza virus, ascorbic acid, and hyperthermia. *J Immunol.* 1979 Nov;123(5):1940-4.
50. Smith, J.B., Knowlton, R.P., Agarwal, S.S., Human Lymphocyte responses are enhanced by culture at 40°C. *J Immunol.* 1978 Aug;121(2):691-4.

51. Roberts, N.J., Sandberg, K., Hyperthermia and Human Leukocyte Function: II. Enhanced Production of and Response to Leukocyte Migration Inhibition Factor (LIF). *J Immunol.* 1979 May 1;122(5):1990-3.
52. Duff, G.W., Durum, S.K., The pyrogenic and mitogenic actions of interleukin -1 are related. *Nature.* 1983 Aug 4-10;304(5925):449-51.
53. Duff, G.W., Durum, S.K., Fever and immunoregulation: hyperthermia, interleukins 1 and 2, and T cell proliferation. *Yale J Biol Med.* 1982 Sep-Dec;55(5-6):437-42.
54. Hanson, D.F., Murphy, P.A., et al., The effect of temperature on the activation of thymocytes by interleukins I and II. *J Immunol.* 1983 Jan;130(1):216-21.
55. Mackowiak, P.A., Marling-Cason, M., Cohen, R.L., Effects of Temperature on Antimicrobal Susceptibility of Bacteria. *J Infect Dis.* 1982 Apr;145(4):550-3.
56. Sande, M.A., Sande, E.R., et al., The Influence of Fever on the Development of Experimental Streptococcus Pneumoniae Meningitis. *J Infect Dis.* 1987 Nov;156(5):849-50.
57. Kluger, J.M., Ringler, D.H., Anver, M.R., Fever and Survival. *Science.* 1975 Apr 11;188(4184):166-8.
58. Carmichael, L.E., Barnes, F.D., Percy, D.H., Temperature as a Factor in Resistance of Young Puppies to Canine Herpesvirus. *J Infect Dis.* 1969 Dec;120(6):669-78.
59. Bernheim, H.A., Kluger, M.J., Fever: Effect of Drug-Induced Antipyresis on Survival. *Science.* 1976 Jul 16;193(4249):237-9.
60. Vaughn, L.K., Veale, W.L., Cooper, K.E., Antipyresis: Its effect on mortality rate of bacterially infected rabbits. *Brain Res Bull.* 1980 Jan-Feb;5(1):69-73.
61. Schulman, C.I., Namias, N., Doherty, J., et al. The effect of antipyretic therapy upon outcomes in critically ill patients: a randomized, prospective study. *Surg Infect (Larchmt).* 2005 Winter;6(4):369-75.
62. Kiekkas, P., Fever treatment in critical care: when available evidence does not support traditional practice. *Nurs Crit Care.* 2012 Jan-Feb;17(1):7-8.
63. Saxena, M., Young, P., et al., Early peak temperature and mortality in critically ill patients with or without infection. *Crit Care.* 2011;15(Suppl 3):24.
64. Schmitt, B.D., Fever Phobia: Misconceptions of Parents About Fevers *Am J Dis Child.* 1980 Feb;134(2):176-81.
65. Schmitt, B.D., Fever in Childhood. *Pediatrics.* 1984 Nov;74(5 Pt 2):929-36.
66. Crocetti, M., Moghbeli, N., Serwint, J., Fever Phobia Revisited: Have Parental Misconceptions About Fever Changed in 20 Years? *Pediatrics.* 2001 Jun;107(6):1241-6.
67. Lenhardt, R., Negishi, C., et al., The effects of physical treatment on induced fever in humans. *Am J Med.*1999 May;106(5):550-5.
68. Doran, T.F., De Angelis, C., et al., Acetaminophen: More harm than good for chickenpox? *J Pediatr.* 1989 Jun;114(6):1045-8. (Acetaminophen and paracetamol are the same thing.)

69. Graham, N.M., Burrell, C.J., et al., Adverse effects of aspirin, acetaminophen, and ibuprofen on immune function, viral shedding, and clinical status in rhinovirus-infected volunteers. *J Infect Dis.* 1990 Dec;162(6):1277-82.
70. Shalabi, E.A., Acetaminophen inhibits the human polymorphonuclear leukocyte function in vitro. *Immunopharmacology.* 1992 Jul-Aug;24(1):37-45.
71. Carr, D.J.J., Gebhardt, B.M., Paul, D., a-Adrenergic and m2 opioid receptors are involved in morphine-induced suppression of splenocyte natural killer activity. *J Pharmacol Exp Ther.* 1993 Mar;264(3):1179-86.
72. Carpenter, G.W., Breeden, L., Carr, D.J.J., Acute exposure to morphine suppresses cytotoxic T-lymphocyte activity. *Int J Immunopharmacol.* 1995 Dec;17(12):1001-6.
73. Sacerdote, P., Manfredi, B., et al., Antinociceptive and immunosuppressive effects of opiate drugs: a structure-related activity study. *Br J Pharmacol.* 1997 Jun;121(4):834-40.
74. Bancos, S., Bernard, M.P., et al., Ibuprofen and other widely used non-steroidal anti-inflammatory drugs inhibit antibody production in human cells. *Cell Immunol.* 2009;258(1):18-28.
75. Poston, R.N., *Nutrition and Immunity,* in, Jarrett, R.J., (ed), *Nutrition and Disease*. Croom Helm, London, 1979, 199.
76. Scrimshaw, N.S., Béhar, M., Malnutrition in Underdeveloped Countries. *New Engl J Med.* 1965 Jan 28;272(4):193-8.
77. Ebrahim, G.J., *The Problems of Undernutrition,* in, Jarrett, R.J., (ed), *Nutrition and Disease.* Croom Helm, London, 1979, 85-6.
78. Hanson, D.F., Fever, Temperature and the Immune Response. *Ann NY Acad Sci.* 1997 mar 15;813:453-64.
79. Stuart, J., and Malcolm, D.McK., (eds), *The Diary of Henry Francis Fynn.* Shuter and Shooter, Pietermaritzburg, 1969, 42-43. There was international distribution of a TV mini series called *Shaka Zulu*, which was claimed to have been based on the diaries of Dr. Fynn, but was actually a racist corruption of Fynn's diary. Made by the Botha regime in 1986, it was based on a Stalinesque "history" penned during the Verwoerd era. Not to be confused with the films called *Zulu, Zulu Dawn* nor *Shaka.*
80. Arnold, Nell, *Rye - A book of Memories*. Rye - Tootagarook Area Committee, 1989, 27.
81. Kluger, M.J., Kozak, W., et al., The adaptive value of fever. *Infect Dis Clin North Am.* 1996 Mar;10(1):1-20.
82. Spock, Benjamin, *Baby and Child Care.* W. H. Allen and Co, London,1983, 497-502.
83. Stanton, A.N., Scott, D.J., Downham, M.A., Is overheating a factor in some unexpected infant deaths? *Lancet.* 1980 May 17;1(8177):1054-7.
84. Fleming, P.J., Gilbert, R., et al., Interaction between bedding and sleeping position in the sudden infant death syndrome: a population based case-control study. *BMJ.* 1990 Jul 14;301(6743):85-9.
85. Ponsonby, A.L., Dwyer, T., et al., Thermal environment and sudden infant

death syndrome: case-control study. *BMJ.* 1992 Feb 1;304(6822):277-82.
86. Nelson, K.B., Ellenberg, J.H., Prognosis in Children with Febrile Seizures. *Pediatrics.* 1978 May;61(5):720-7.
87. Verity, C.M., Greenwood, R., Golding, J., Long-term Intellectual and Behavioral Outcomes of Children with Febrile Convulsions. *N Eng J Med.* 1998 Jun;338(24):1723-8.
88. Annergers, J.H., Hauser, W.A., et al., The risk of epilepsy following febrile convulsions. *Neurology.* 1979 Mar;29(3):297-303.
89. Camfield, P., Camfield, C., et al., What types of epilepsy are preceded by febrile seizures? A population based study of children. *Dev Med Child Neurol.* 1994 Oct;36(10):887-92.
90. Sofijanov, N., Sadikario, A., et al., Febrile Convulsions and Later Development of Epilepsy. *Am J Dis Child.* 1983 Feb;137(2):123-6.
91. Verity, C.M., Golding, J., Risk of epilepsy after febrile convulsions; a national cohort study. *BMJ.* 1991 Nov 30;303(6814):1373-6.
92. Knüdsen, F.U., Paerregaard, A., et al., Long term outcome of prophylaxis for febrile convulsions. *Arch Dis Child.* 1996 Jan;74(1):13-8.
93. Hirtz, D.G., Febrile Seizures. *Pediatr in Rev.* 1997 Jan;18(1):5-8.
94. Mole, B., Cold viruses thrive in frosty conditions: Icy temperatures chill the immune response that thwarts the common cold. *Nature.* 20 May 2013.
95. Johnson, C., and Eccles, R., Acute cooling of the feet and the onset of common cold symptoms. *Fam Prac.* 2005 Dec;22(6):608-13.
96. Baerheim, A., Laerum, E., Symptomatic lower urinary tract infection induced by cooling of the feet. A controlled experimental trial. *Scand J Prim Health Care.* 1992 Jun;10(2):157-60.
97. Kiser, W.R., Nusbaum, M.R., et al., Symptomatic lower urinary tract infection induced by cooling of the feet. *Scand J Prim Health Care.* 1993 Dec;11(4):289-90.
98. Engel, P., Ueber den Infektionsindex der Krebskranken. *Wien Klin Wsch*r. 1934;47:1118-9.
99. Engel, P., Ueber den Einfluss des Alters auf den Infektionsindex der Krebskranken. *Wien Klin Wschr.* 1935;48:112-3.
100. Sinek, F., Versuch einer statistischen Erfassung endogener Faktoren bei Carcinomkranken. *Z Krebsforsch.* 1936;44:492-527.
101. Witzel, L., Anamnese und Zweiterkrankungen bei Patienten mit bsartigen Neubildungen. *Med Klin.* 1970;65:876-9.
102. Remy, W., Hammerschmidt, K., et al. Tumorträger haben selten Infekte in der Anamnese. *Med Min.* 1983;78:95-8.
103. Albonico, H.U., Bräker, H.U., Hüsler, J., Febrile infectious childhood diseases in the history of cancer patients and matched controls. *Med Hypotheses.* 1998 Oct;51(4):315-20.
104. Montella, M., Maso, L.D., et al., Do childhood diseases affect NHL and HL risk? A case-control study from northern and southern Italy. *Leuk Res.* 2006 Aug;30(8):917-22.
105. Hoption Cann, S.A., van Netten, J.P., van Netten C., Acute infections as a

means of cancer prevention: opposing effects to chronic infections? *Cancer Detect Prev.* 2006;30(1):83-93.
106. West, R., Epidemiologic study of malignancies of the ovaries. *Cancer.* 1966 Jul;19(7):1001-7.
107. Newhouse, M.L., Pearson, R.M., et al., A case control study of carcinoma of the ovary. *Brit J Prev Soc Med.* 1977 Sep;31(3):148-53.
108. Cramer, D.W., Vitonis, A.F., et al., Mumps and ovarian cancer: modern interpretation of an historic association. *Cancer Causes Control.* 2010 Aug;21(8):1193-201.
109. Wrensch, M., Lee, M., et al., Familial and personal medical history of cancer and nervous system conditions among adults with glioma and controls. *Am J Epidemiol.* 1997 Apr 1;145(7):581-93.
110. Wrensch, M., Weinberg, A., et al., Does prior infection with varicella-zoster virus influence risk of adult glioma? *Am J Epidemiol.* 1997 Apr 1;145(7):594-7.
111. Wrensch, M., Weinberg, A., et al., Prevalence of antibodies to four herpes viruses among adults with glioma and controls. *Am J Epidemiol.* 2001 Jul 15;154(2):161-5.
112. Wrensch, M., Weinberg, A., et al., History of chickenpox and shingles and prevalence of antibodies to varicella-zoster virus and three other herpesviruses among adults with glioma and controls. *Am J Epidemiol.* 2005 May 15;161(10):929-38.
113. Pesonen E, Andsberg E, et al. Dual role of infections as risk factors for coronary heart disease. *Atherosclerosis.* 2007 Jun;192(2):370-5.
114. Kubota, Y., Iso, H., Tamakoshi, A.; JACC Study Group. Association of measles and mumps with cardiovascular disease: The Japan Collaborative Cohort (JACC) study. *Atherosclerosis*, 2015 Aug;241(2):682-6.
115. Sasco, A.J., Paffenbarger, R.S., Measles infection and Parkinson's disease. *Am J Epidemiol.* 1985 Dec;122(6):1017-31.
116. Silverberg, J.I., Kleiman, E., et al., Chickenpox in childhood is associated with decreased atopic disorders, IgE, allergic sensitization, and leukocyte subsets. *Pediatr Allergy Immunol.* 2012 Feb;23(1):50-8.
117. Silverberg, J.I., Norowitz, K.B., et al., Varicella zoster virus (wild-type) infection, but not varicella vaccine, in late childhood is associated with delayed asthma onset, milder symptoms, and decreased atopy. *Pediatr Asthma Allergy Immunol.* 2009 Mar; 22:15-20.
118. Farooqi, I.S., Hopkin, J.M., Early childhood infection and atopic disorder. *Thorax.* 1998 Nov;53(11):927-32.
119. Kucukosmanoglu, E., Cetinkaya, F., et al., Frequency of allergic diseases following measles. *Allergol Immunopathol (Madr).* 2006 Jul-Aug;34(4):146-9.
120. Rosenlund, H., Bergström, A., et al., Allergic disease and atopic sensitization in children in relation to measles vaccination and measles infection. *Pediatrics.* 2009 Mar;123(3):771-8.
121. Shaheen, S.O., Aaby, P., et al. Measles and atopy in Guinea-Bissau. *Lancet.*

1996 Jun 29;347(9018):1792-6
122. Paunio, M., Heinonen, O.P, et al. Measles history and atopic diseases: a population-based cross-sectional study. *JAMA*. 2000 Jan 19;283(3):343-6.
123. Burgess, J.A., Abramson, M.J., et al., Childhood infections and the risk of asthma: a longitudinal study over 37 years. *Chest.* 2012 Sep;142(3):647-54.
124. Chakravarti, V.S., Lingam, S., Measles induced remission of psoriasis. *Ann Trop Paediatr.* 1986 Dec;6(4):293-4.
125. Lintas, N., Case of psoriasis cured after intercurrent measles. *Minerva Dermatol.* 1959 Apr;34(4):296-7.
126. Fomin, K.F., Cure if psoriasis after co-existing measles. *Vestn Dermatol Venerol.* 1961 Jun;35:66-8.
127. Bonjean, M., Prime, A., Suspensive effect of measles on psoriasic erythroderma of 12 years' duration. *Lyon Med.* 1969 Nov 9;222(40):839.
128. Thiers, H., Normand, J., Fayolle, J., Suspensive effect of measles on chronic psoriasis in children: 2 cases *Lyon Med.* 1969 Nov 9;222(40):839-40.
129. Agarwal, V., Singh, R., Chauhan, S., Remission of rheumatoid arthritis after acute disseminated varicella-zoster infection. *Clin Rheumatol.* 2007 May;26(5):779-80.
130. Urbach, J., Schurr, D., Abramov, A., Prolonged remission of juvenile rheumatoid arthritis (Still's disease) following measles. *Acta Paediatr Scand.* 1983 Nov;72(6):917-8.
131. Pasquinucci, G., Possible Effect of Measles on Leukaemia. *Lancet.* 1971 Jan 16;1(7690):136.
132. Gross, S., Measles and Leukaemia. *Lancet.* 1971 Feb 20;1(7695):397-8.
133. Hutchins, G., Observations on the relationship of measles and remissions in the nephrotic syndrome. *Am J Dis Child.* 1947 Feb;73(2):242-3.
134. Blumberg, R.W., Cassady, H.A., Effect of Measles on the Nephrotic Syndrome. *Am J Dis Child.* 1947 Feb;73(2):151-66.
135. Barnett, H.L., Forman, C.W., Lauson, H.D., The nephrotic syndrome in children. *Adv Pediatr.* 1952 Jan;5:53-128.
136. Saeed, M.A., Varicella-Induced Remission of Steroid-Resistant Nephrotic Syndrome in a Child. *Saudi J Kidney Dis Transpl.* 2004 Oct-Dec;15(4):486-8.
137. Zygiert, Z., Hodgkin's disease: remissions after measles. *Lancet.* 1971 Mar 20;1(7699):593.
138. Taqi, A.M., Abdurrahman, M.B., et al., Regression of Hodgkin's disease after measles. *Lancet.* 1981 May 16;1(8229):1112.
139. Hernández, S.A., Observación de un caso de enfermedad de Hodgkin, con regresion at los sitomas e infartos ganglionares, post-sarampión. *Arch Cubanos Cancer.* 1949;8:26-31.
140. Mota, H.C., Infantile Hodgkin's disease: remission after measles. *Br Med J.* 1973 May 19;2(5863):421.
141. Ziegler JL. Spontaneous remission in Burkitt's lymphoma. *Natl Cancer Inst Monogr*. 1976 Nov;44:61-5.
142. Bluming, A.Z., Ziegler, J.L., Regression of Burkitt's Lymphoma in

association with measles infection. *Lancet.* 1971 July 10;2(7715)105-6.
143. Burnet, F.M., Measles as an Index of Immunological Function. *Lancet.* 1968 Sep 14;2(7568):610-3.
144. Olding-Stenkvist, E., Bjorvatn, B., Rapid Detection of Measles Virus in Skin Rashes by Immunoflourescence. *J Infect Dis.* 1976 Nov;134(5):463-9.
145. Dossetor, J., Whittle, H.C., Greenwood, B.M., Persistent measles infection in malnourished children. *Brit Med J.* 1977 Jun 25;1(6077):1633-5.
146. Personal communication, Dr. J. Anthony Morris.
147. Pharmacy Guild of New Zealand (Inc.), *Your Health Update*, Issue No.3. Undated.
148. Cantacuzène, J., *Ann Inst Pasteur.* 1898, 12: Paris, 273, cited in Silverstein, A.M., *A History of Immunology,* Academic Press Inc., San Diego, 1989, 49.
149. Graham, N.M, Burrell, C.J., et al, Adverse effects of aspirin, acetaminophen, and ibuprofen on immune function, viral shedding, and clinical status in rhinovirus-infected volunteers. *J Infect Dis.* 1990 Dec;162(6):1277-82.
150. Viken, K.E., Effect of Sosium-salicylate on the function of cultured, human mononuclear cells. *Acta Pathol Microbiol Scand [C].* 1976 Dec;84C(6):465-70.
151. van Zyl, J.M., Basson, K., van der Walt, B.J., The inhibitory effect of acetaminophen on the myeloperoxidase-induced antimicrobal system of the polymorphonuclear leukocyte. *Biochem Pharmacol.* 1989 Jan 1;38(1):161-5.
152. Opelz, G., Terasaki, P.L., Hirata, A.A., Suppression of lymphocyte transformation by aspirin. *Lancet.* 1973 Sep 1;2(7827):478-480.
153. Crout, J.E., Hepburn, B., et al, Suppression of lymphocyte transformation after aspirin ingestion. *New Engl J Med.* 1975 Jan 30;292(5):221-3.
154. Morely, D., Severe Measles in the Tropics. - I. *Brit Med J.* 1969 Feb 1;1(5639)297-300.
155. Hardy, I.R.B., Lennon, D.R., Mitchell, E.A., Measles epidemic in Auckland 1984-85. *NZ Med J.* 1987 May 13;100(823)273-5.
156. Lydall, W., Scaremongering about measles. *Soil and Health* 1992;51(1):55.
157. Sanchez, A., Reeser, J.L., et al., Role of sugars in human neutrophilic phagocytosis. *Am J Clin Nutr.* 1973 Nov;26(11):1180-4.
158. Ronne, T., Measles virus infection without rash in childhood is related to disease in adult life. *Lancet.* 1985 Jan 5;1(8419)1-5.
159. Kalokerinos, Archie, *Every Second Child.* Keats Publishing, Inc., New Canaan, Connecticut, 1981.
160. Kalokerinos, Archie, *Science Friction.* International Symposium, The Vaccination Dilemma, Auckland, 1992.
161. Kalokerinos, Archie, *Experience with Immunisation Reactions.* International Symposium, The Vaccination Dilemma II, Auckland,1995.
162. Zahorsky, J., Roseola Infantum. *JAMA.* 1913 Oct 18;61(16):1446-50.
163. Koplik, H., The Diagnosis of the Invasion of Measles from a Study of the Exanthema as it Appears on the Buccal Membrane. *Arch Pediatr.* 1896;12:918-22.

164. Beckford, A.P., Kaschula, R.O., Stephen, C., Factors associated with fatal cases of measles. A retrospective autopsy study. *S Afr Med J.* 1985 Dec 7;68(12):858-63.
165. Hussey, G.D., Clements, C.J., Clinical problems in measles case management. *Ann Trop Paediatr.* 1996;16(307):17.
166. Cole, T.J., Relating Growth Rate to Environmental Factors -Methodological Problems in the Study of Growth-Infection Interaction. *Acta Paediatr Suppl.* 1989;350:14-20.
167. Ebrahim, G.J., *The Problems of Undernutrition*, in, Jarrett, R.J., (ed), *Nutrition and Disease*. Croom Helm, London, 1979, 60 & 74.
168. Von Pirquet, C., Verhalten der kutanentuberkulin-reaktionwahrend der Masern. *Deutsch Med Wochenschr*. 1908;34(30):1297–1300.
169. Griffin, D.E., Measles virus-induced suppression of immune responses. *Immunol Rev.* 2010 Jul;236:176-89.
170. Griffin, D.E., Ward, B.J., et al., Natural killer cell activity during measles. *Clin Exp Immunol.* 1990 Aug;81(2):218-24.
171. Ellison, J., Intensive vitamin therapy in measles. *Brit Med J.* 1932 Oct 15;II(3745):708-11.
172. Fawzi, W.W., Chalmers, T.C., et al., Vitamin A supplementation and child mortality, a meta-analysis. *JAMA.* 1993 Feb 17;269(7):899-903.
173. Barclay, A.J., Foster, A., Sommer, A., Vitamin A supplements and mortality related to measles: a randomised clinical trial. *Br Med J (Clin Res Ed.).* 1987 Jan 31;294(6567):294-6.
174. Hussey, G.D., Klein, M., Routine high-dose vitamin A therapy for children hospitalized with measles. *J Trop Pediatr.* 1993 Dec;39(6):342-5.
175. D'Souza, R. M., D'Souza, R., Vitamin A given to children with measles - Does dose make a difference? *8th Cochrane Colloquium*, Cape Town, 25-29 October 2000.
176. Hussey, G.D., Klein, M., A randomized, controlled trial of vitamin A in children with severe measles. *N Engl J Med.* 1990 Jul 19;323(3):160-4.
177. Florentino, R.F., Tanchoco, C.C., et al., Tolerance of preschoolers to two dosage strengths of vitamin A preparation. *Am J Clin Nutr.* 1990 Oct;52(4):694-700.
178. Imdad, A., Herzer, K., et al., Vitamin A supplementation for preventing morbidity and mortality in children from 6 months to 5 years of age. *Cochrane Database Syst Rev.* 2010 Dec 8;(12):CD008524.
179. Harris, H.F., A Case of Diabetes Mellitus Quickly Following Mumps. *Boston Med Surg J.* 1899;140(20):465-9.
180. Swartout, H.O., *Modern Medical Counsellor.* Signs Publishing Company, Warburton, Australia, 1958, 715.
181. Das, B.D., Lakhani, P., et al., Congenital rubella after previous maternal immunity. *Arch Dis Child.* 1990 May;65(5):545-6.
182. Partridge, J.W., Flewett, T.H., Whitehead, J.E., Congenital rubella affecting an infant whose mother had rubella antibodies before conception. *Brit Med J (Clin Res Ed).* 1981 Jan 17;282(6259):187-8.

183. Bott, L.M., Eizenberg, D.H., Congenital rubella after successful vaccination. *Med J Aust.* 1982 Jun 12;1(12):514-5.
184. Strannegård, Ö., Holm, S.E., et al., Case of Apparent Reinfection with Rubella. *Lancet.* 1970 Jan 31;1(7640)240-1.
185. Ushida, M., Katow, S., Furukawa, S., Congenital Rubella Syndrome due to Infection after Maternal Antibody Conversion with Vaccine. *Jpn J Infect Dis.* 2003 Apr;56(2):68-9.
186. Numazaki, K., Fujikawa, T., Intracranial calcification with congenital rubella syndrome in a mother with serologic immunity. *J Child Neurol.* 2003 Apr;18(4):296-297.
187. American College of Obstetricians and Gynecologists, ACOG Committee Opinion: number 281, December 2002. Rubella vaccination. *Obstet Gynecol.* 2002 Dec;100(6):1417.
188. Tingle, A.J., Mitchell, L.A., et al., Randomised double-blind placebo controlled study on adverse effects of rubella immunisation in seronegative women. *Lancet.* 1997 May 3;349(9061):1277-81.
189. Geier, D.A., Geier, M.R., A one year follow up of chronic arthritis following rubella and hepatitis B vaccination based upon analysis of the Vaccine Adverse Events Reporting System (VAERS) database. *Clin Exp Rheumatol.* 2002 Nov-Dec;20(6):767-71.
190. Plotkin, S.A., Cornfeld, D., Ingalls, T.H., Studies of Immunization with Living Rubella Virus. *Amer J Dis Child.* 1965 Oct;110(4):381-9.
191. Plotkin, S.A., Farquhar, J.D., et al., Attenuation of RA 27/3 Rubella Virus in WI-38 Human Diploid Cells. *Amer J Dis Child.* 1969 Aug;118(2):178-85.
192. Bell, J.A., Pittman, M., Olson, B.J., Pertussis and aureomycin. *Public Health Rep.* 1949 May 13;64(19):589-98.
193. Bass, J.W., Erythromycin for treatment and prevention of pertussis. *Ped Infect Dis J.* 1986 Jan-Feb;5(1):154-7.
194. Altunaiji, S., Kukuruzovic, R., et al., Antibiotics for whooping cough (pertussis). *Cochrane Database Syst Rev.* 2007 Jul 18;(3):CD004404.
195. Bartkus, J.M., Juni, B.A., et al., Identification of mutation associated with erythromycin resistance in Bordetella pertussis: implications for surveillance of antimicrobial resistance. *J Clin Microbiol.* 2003 Mar;41(3):1167-72.
196. Silver, H.K., Kempe, C.H., Bruyn, H.B., *Handbook of Pediatrics,* 14th Edition. Lange Medical Publications, Los Altos, California, 1977, 507.
197. Cherry, J.D., Xing, D.X., et al. Determination of serum antibody to Bordetella pertussis adenylate cyclase toxin in vaccinated and unvaccinated children and in children and adults with pertussis. *Clin Infect Dis.* 2004 Feb 15;38(4):502-7.
198. Cherry, J.D., Heininger, U., et al. Antibody response patterns to Bordetella pertussis antigens in vaccinated (primed) and unvaccinated (unprimed) young children with pertussis. *Clin Vaccine Immunol.* 2010 May;17(5):741-7.
199. Mullan, B., *The Enid Blyton Story*. Boxtree Ltd., London, 1987, 15.
200. Otani, T., Concerning the vitamin C therapy of whooping cough. *Klinische*

Wochenschrift. 1936 Dec 19;15(51):1884-5.
201. Personal communication, Dr. Suzanne Humphries.
202. Theilen, U., Johnston, E.D., Robinson, P.A., Rapidly fatal invasive pertussis in young infants - how can we change the outcome? *BMJ.* 2008 Nov 27;337:a343.
203. 60 Minutes, New Zealand TV. The Alan Smith Story; recovery from terminal viral pneumonia with high dose IV Vitamin C, Denying the Obvious.
204. Centers for Disease Control, Pertussis Surveillance - United States, 1986 - 1988. *MMWR Morb Mortal Wkly Rep.* 1990 Feb 2;39(4):57-66.
205. Taranger, J., Mild Clinical Course of Pertussis in Swedish Infants of Today. *Lancet.* 1982 June 12;1(8283):1360.
206. Pollock, T.M., Miller, E., Lobb, J., Severity of whooping cough in England before and after the decline in pertussis immunisation. *Arch Dis Child.* 1984 Feb;59(2):162-5.
207. Marin, M., Güris, D., et al., Prevention of varicella: recommendations of the Advisory Committee on Immunization Practices (ACIP). Advisory Committee on Immunization Practices, Centers for Disease Control and Prevention (CDC) *MMWR Recomm Rep.* 2007 Jun 22;56(RR-4):1-40.
208. Meyer, P.A., Seward, J.F., et al., Varicella mortality: trends before vaccine licensure in the United States, 1970-1994. *J Infect Dis.* 2000 Aug;182(2):383-90.
209. Takahashi, M., Okuno, Y., et al., Development of a Live Attenuated Varicella Vaccine. *Biken J.* 1975 Mar;18(1):25-33.
210. Takahashi, M., Development and Characterization of a Live Varicella Vaccine (Oka strain). *Biken J.* 1984 Sep;27(2-3):31-6.
211. Krause, P.R., Klinman, D.M., Efficacy, immunogenicity, safety, and use of live attenuated chickenpox vaccine. *J Pediatr.* 1995 Oct;127(4):518-25.
212. Goldman, G.S., Adverse effects of varicella vaccination are under-reported in VAERS, mitigating against discovery of the true-cost benefit. *Medical Veritas.* 2005 2:1;406-8.
213. Goldman, G.S., The case against universal varicella vaccination. *Int J Toxicol.* 2006 Sep-Oct;25(5):313-7.
214. Guris D, Jumaan AO, Mascola L, et al. Changing varicella epidemiology in active surveillance sites - United States, 1995-2005. *J Infect Dis.* 2008 Mar 1;197 Suppl 2:S71-5.
215. Redondo Granado, M.J., Vizcaíno López, I., et al., Early presentation of breakthrough varicella in vaccinated children. *An Pediatr (Barc).* 2013 May;78(5):330-4.
216. Zhou, F., Ortega-Sanchez, I.R., An economic analysis of the universal varicella vaccination program in the United States. *J Infect Dis.* 2008 Mar 1;197 Suppl 2:S156-64.
217. Lopez, A.S., Guris, D., et al., One dose of varicella vaccine does not prevent school outbreaks: is it time for a second dose? *Pediatrics.* 2006 Jun;117(6):e1070-7.

218. Kelly, H., Grant, K., et al., Decreased varicella and increased herpes zoster incidence at a sentinel medical deputising service in a setting of increasing varicella vaccine coverage in Victoria, Australia, 1998 to 2012. *Euro Surveill.* 2014 Oct 16;19(41).
219. Nowgesic, E., Skowronski, D., et al., 1999. Direct costs attributed to chickenpox and herpes zoster in British Columbia - 1992 to 1996. *Can Commun Dis Rep.* 1999 Jun 1;25(11):100-4.
220. Rolfe, M., Measles immunization in the Zambian Copperbelt: cause for concern. *Trans Royal Soc Trop Med Hyg.* 1982;76(4):529-30.
221. Poland, G.A., Jacobson, R.M., Failure to Reach the Goal of Measles Elimination. *Arch Intern Med.* 1994 Aug 22;154(16):1815-20.
222. Hartley, P., Tulloch, W.J., et al., *A Study of Diphtheria in Two Areas of Great Britain.* Medical Research Council, Special Report Series No 272, His Majesty's Stationary Office, London, 1950, 4.
223. The official statistics collected for England and Wales from 1866 record the ages of victims.
224. Joint Committee on Vaccination and Immunisation, *Immunisation against Infectious Disease.* Her Majesty's Stationary Office, London, 1988, 19.
225. Ibid., 22.
226. Hartley, P., Tulloch, W.J., et al., *A Study of Diphtheria in Two Areas of Great Britain.* Medical Research Council, Special Report Series No 272, His Majesty's Stationary Office, London, 1950.
227. Linklater, A., *An Unhusbanded Life, Charlotte Despard, Suffragette, Socialist and Sinn Feiner.* Hutchinson, London, 1980.
228. Ibid., 98-99.
229. Ibid., 99.
230. Douglas Hume, Ethel, *Béchamp or Pasteur? A Lost Chapter in the History of Biology.* C. W. Daniel, Ashingdon, Rochford, Essex, Fourth Edition, 1963, 217-8.
231. Ibid., 207.
232. Centers for Disease Control, Diphtheria Outbreak - Russian Federation, 1990 - 1993. *MMWR Morb Mortal Wkly Rep.* 1993 Nov 5;42(43):840-1 & 847.
233. Centers for Disease Control, Diphtheria Epidemic - New Independent States of the Former Soviet Union, 1990-1994. *MMWR Morb Mortal Wkly Rep.* 1995 Mar 17;44(10):177-81.

Bibliography re bubonic plague and cholera;

Philip Ziegler, The Black Death. Collins, London, 1969.
Arthur M. Silverstein, A History of Immunology. Academic Press, Inc., San Diego, 1989.
Stanley L. Robbins, M.D., The Pathologic Basis of Disease. W. B. Saunders Company, Philadelphia, 1974.
Folke Henschen, The History of Disease. Longmans Green and Co. Ltd.,

London, 1966.
Norman Longmate, King Cholera. Hamish Hamilton, London, 1966.
George Deaux, The Black Death. Hamish Hamilton, London, 1969.
Charles E. Rosenberg, The Cholera Years. University of Chicago Press, Chicago, 1962.

234. Hedrich, A.W., The corrected average attack rate from measles among city children. *Amer J Hyg.* 1930;11:576-600.
235. Cherry, J.D., The 'New' Epidemiology of Measles and Rubella. *Hospital Practice.* July 1980;49-57. With regard to herd immunity, Cherry not only twists the meaning of the research finding, he also changes the percentage to 68%. Cherry dishonestly says, "He (Hedrich) reported that when 68% of the children less than 15 years of age were immune to measles, epidemics did not develop." What Hedrich actually reported is that when measles epidemics die out, the percentage of children who have had measles is never higher than 53%, and never lower than 32%. The research done by Hedrich shows that when an outbreak comes to an end, the number of immune people in a community has absolutely nothing to do with the fact that the measles virus has declined in virulence. In fact Hedrich states very clearly that measles epidemics do not eliminate the non-immune population. The data collected by Hedrich shows that the concept of herd immunity is fundamentally flawed, and that herd immunity does not exist.
236. Fine, P.E.M., Herd Immunity: History, Theory, Practice. *Epidemiol Rev.* 1993;15(2):265-302.
237. Centers for Disease Control, Measles Outbreak among Vaccinated High School Students - Illinois. *MMWR Morb Mortal Wkly Rep.* 1984 June 22;33(24):349-51.
238. Wang, Z., Yan, R., et al., Difficulties in Eliminating Measles and Controlling Rubella and Mumps: A Cross-Sectional Study of a First Measles and Rubella Vaccination and a Second Measles, Mumps, and Rubella Vaccination. PLoS One. 2014 Feb 20;9(2):e89361.
239. Davis, R.M., Whitman, E.D., et al., A persistent outbreak of measles despite appropriate prevention and control measures. *Am J Epidemiol.* 1987 Sep;126(3):438-49.
240. Gustafson, T.L., Brunell, P.A., et al., Measles outbreak in a 'fully immunized' secondary school population. *New Eng J Med.* 1987 Mar 26;316(13):771-4.
241. Nkowane, B.M., Bart, S.W., et al., Measles outbreak in a vaccinated school population: epidemiology, chains of transmission and the role of vaccine failures. *Am J Pub Health.* 1987 Apr;77(4):434-8.
242. Chen, R.T., Goldbaum, G.M., et al., An explosive point-source measles outbreak in a highly vaccinated population: modes of transmission and risk factors for disease. *Am J Epidemiol.* 1989 Jan;129(1):173-82.
243. Boulianne, N., De Serres, G., Major measles epidemic in the region of

Quebec despite a 99% vaccine coverage. *Can J Public Health.* 1991 May-Jun;82(3):189-90.
244. Anderson, R.M., May, R. M., Immunisation and herd immunity. *Lancet.* 1990 March 17;335(8690):641-5.
245. Paunio, M., Peltola, H., et al., Explosive school-based measles outbreak: intense exposure may have resulted in high risk, even among revaccinees. *Am J Epidemiol.* 1998 Dec 1;148(11):1103-10.
246. Centers for Disease Control, International Notes: Measles - Hungary. *MMWR Morb Mortal Wkly Rep.* 1989 Oct 6;38(39):665-8.
247. Williams, P.J., and Hull, H.F., Status of Measles in the Gambia, 1981. *Rev Infect Dis.* 1983 May-Jun;5(3):391-4.
248. Lamb, W.H., Epidemic Measles in a Highly Immunized Rural West African (Gambian) Village. *Rev Infect Dis.* 1988 Mar-Apr;10(2):457-62.
249. Norby, E., The Paradigms of Measles Vaccinology. *Curr Top Microbiol Immunol.* 1995;191:167-80.
250. Markowitz, L.E., Preblud, S.R., et al., Patterns of Transmission in Measles Outbreaks in the United States, 1985 - 1986. *New Engl J Med.* 1989 Jan 12;320(2):75-81.
251. Cogger, H.G., *Reptiles and Amphibians of Australia*, 5th Edition. Reed Books of Australia, 1996, 121-2.
252. Gay, N.J., Eliminating measles - no quick fix. *Bull World Health Organ.* 2000;78(8):949.
253. *Global measles and rubella strategic plan : 2012-2020.* World Health Organization, 2012.
254. World Health Organisation, Global Eradication of Poliomyelitis by the Year 2000. *Wkly Epidemiol Rec.* 1988;63:161-2.
255. Personal communication, Ministry of Health, Fiji.
256. Samuel, R., Balraj, V., John, T.J., Persisting poliomyelitis after high coverage with oral polio vaccine. *Lancet.* 1993 Apr 3;341(8849):903.
257. Sutter, R.W., Patriarca, P.A., et al., Outbreak of paralytic poliomyelitis in Oman: evidence for widespread transmission among fully vaccinated children. *Lancet.* 1991 Sep 21;338(8769):715-20.
258. Williams, G.D., Matthews, N.T., et al., Infant pertussis deaths in New South Wales 1996-1997. *Med J Aust.* 1998 Mar 16;168(6):281-3.
259. Stewart, G.T., Whooping cough and whooping cough vaccine: the risks and benefit debate. *Am J Epidemiol.* 1984;119(1):135-7.
260. Fine, P.E.M., Clarkson, J.A., The recurrence of whooping cough: possible implications for assessment of vaccine efficacy. *Lancet.* 1982 Mar 20;1(8273):666-9. The writers state, "Since epidemic frequency is a function of the rate of influx of susceptibles, it is surprising that the inter-epidemic period did not decrease after the 1974 fall in vaccine uptake." Epidemic frequency is not a function of the rate of influx of susceptibles. This delusion is absolute nonsense.
261. Stewart, G.T., Whooping cough and pertussis vaccine: A comparison of risks and benefits in Britain during the period 1968 - 83. *Dev Biol Stand.*

1985;61:395-405.
262. Romanus, V., Jonsell, R., Bergquist, S., Pertussis in Sweden after the cessation of general immunization in 1979. *Ped Infect Dis J.* 1987 Apr;6(4):364-71.
263. Trollfors, B., Rabo, E., Whooping cough in adults. *Brit Med J (Clin Res Ed).* 1981 Sep 12;283(6293):696-7.
264. Miller, E., Acellular pertussis vaccines. *Arch Dis Child.* 1995 Nov;73(5):390-1.
265. Nielsen, A., Larsen, S.O., Epidemiology of Pertussis in Denmark: The Impact of Herd Immunity. *Int J Epidemiol.* 1994 Dec;23(6):1300-7.
266. Mortimer, E.A., Immunization Against Infectious Disease. *Science.* 1978 May 26;200(4344):902-7.
267. *What Doctors Don't Tell You*, 4(4):10. 4 Wallace Rd, LondonN1 2PG,UK.
268. van Rensburg, J.W.J., Whooping Cough in Cape Town. *Epidemiological Comments.* April 1992;19(4):69-75.
269. The historical details of this story are based on chapter 3 of Silverstein, A.M., *A History of Immunology,* Academic Press Inc., San Diego, 1989, but the interpretation of the commercial significance is my own.
270. Hartley, P., Tulloch, W.J., et al., *A Study of Diphtheria in Two Areas of Great Britain.* Medical Research Council, Special Report Series No272, His Majesty's Stationary Office, London, 1950, 1.
271. Ibid., 16.
272. Ibid., 81.
273. Ibid., 37.
274. Ibid., 39.
275. Nossal, G.J.V., *Antibodies and Immunity.* Basic Books Inc., New York,1978.
276. Burnet, M., *The Integrity of the Human Body.* Harvard University Press, Cambridge, 1962, 42-3.
277. Good, R.A., Zak, S.J., Disturbances in Gamma Globulin Synthesis as "Experiments of Nature". *Pediatrics.* 1956 Jul;18(1):109-49.
278. Ruata, C., Vaccination in Italy. *NY Med J.* 1899 July 22;133-4.
279. Johnson, S., Schoub, B.D., et al., Poliomyelitis outbreak in South Africa, 1982. II. Laboratory and vaccine aspects. *Trans R Soc Trop Med Hyg.* 1984;78(1):26-31.
280. Connor, J.D., Evidence for an etiologic role of adenoviral infection in pertussis syndrome. *N Engl J Med.* 1970 Aug 20;283(8):390-4.
281. Measles Striking More Under Age 1. *Washington Post,* November 22, 1992;a17.
282. Albonico, H., Klein, P., Grob, Ch., Pewsner, D., Vaccination against measles, mumps and rubella. A constraining project for a dubious future? *IAS Newsletter.* December 1991;4(3):4.
283. Waaijenborg, S., Hahné, S.J., et al., Waning of maternal antibodies against measles, mumps, rubella, and varicella in communities with contrasting vaccination coverage. *J Infect Dis.* 2013 Jul;208(1):10-6.

284. Gans, H.A., Maldonado, Y.A., Loss of passively acquired maternal antibodies in highly vaccinated populations: an emerging need to define the ontogeny of infant immune responses. *J Infect Dis.* 2013 Jul;208(1):1-3.
285. Douglas Hume, Ethel, *Béchamp or Pasteur? A Lost Chapter in the History of Biology.* C. W. Daniel, Ashingdon, Rochford, Essex, Fourth Edition, 1963, 198.
286. Campos-Outcalt, D., Measles Outbreak in an Immunized School Population. *New Engl J Med.* 1987 Sep 24;317(13):834-5.
287. Panum, P.L., *Observations Made During The Epidemic Of Measles On The Faroe Islands In The Year 1846.* Originally published in the Bibiliothek for Laeger, Copenhagen, 3R., 1:270-344, 1847, translated by Ada S. Hatcher.
288. Dew, Kevin, *The Measles Vaccination Campaigns In New Zealand,1985 and 1991: The Issues Behind the Panic.* Department of Sociology and Social Policy, Working Papers No 10, 1995, Victoria University of Wellington.
289. Measles end Nikki's hopes for Olympics. *North Shore Times Advertiser,* September 12 1991; 1.
290. Galloway, Y., Stehr-Green, P., Measles in New Zealand, 1991. *CDNZ:communicable disease New Zealand.* December 1991;91(12):107-9.
291. Markowitz, L.E., Preblud, S.R., et al., Duration of live measles vaccine-induced immunity. *Pediatr Infect Dis J.* 1990 Feb 9;9(2):101-10.
292. Ammari, L.K., Bell, L.M., Hodinka, R.L., Secondary measles vaccine failure in healthcare workers exposed to infected patients. *Infect Control Hosp Epidemiol.* 1993 Feb;14(2):81-6.
293. American Academy of Pediatrics: Committee on Infectious Diseases, Age for Routine Administration of the Second Dose of Measles-Mumps-Rubella Vaccine. *Pediatrics.* 1998 Jan;101(1 Pt 1):129-33.
294. Markowitz, L.E., Albrecht, P., Persistence of Measles Antibody after revaccination. *J Infect Dis.* 1992 Jul;166(1)205-8.
295. Huiss, S., Damien, B., et al., Characteristics of asymptomatic secondary immune responses to measles virus in late convalescent donors. *Clin Exp Immunol.* 1997 Sep;109(3):416-20.
296. Pedersen, I.R., Mordhorst, C.H., et al., Subclinical measles infection in vaccinated seropositive individuals in arctic Greenland. *Vaccine.* 1989 Aug;7(4):345-8.
297. Damien, B., Huiss, S., et al., Estimated susceptibility to asymptomatic secondary immune response against measles in late convalescent and vaccinated persons. *J Med Virol.* 1998 Sep;56(1):85-90.
298. Lambert, S., Lynch, P., Measles Outbreak - Young Adults at High Risk. *Victorian Infectious Diseases Bulletin* May 1999;2(2):21-2.
299. Another Measles Outbreak in Young Adults in Melbourne. *Victorian Infectious Diseases Bulletin* December 2001;4(4):52.
300. Guidelines for the control of measles outbreaks in Australia. *Communicable Diseases Intelligence.* Technical Report Series No. 5,2000, 10.
301. Stewart, G.T., Vaccination against whooping-cough. Efficacy versus risks.

Lancet. 1977 Jan 29;1(8005):234-7.

302. Mansoor, O., and Durham, G., Does Control of Pertussis Need Rethinking? *CDNZ: communicable disease New Zealand.* April1991;91(4):43-5,48.
303. Centers for Disease Control, Pertussis Outbreak - Oklahoma. *MMWR Morb Mortal Wkly Rep.* 1984 Jan 13;33(1):2-10.
304. Centers for Disease Control, Pertussis Outbreaks - Massachusetts and Maryland, 1992. *MMWR Morb Mortal Wkly Rep.* 1993 Mar 26;42(11):197-200.
305. Keitel, W.A., Edwards, K.M., Acellular Pertussis Vaccines in Adults. *Infectious Dis Clin North Am.* 1999 Mar 1;13(1):83-94.
306. Laing, J., Hay, M., Whooping-cough: Its prevalence and mortality in Aberdeen *Public Health.* 1902;14:584-99.
307. Versteegh, F.G., Schellekens, J.F., et al., Laboratory-confirmed reinfections with Bordetella pertussis. *Acta Paediatr.* 2002;91(1):95-7.
308. Wirsing von König, C.H., Postels-Multani, S., et al., Pertussis in adults: frequency of transmission after household exposure. *Lancet.* 1995 Nov 18;346(8986):1326-9.
309. Broutin, H., Rohani, P., et al. Loss of immunity to pertussis in a rural community in Senegal. *Vaccine.* 2004 Jan 26;22(5-6):594-6.
310. Wendelboe, A.M., Van Rie, A., et al. Duration of immunity against pertussis after natural infection or vaccination. *Pediatr Infect Dis J.* 2005 May;24(5 Suppl):S58-61.
311. Wearing, H.J., Rohani, P., Estimating the duration of pertussis immunity using epidemiological signatures. *PLoS Pathog.* 2009 Oct;5(10):e1000647.
312. Dajani, N.A., Scheifele, D., How long can we expect pertussis protection to last after the adolescent booster dose of tetanus-diphtheria-pertussis (Tdap) vaccines? *Paediatr Child Health.* 2007 Dec;12(10):873-4.
313. Mills, K.H., Immunity to Bordetella pertussis. *Microbes Infect.* 2001 Jul;3(8):655-77.
314. Department of National Health and Population Development - Pretoria, Poliomyelitis Epidemic in Natal and Kwazulu. *Epidemiological Comments.* March 1988;15(3):28-9.
315. Schoub, B., Johnson, S., McAnerney, J.M., Immunity to poliomyelitis. *Lancet.* July 14 1990;336(8707):126.
316. Slater, P.E., Orenstein, W.A., et al., Poliomyelitis outbreak in Israel in1988: a report with two commentaries. *Lancet.* 1990 May 19;335(8699):1192-8.
317. Cello, J., Paul, A.V., Wimmer, E., Chemical synthesis of poliovirus cDNA: generation of infectious virus in the absence of natural template. *Science.* 2002 Aug 9;297(5583):1016-8.
318. Wimmer, E., The test-tube synthesis of a chemical called poliovirus: The simple synthesis of a virus has far-reaching societal implications. *EMBO Rep.* 2006 Jul;7(SI):S3-S9.
319. Douglas Hume, Ethel, *Béchamp or Pasteur? A Lost Chapter in the History of Biology.* C. W. Daniel, Ashingdon, Rochford, Essex, Fourth Edition, 1963, 198 & 201.

320. Ibid., 201.
321. Wilson, Graham S., *The Hazards of Immunization.* The Athlone Press, London, 1967, 180.
322. Douglas Hume, Ethel, *Béchamp or Pasteur? A Lost Chapter in the History of Biology.* C. W. Daniel, Ashingdon, Rochford, Essex, Fourth Edition, 1963, 202.
323. D'Arcy Hart, P., et al., *B.C.G. and Vole Bacillus Vaccines in the Prevention of Tuberculosis in Adolescence and Early Adult Life.* Third Report to the Medical Research Council by their Tuberculosis Vaccines Clinical Trials Committee, Fisher, Knight and Co, Ltd., Gainsborough Press, St Albans, undated.
324. James, E.F., B.C.G. and Vole Bacillus Vaccines. *Br Med J.* 1956 Oct 6;2:826-7.
325. Tuberculosis Prevention Trial, Madras. Trial of BCG vaccines in South India for tuberculosis prevention. *Indian J Med Res.* 1979;70:349-63.
326. Tuberculosis Prevention Trial, Madras. Trial of BCG vaccines in South India for tuberculosis prevention. *Indian J Med Res.* 1980;72:suppl.,1-74.
327. Editorial, BCG: Bad News from India. *Lancet.* 1980 Jan 12;(8159):73-4.
328. Editorial, BCG Vaccination after the Madras Study. *Lancet.* February 7 1981 Feb 7;1(8215):309-10.
329. Editorial, Is BCG Vaccination Effective? *Tubercle.* 1981 Sep;62(3):219-21.
330. Böttiger, M., Romanus, V., et al., Osteitis and Other Complications Caused by Generalised BCG-itis: Experiences in Sweden. *Acta Paediatr Scand.* 1982 May;71(3):471-8.
331. Daoud, W., Control of an outbreak of BCG complications in Gaza. *Respirology.* 2003 Sep;8(3):376-8.
332. Here are four examples of trials that show homoeopathy to be effective:
Jacobs, J., Jonas, W.B., et al., Homeopathy for childhood diarrhea: combined results and metaanalysis from three randomized, controlled clinical trials. *Pediatr Infect Dis J.* 2003 Mar;22(3):229-34.
Bell, I.R., Lewis, D.A., et al., Improved clinical status in fibromyalgia patients treated with individualized homeopathic remedies versus placebo. *Rheumatology (Oxford).* 2004 May;43(5):577-82.
Kundu, T., Shaikh, A., et al., Homeopathic medicines substantially reduce the need for clotting factor concentrates in haemophilia patients: results of a blinded placebo controlled cross over trial. *Homeopathy.* 2012 Jan;101(1):38-43.
Danno, K., Colas, A., et al., Homeopathic treatment of migraine in children: results of a prospective, multicenter, observational study. *J Altern Complement Med.* 2013 Feb;19(2):119-23.
333. Personal communication, Dr. Boiron.
334. Dennehy, P.H., Transmission of rotavirus and other enteric pathogens in the home. *Pediatr Infect Dis J.* 2000 Oct;19(10 Suppl):S103-5.
335. The information about how Hahnemann discovered homoeopathy comes from; Cook, T.M., *Samuel Hahnemann, The Founder of Homoeopathic*

Medicine. Thorsons Publishers Ltd., Wellingborough, Northamptonshire, 1981. Another book on Hahnemann's life (in two volumes) is Haehl, Richard, *Samuel Hahnemann: His Life and Work*. London, Homoeopathic Publishing Co., 1922.
336. Hahnemann, Samuel, *Organon of Medicine*, 6th edition. 10, J P Tarcher, Inc., 9110 Sunset Blvd, Los Angeles, CA90069, USA, 1982.
337. Pauling, Linus, *Vitamin C, the Common Cold and the Flu*. Berkley Books, New York, 1983, 167-8.
338. Stone, Irwin, *The Healing Factor, Vitamin C against Disease*. Grosset and Dunlap, New York, 1972.
339. Cheraskin, E., Ringsdorf, W.M., Sisley, E.L., *The Vitamin C Connection: Getting well and staying well with Vitamin C*. Thorsons, Wellingborough, Northamptonshire, 1983.
340. Chan, R.C., Penney, D.J., et al., Hepatitis and death following vaccination with 17D-204 yellow fever vaccine. *Lancet*. 2001 Jul 14;358(9276):121-2.
341. Ayvazian, L.F., Risks of Repeated Immunization. *Ann Intern Med*. 1975 Apr;82(4):589.
342. Thomas, R.E., Lorenzetti, D.L., et al., Reporting rates of yellow fever vaccine 17D or 17DD-associated serious adverse events in pharmacovigilance data bases: systematic review. *Curr Drug Saf*. 2011 Jul;6(3):145-54.
343. Dye, C., Scheele, S., et al., Consensus statement. Global burden of tuberculosis: estimated incidence, prevalence, and mortality by country. WHO Global Surveillance and Monitoring Project. *JAMA*. 1999 Aug 18;282(7):677-86.
344. Balasubramanian, R., Garg, R., et al. Gender disparities in tuberculosis: report from a rural DOTS programme in south India. *Int J Tuberc Lung Dis*. 2004 Mar;8(3):323-32.
345. Lin, P.L., Flynn, J.L., Understanding latent tuberculosis: A moving target. *J Immunol*. 2010 Jul 1;185(1):15-22.
346. Lönnroth, K., Raviglione, M., Global epidemiology of tuberculosis: prospects for control. *Semin Respir Crit Care Med*. 2008 Oct;29(5):481-91.
347. Horsburgh, C.R., Priorities for the treatment of latent tuberculosis infection in the United States. *N Engl J Med*. 2004 May 13;350(20):2060-7.
348. Koch, R., Die Aetiologie der Tuberculose. *Berl Klin Wochenschr. 1882* 19;221-30.
349. Bhargava, A., Chatterjee, M., et al. Nutritional status of adult patients with pulmonary tuberculosis in rural central India and its association with mortality. *PLoS One*. 2013 Oct 24;8(10):e77979.
350. Cegielski, J.P., McMurray, D.N., The relationship between malnutrition and tuberculosis: evidence from studies in humans and experimental animals. *Int J Tubercul Lung Dis*. 2004 Mar;8(3):286-98.
351. Onwubalili, J.K., Malnutrition among tuberculosis patients in Harrow, England. *Eur J Clin Nutr*. 1988 Apr;42(4):363-6.
352. Karyadi, E., Schultink, W., et al., Poor Micronutrient Status of

Active Pulmonary Tuberculosis Patients in Indonesia. *J Nutr.* 2000 Dec;130(12):2953-8.
353. Tshabalala, R.T., Anaphylactic Reactions to BCG in Swaziland. *Lancet.* 1983 Mar 19;1(8325):653.
354. Pichat, P., Reveilleau, A., Bactericidal action for Koch's bacilli of massive doses of vitamin C; comparison of its action on a certain number of other microbes. *Ann Inst Pasteur (Paris).* 1950 79;342-4.
355. Pichat, P., Reveilleau, A., Comparison between the in vivo and in vitro bactericidal action of vitamin C and its metabolite, and ascorbic acid level. *Ann Inst Pasteur (Paris).* 1951 80;212-3.
356. Vilchèze, C., Hartman, C., et al., Mycobacterium tuberculosis is extraordinarily sensitive to killing by a vitamin C-induced Fenton reaction. *Nat Commun.* 2013 May 21; 4:1881.
357. Albrecht, E., Vitamin C as an Adjuvant in the Therapy of Pulmonary Tuberculosis. *Med Klin.* 1938;39:972-3.
358. Deerr, Noel, *The History of Sugar*. Chapman and Hall, London, 1949.
359. Sheridan, Richard, Sugar and Slavery: An Economic History of the British West Indies, 1623 – 1775. The John Hopkins University Press, 1974.
360. Dunbabin, Thomas, *Slavers of the South Seas.* Angus and Robertson, Sydney, 1935.
361. Docker, Edward, *The Blackbirders: A brutal story of the Kanaka Slave Trade.* Angus and Robertson, London, 1970.
362. Huggins, Hal, *Why Raise Ugly Kids?* Arlington House, Westport, Connecticut, 1981.
363. Price, Weston, *Nutrition and Physical Degeneration.* The Price-Pottinger Nutrition Foundation, Inc, La Mesa, California, 1982. I loaned this book to an orthodontist, and after he had read it he said, "But he doesn't give any evidence." Denialus supremus.
364. Smith, Lendon, *Feed Your Kids Right.* Dell Publishing Co, New York, 1981.
365. Yudkin, John, *Sweet and Dangerous.* Bantam Books, New York, 1977.
366. Yudkin, John, *Pure, White and Deadly: The Problem of Sugar.* Davis-Poynter Ltd, London, 1972.
367. Smith, Lendon, *Improving Your Child's Behaviour Chemistry.* Pocket Books, New York, 1977.
368. Jarrett, R.J., (ed), *Nutrition and Disease.* Croom Helm, London, 1979.
369. Atkins, Robert C., Linde, Shirley, *Dr. Atkins' Super-Energy Diet.* Bantam Books, New York, 1978, 279-89.
370. Weinstein, L., Aycock, W.L., Feemster, R.F., The relation of sex, pregnancy and menstruation to susceptibility in poliomyelitis. *N Engl J Med.* 1951 Jul 12;245(2):54-8.
371. Paffenbarger, R.S., Wilson, V.O., Previous tonsillectomy and current pregnancy as they affect risk of poliomyelitis. *Ann N Y Acad Sci.* 1955 Sep 27;61(4):856-68.
372. Anderson, G.W., Anderson, G., et al., Poliomyelitis in pregnancy. *Am J*

Hyg. 1952 Jan;55(1):127-39.
373. Horstmann, D.M., Acute poliomyelitis. Relation of physical activity at the time of onset to the course of the disease. *JAMA.* 1950 Jan 28;142(4):236-41.
374. Russell, W.R., Poliomyelitis: The Pre-Paralytic Stage, and the Effect of Physical Activity on the Severity of Paralysis. *Br Med J.* 1947 Dec 27;2(4538):1023-8.
375. Russell, W.R., Paralytic poliomyelitis: The early symptoms, and the effect of physical activity on the course of disease. *Br Med J.* 1949 Mar 19;1(4602):465-471.
376. Hargreaves, E. R., Poliomyelitis: Effect of Exertion During the Pre-Paralytic Stage. *Br Med J.* 1948 Dec 11;2(4588):1021-2.
377. Churchill, Allen, *The Roosevelts.* Frederick Muller Limited, London,1966.
378. Wright, A.E., The Changes Effected by Anti-typhoid Inoculation in the Bactericidal Power of the Blood: with Remarks on the Probable Significance of These Changes. *Lancet.* 1901 Sep 14;2(4072):715-23.
379. Wilson, Graham S., *The Hazards of Immunization.* The Athlone Press, London, 1967, 265.
380. Hill, A.B., Knowelden, J., Inoculation and Poliomyelitis: A statistical investigation in England and Wales in 1949. *Br Med J.* 1950 Jul 1;2(4669):1-6.
381. Shelton, H.N., *Serums and Polio.* Dr Shelton's Hygienic Review, August 1951, reprinted in McBean, E., *The Poisoned Needle.* Health Research, 1974, 164.
382. Shepherd, Dorothy, *Homoeopathy in Epidemic Diseases.* Health Science Press, Rustington, Sussex, 1967, 76.
383. Shelton, H.N., *Serums and Polio*, Dr Shelton's Hygienic Review, August 1951, reprinted in McBean, E., *The Poisoned Needle.* Health Research, 1974, 165.
384. Wilson, Graham S., *The Hazards of Immunization.* The Athlone Press, London, 1967, 273.
385. Sutter, R.W., Patriarca, P.A., et al., Attributable Risk of DPT (Diphtheria and Tetanus Toxoids and Pertussis Vaccine) Injection in Provoking Paralytic Poliomyelitis during a Large Outbreak in Oman. *J Infect Dis.* 1992 Mar;165(3):444-9.
386. Aycock, W.L., Tonsillectomy and poliomyelitis. *Medicine.* 1942;21(65):65-94.
387. Weinstein, L., Vogel, M.L., Weinstein, N., A study of the relationship of the absence of tonsils to the incidence of bulbar poliomyelitis. *J Pediatr.* 1954 Jan;44(1):14-9.
388. Southcott, R.V., Studies on a long range association between bulbar poliomyelitis and previous tonsillectomy. *Med J Aust.* 1953 Aug 22;2(8):281-98.
389. Mills, C. K., The tonsillectomy-poliomyelitis problem; a review of the literature. *Laryngoscope.* 1951 Dec;61(12):1188-96.
390. Shepherd, Dorothy, *Homoeopathy in Epidemic Diseases.* Health Science Press, Rustington, Sussex, 1967, 76-8.

391. Honorof, I., McBean, E., *Vaccination the Silent Killer: A Clear and Present Danger. Honor Publications,* Sherman Oaks, California, 1977,32-3.
392. Jungeblut, C.W., Inactivation of Poliomyelitis Virus by Crystalline Vitamin C (Ascorbic Acid). *J Exp Med.* 1935 Sep 30;62(4):517-21.
393. Pauling, Linus, *Vitamin C and the Common Cold and the Flu.* Berkley Books, New York, 1983, 52. Linus Pauling gives 11 references to Klenner's documentation of the treatment in medical journals.
394. Davis, Adelle, *Let's Eat Right to Keep Fit.* Unwin Paperbacks, London, 1984, 111-2.
395. Klenner, F.R., The treatment of poliomyelitis and other virus diseases with vitamin C. *South Med Surg.* 1949 Jul;111(7):209-14.
396. Klenner, F.R., Massive doses of vitamin C and the virus diseases. *South Med Surg.* 1951 Apr;103(4):101-7. (PubMed gives the wrong volume number.)
397. Greer, E., Vitamin C In Acute Poliomyelitis. *Med Times.* 1955 Nov;83(11):1160-1.
398. Pauling, Linus, *Vitamin C, the common cold and the flu.* Berkley Books, New York, 55.
399. Jahan, K., Ahmad, K., Ali, M.A., Effect of Ascorbic Acid in the Treatment of Tetanus. *Bangladesh Med Res Counc Bull.* 1984 June;10(1):24-8.
400. Judd, L.D., Calomel as a curative agent in diphtheria. *Trans Am Climatol Assoc.* 1897;13:206-13. Calomel is another word for mercury.
401. Judd, L.D., Remarks based upon a further experience with calomel in diphtheria. *Trans Am Climatol Assoc.* 1899;15:197-202.
402. Lagget, M., Rizetto, M., Current pharmacotherapy for the treatment of chronic hepatitis B. *Expert Opin Pharmacother.* 2003 Oct;4(10):1821-7.
403. Statement of the Association of American Physicians and Surgeons to the Subcommittee on Criminal Justice, Drug Policy, and Human Resources of the Committee on Government Reform U.S. House of Representatives Re: Hepatitis B Vaccine. Submitted by Jane Orient, M.D. June 14, 1999.
404. Hernán, M.A., Jick, S.S., et al., Recombinant hepatitis B vaccine and the risk of multiple sclerosis – A prospective study. *Neurology.* 2004 Sep 14;63(5):838-42.
405. Le Houézec, D. Evolution of multiple sclerosis in France since the beginning of hepatitis B vaccination. *Immunol Res.* 2014 Dec;60(2-3):219-25
406. Langer-Gould, A., Qian, L., et al., Vaccines and the risk of multiple sclerosis and other central nervous system demyelinating diseases. *JAMA Neurol.* 2014 Dec;71(12):1506-13.
407. Wood, H., Demyelinating disease: new study refutes link between vaccines and demyelination. *Nat Rev Neurol.* 2014 Dec;10(12):673.
408. Girard, M, Autoimmune hazards of hepatitis B vaccine. *Autoimmun Rev.* 2005 Feb;4(2):96-100.
409. Lee, C., Gong, Y., et al., Effect of hepatitis B immunisation in newborn infants of mothers positive for hepatitis B surface antigen: systematic

review and meta-analysis. *BMJ.* 2006 Feb 11;332(7537):328-36.
410. Sarter, B., Banerji, P., Banerji, P., Successful Treatment of Chronic Viral Hepatitis with High-dilution Medicine. *Glob Adv Health Med.* 2012 Mar;1(1):26–29.
411. Roy, S.K., Hossain, M.J., et al., Zinc supplementation in children with cholera in Bangladesh: randomised controlled trial. *BMJ.* 2008 Feb 2;336(7638):266-8.
412. Cook, T.M., *Samuel Hahnemann, The Founder of Homoeopathic Medicine.* Thorsons Publishers Ltd., Wellingborough, Northamptonshire, 1981, 146.
413. Blackie, Margery G., *The Patient, Not The Cure.* Macdonald and Jane's, London, 1976, 32.
414. Ibid., 1976, 31.
415. Cook, T.M., Samuel Hahnemann, *The Founder of Homoeopathic Medicine.* Thorsons Publishers Ltd., Wellingborough, Northamptonshire, 1981, 148.
416. Blackie, Margery G., *The Patient, Not The Cure.* Macdonald and Jane's, London, 1976, 34.
417. Fisher, P., The World's Most Famous Homoeopathic Hospital. *Homoeopathy Today.* 1989;2(12):6.
418. Butler, A.G., *The Australian Army Medical Services in the war of 1914-1918.* Australian War Memorial, Melbourne, 1930.
419. Hurst, A., *Diseases of the War.* London, Arnold, 1917.
420. Martin, C.J., Upjohn, W.G.D., The distribution of typhoid and paratyphoid infections amongst enteric fevers at Mudros. *Br Med J.* 1916 Sep 2;2(2905):313-6.
421. Engels, E.A., Falagas, M.E., et al. Typhoid fever vaccines: a meta-analysis of studies on efficacy and toxicity. *BMJ.* 1998 Jan 10;316(7125):110-6.
422. Butler, A.G., *The Australian Army Medical Services in the War of 1914-1918.* Australian War Memorial, Melbourne, 1930, 364.
423. Cook, T.M., *Samuel Hahnemann, The Founder of Homoeopathic Medicine.* Thorson's Publishers, 1981, 103-4.
424. Swartout, H.O., *Modern Medical Counsellor.* Signs Publishing Company, Warburton, Victoria, Australia. 1958, 763.
425. Clarke, John Henry, *Dictionary of Materia Medica.* Health Science Press, Bradford, Holsworthy, Devon, 1977, 211. (First printed in 1901.)
426. Blackie, Margery G., *The Patient, Not the Cure.* MacDonald and Jane's, London, 1976, 39 & 81-2.
427. Carmichael, A.E., Silverstein, A.M., Smallpox in Europe before the Seventeenth Century: Virulent Killer or Benign Disease? *J Hist Med Allied Sci.* 1987;42(2):147-68.
428. Observations by Mr. Fosbrooke. *Lancet.* 1829 Aug 8;2(310):582-5.
429. Douglas Hume, Ethel, *Béchamp or Pasteur? A Lost Chapter in the History of Biology.* C. W. Daniel, Ashingdon, Rochford, Essex, Fourth Edition, 1963, 171.
430. Jenner, E., *Facts, for the most part unobserved, or not duly noticed, respecting variolous contagion.* S. Gosnell, London, 1808. There is an

original copy of this in Melbourne on which Jenner has written, "A. Cooper Esq, with the best wishes of the Author."
431. Vaccination Tracts: Opinions of Statesmen, Politicians, Publicists, Statisticians, and Sanitarians. No 1. Second Edition. William Young, London, 1879.
432. Wilson, Graham S., *The Hazards of Immunization.* The Athlone Press, London, 1967, 256.
433. Marmelzat, W.L., Malignant tumors in smallpox vaccination scars: a report of 24 cases. *Arch Dermatol.* 1968 Apr;97(4):400-6.
434. Lane, J.M., Ruben, F.L., et al., Complications of Smallpox Vaccination, 1968: Results of Ten Statewide Surveys. *J Infect Dis.* 1970 Oct;122(4):303-9.
435. Rich, J.D., Shesol, B.F., Horne, D.W., Basal cell carcinoma arising in a smallpox vaccination site. *J Clin Pathol.* 1980 Feb;33(2):134-5.
436. Crookshank, E.M., *History and Pathology of Vaccination.* Vol 1. H. K. Lewis, 1889, 74.
437. Stickl, H., Die Nichtenzephalitischen Erkrankungen nach der Pockenschutzimpfung. *Deutsche Medizinische Wochenschrift.* 1968;93:511-7.
438. Wolfe, R.M., Sharp, L.K., Anti-vaccinationists past and present. *BMJ.* 2002 August 24;325(7361):430-2.
439. The manuscript of the article which Jenner submitted to the Royal Society in the hopes that they would publish it in their Transactions of the Royal Society was left lying in a drawer until it was shown to E.M. Crookshank by the librarian at the Royal College of Surgeons in January 1888. E.M. Crookshank ensured "that it has been carefully preserved, and entered in the catalogue of the Library, and may be consulted by anyone desiring to do so." Crookshank, E.M., *History and Pathology of Vaccination.* Vol 1. H. K. Lewis, 1889, page viii. It was later published in the Lancet of 20th January 1923, on pages 137-41.
440. Jenner, Edward, *An Inquiry into the Causes and Effects of the Variolae Vaccinae, a disease discovered in some of the western counties of England, particularly Gloucestershire, and known by the name of the Cow Pox.* Sampson Low, London, 1798. Facsimile Reprint, An Inquiry into the Causes and Effects of the Variolae Vaccinae. Dawsons of Pall Mall, London, 1966.
441. Ibid., 37.
442. Crookshank, E.M., *History and Pathology of Vaccination.* H. K. Lewis, 1889, 1:270.
443. Ibid., 269-73.
444. Further Observations on the Variole Vaccinae, or Cow Pox. Edward Jenner, M.D., F.R.S., &c, in Crookshank, E.M., *History and Pathology of Vaccination.* Vol 1. H. K. Lewis, 1889, 2:155-190. Page 169 is where the death is mentioned.
445. Fenner, F., Henderson, D.A., et al., *Smallpox and its Eradication.* World

Health Organization, Geneva, 1988.
446. Jenner, Edward, *An Inquiry into the Causes and Effects of the Variolae Vaccinae, a disease discovered in some of the western counties of England, particularly Gloucestershire, and known by the name of the Cow Pox.* Sampson Low, London, 1798. Facsimile Reprint, An Inquiry into the Causes and Effects of the Variolae Vaccinae. Dawsons of Pall Mall, London, 1966, 6.
447. Fenner, F., Henderson, D.A., et al., *Smallpox and its Eradication.* World Health Organization, Geneva, 1988, 271.
448. Ibid., 273.
449. Thagard, Paul, *How Scientists Explain Disease.* Princeton University Press, Princeton, 1999, 155-6.
450. Trusted, Jennifer, Theories and Facts, Unit 7, *The Germ Theory of Disease.* The Open University Press, Milton Keynes, 1981, 10.
451. Dobell, C., *Antony van Leewenhoek and his "Little Animals".* Russel and Russel Inc., New York, 1958.
452. Geison, G.L., *The Private Science of Louis Pasteur.* Princeton University Press, Princeton, New Jersey, 1995, 267.
453. Ibid., 267-9.
454. Douglas Hume, Ethel, *Béchamp or Pasteur? A Lost Chapter in the History of Biology.* C. W. Daniel, Ashingdon, Rochford, Essex, Fourth Edition, 1963.
455. Geison, G. L., *The Private Science of Louis Pasteur.* Princeton University Press, Princeton, New Jersey, 1995.
456. Katz Miller, S., The Daring and Devious Father of Vaccines. *New Sci.* 20 February 1993;137:10.
457. Anderson, C., Pasteur Notebooks Reveal Deception. *Science.* 19 February 1993;259:1117.
458. Geison, G. L., *The Private Science of Louis Pasteur.* Princeton University Press, Princeton, New Jersey, 1995, 3.
459. Douglas Hume, Ethel, *Béchamp or Pasteur? A Lost Chapter in the History of Biology.* C. W. Daniel, Ashingdon, Rochford, Essex, Fourth Edition, 1963, 38.
460. Ibid., 58.
461. Ibid., 101.
462. Ibid., 90.
463. Ibid., 92.
464. Ibid., 93.
465. The World Book Encyclopedia 1994;15:212. World Book International.
466. Geison, G. L., *The Private Science of Louis Pasteur.* Princeton University Press, Princeton, New Jersey, 1995, 145-76.
467. Douglas Hume, Ethel, *Béchamp or Pasteur? A Lost Chapter in the History of Biology.* C. W. Daniel, Ashingdon, Rochford, Essex, Fourth Edition, 1963, 185-6.
468. Ibid., 191-2.

469. Ibid., 192.
470. Nass, M., Anthrax Vaccine; Model of a Response to the Biologic Warfare Threat. *Infect Dis Clin North Am.* 1999 Mar;13(1):187-208.
471. Pearson, R.B., *Pasteur, Plagiarist, Imposter.* 1942. Reprinted by Health Research, Mokelumne Hill, California, 1964, 95.
472. Ad Hoc Group for the study of pertussis vaccines, Placebo-Controlled Trial of two acellular pertussis vaccines in Sweden - Protective Efficacy and Adverse Events. *Lancet.* April 30 1988;955-60.
473. Geison, G. L., *The Private Science of Louis Pasteur.* Princeton University Press, Princeton, New Jersey, 1995, 240-5.
474. Ibid., 240.
475. Ibid., 240-1.
476. Ibid., 241.
477. Ibid., 243.
478. Ibid., 189.
479. Ibid., 191.
480. Ibid., 213.
481. Ibid., 213-4.
482. Douglas Hume, Ethel, *Béchamp or Pasteur? A Lost Chapter in the History of Biology.* C. W. Daniel, Ashingdon, Rochford, Essex, Fourth Edition, 1963, 196.
483. Human Viral and Rickettsial Vaccines. *Wld Hlth Org Tech Rep Ser.* 1966;325:31.
484. Dole, Lionel, *The Blood Poisoners.* Gateway Book Company, Croydon, Surrey, 1965, 58.
485. Douglas Hume, Ethel, *Béchamp or Pasteur? A Lost Chapter in the History of Biology.* C. W. Daniel, Ashingdon, Rochford, Essex, Fourth Edition, 1963, 195.
486. Ibid., 200.
487. Geison, G. L., *The Private Science of Louis Pasteur.* Princeton University Press, Princeton, New Jersey, 1995, 221.
488. McBean, E., *The Poisoned Needle.* Health Research, 1974, 188.
489. Plotkin, S.A., Vaccine production in human diploid cell strains. *Am J Epidemiol.* 1971 Oct;94(4):303-6.
490. Koprowski, H., Laboratory techniques in rabies: vaccine for man prepared in human diploid cells. *Monogr Ser World Health Organ.* 1973;(23):256-60.
491. Plotkin, S.A., Wiktor, T.J., et al., Immunization Schedules for the new human diploid cell vaccine against rabies. *Am J Epidemiol.* 1976 Jan;103(1):75-80.
492. Oelofsen, M.J., Gericke, A., et al., Immunity to rabies after administration of prophylactic human diploid cell vaccine. *S Afr Med J.* 1991 Aug 17;80(4):189-90.
493. Mansour, A.B., Abrous, M., Properties and potency of a rabies vaccine produced on the brain matter of young goats and inactivated by betapropiolactone. *Dev Biol Stand.* 1978;41:217-24.

494. Lin, F., Zeng, F., et al., The primary hamster kidney cell rabies vaccine: adaptation of viral strain, production of vaccine and pre- and post exposure treatment. *J Infect Dis*. 1983 Mar;147(3):467-73.
495. Wasi, C., Chaiprasithikul, P., et al., Purified chick embryo cell rabies vaccine. *Lancet*. 1986 Jan 4;1(8471):40.
496. van Wezel, A. L., van Steenis, G., Production of an inactivated rabies vaccine in primary dog kidney cells. *Dev Biol Stand.* 1978;40:69-75.
497. Wilson, Graham S., *The Hazards of Immunization*. The Athlone Press, London, 1967, 255.
498. Kaufmann S.H.E., Robert Koch's highs and lows in the search for a remedy for tuberculosis. *Nature Medicine*. 2000. Special Web Focus: Tuberculosis.
499. Coulter, H.L., Loe Fisher, B., *DPT A Shot in the Dark.* Warner Books, New York, March 1986, 294.
500. Ibid. 298.
501. Ibid. 296.
502. Gary Hughes, Polio vaccine tested at orphanages. *The Age*, October 25, 2004.
503. Coulter, H.L., Loe Fisher, B., *DPT A Shot in the Dark.* Warner Books, New York, March 1986, 44.
504. Whooping Cough Immunization Committee of the Medical Research Council, Vaccination Against Whooping-Cough. *Br Med J.* 1956 Aug 25;2(4990):454-62.
505. Coulter, H.L., Loe Fisher, B., *DPT A Shot in the Dark.* Warner Books, New York, March 1986, 34.
506. Ibid., 32.
507. Cody, C.L., Baraff, L.J., et al., Nature and Rates of Adverse Reactions Associated with DTP and DT Immunizations in Infants and Children. *Pediatrics.* 1981 Nov;68(5):650-60.
508. Coulter, H.L., Loe Fisher, B., *DPT A Shot in the Dark.* Warner Books, New York, March 1986, 243-54.
509. Dellepiane, N., Griffiths, E., Milstien, J.B., New Challenges in assuring vaccine quality. *Bull World Health Organ*. 2000;78(2):155-62.
510. Coulter, H.L., Loe Fisher, B., *DPT A Shot in the Dark.* Warner Books, New York, March 1986, 28-31.
511. Pittman, M., *Bordatella Pertussis - Bacterial and Host Factors in the Pathogenesis and Prevention of Whooping Cough,* in, Mudd, S., *Infectious Agents and Host Reactions,* W.B. Saunders Co, Philadelphia,1970, 261.
512. Ibid., 259.
513. Dick, G., Convulsive disorders in young children. *Proc Roy Soc Med.* 1974 May;67:371-2.
514. Brian McDonald, Drugs firm withheld key results of vaccine test. *Irish Independent,* 29 June 2001.
515. *Against All Odds - Margaret's Story*, Jan 1994, BBC.
516. Neville Hodgkinson, Mother wins 20-year battle against vaccine drug giant. *The Sunday Times*. 25 April 1993.

517. Stuart-Smith, Lord Justice. Judgement, Susan Jaqueline Loveday v. Dr. GH Renton and The Wellcome Foundation Limited, 29-30 March 1988. London, Chilton Vint and Co.
518. Dyer, C., Judge "not satisfied" that whooping cough vaccine causes permanent brain damage. *Br Med J (Clin Res Ed)*. 1988 Apr 23;296(6630):1189-90.
519. Cutts, F.T., Zaman, S.M., et al., Gambian Pneumococcal Vaccine Trial Group. Efficacy of nine-valent pneumococcal conjugate vaccine against pneumonia and invasive pneumococcal disease in The Gambia: randomised, double-blind, placebo-controlled trial. *Lancet*. 2005 Mar 26-Apr 1;365(9465):1139-46.
520. Golomb, B.A., Erickson, L.C., What's in placebos: who knows? Analysis of randomized, controlled trials. *Ann Intern Med*. 2010 Oct 19;153(8):532-5.
521. Fuhr, U., Tuculanu, D., et al., Bioequivalence between novel ready-to-use liquid formulations of the recombinant human GH Omnitrope and the original lyophilized formulations for reconstitution of Omnitrope and Genotropin. *Eur J Endocrinol*. 2010 Jun;162(6):1051-8.
522. Golomb, B.A., Paradox of Placebo Effect. *Nature*. 1995 Jun 15;375(6532):530.
523. Golomb, B.A., When are medication side effects due to the nocebo phenomenon? *JAMA*. 2002 May 15;287(19):2502-4.
524. Gorman, C., Drug Safety; Can Drug Firms Be Trusted? *Time*. February10, 1992, 33.
525. Coulter, H.L., Loe Fisher, B., DPT; *A Shot in the Dark*. Warner Books, New York, March 1986, 286.
526. Braithwaite, J., *Corporate Crime in the Pharmaceutical Industry*. Routledge and Kegan Paul, London, 1984.
527. Tom Mangold, *The Halcion Nightmare*. Panorama, BBC.
528. McCarthy, M., Conflict of interest taints vaccine approval process, charges US report. *Lancet*. 2000 Sep 2;356(9232):838.
529. *Vaccination, The Choice is Yours* 6(2):2000, 38, quoting Kathi Williams of NVIC. The congressman was Dan Burton of Indiana.
530. Coulter, H.L., Loe Fisher, B., *DPT A Shot in the Dark*. Warner Books, New York, March 1986, 314.
531. *Total Recall*, Four Corners, 11 April 2005.
532. Child vaccine may be delayed. *New Zealand Herald*. 8 September, 1992.
533. Stewart, G.T., Toxicity of pertussis vaccine: frequency and probability of reactions. *J Epidemiol Comm Health*. 1979 Jun;33(2):150-6.
534. Official Line on Vaccine Does U-turn. *New Zealand Herald*. 11 July, 1987.
535. Giarnia Thompson - An Innocent Bystander. Hilary Butler, *IAS Newsletter*. April 1992;4(5):2-6.
536. Hood, A., Edwards, I. R., Meningococcal vaccine - do some children experience side effects? *NZ Med J*. 1989 Feb 22;102(862):65-7.
537. *IAS Newsletter*. August 1989;2(1):12.
538. Personal communication, Hilary Butler, after she had been speaking to the

Medical Assessor.
539. Butler, H., Introducing the New Zealand Department of Health's Meningococcal Meningitis Immunisation Campaign. IRONI, 1987.
540. Ibid., 24.
541. President Reagan Signs Vaccine Injury Compensation and Safety Bill Into Law. *DPT News*, Spring 1987;3(1):1, 10-6.
542. Centers for Disease Control, Vaccine Adverse Events Reporting System – United States. *MMWR Morb Mortal Wkly Rep.* 1990 Oct 19;39(41):730-3.
543. Personal communication, Hilary Butler, after talking on the phone to Dr. Morris.
544. Morris, J. Anthony, *Childhood Vaccine Injury Compensation Programme in the US; Hope Versus Reality*. International Symposium, The Vaccination Dilemma, Auckland, 1992.
545. Annex 1, Q and A's: Vaccine Adverse Event Reporting System (VAERS).
546. NVIC/DPT Investigation Shows That Doctors And Government Fail To Report And Monitor Vaccine Death And Injury Reports. *NVIC News.* August 1994;4(1).
547. National Health and Medical Research Council, *The Australian Immunisation Handbook,* 7th Edition. March 2000, 22.
548. Personal communication, Meryl Dorey.
549. Grimsey, L., Our trip to Canberra. *Vaccination, The Choice is Yours.* 4(2):1998, 22.
550. Mehta, U., Milstien, J.B., et al., Developing a national system for dealing with adverse events following immunization. *Bull World Health Organ.* 2000,78(2):170-5.
551. Kearney, M., Yach, D., et al., Evaluation of a mass measles immunisation campaign in a rapidly growing peri-urban area. *S Afr Med J.* 1989 Aug 19;76(4):157-9.
552. Coulter, H.L., Loe Fisher, B., *DPT; A Shot in the Dark.* Warner Books, New York, March 1986, 100.
553. Offit, P. A., Bell, L.M., *Vaccines: What every parent should know.* IDG Books, New York, 1999, 44.
554. Floersheim, G.L., Facilitation of Tumour Growth by Bacillus pertussis. *Nature.* 1967;216(5121):1235-6.
555. Moskowitz, R., The Case Against Immunizations. Reprinted from the *Journal of the American Institute of Homeopathy*, 1983.
556. Offit, P.A., DeStefano, F., *Vaccine Safety*, in Plotkin, S.A., Orenstein, W., Offit, P.A., (eds.) *Vaccines*, 6th Edition. Elsevier Saunders, 2013, 1468, printed in China.
557. Institute of Medicine, *Childhood Immunization Schedule and Safety: Stakeholder Concerns, Scientific Evidence, and Future Studies*. January 16, 2013.
558. Ibid., 133.
559. Madsen, K.M., Hviid, A., et al., A Population-Based Study of Measles, Mumps, and Rubella Vaccination and Autism. *New Engl J Med.* 2002 Nov

7;347(19):1477-82.
560. Shaw, F.E., Graham, D.J., et al., Postmarketing surveillance for neurologic adverse events reported after Hepatitis B vaccination. Experience of the first three years. *Am J Epidemiol.* 1988 Feb;127(2):337-52.
561. Hepatitis B vaccines: reported reactions. *WHO Drug Inf.* 1990;4(3):129.
562. Herroelen, L., De Keyser, J., Ebinger, G., Central-nervous-system demyelination after immunisation with recombinant hepatitis B vaccine. *Lancet.* 1991 Nov 9;338(8776):1174-5.
563. Kaprowski, H., Lebell, I., The presence of complement-fixing antibodies against brain tissue in sera of persons who had received antirabies vaccine treatment. *Am J Hyg.* 1950 May;51(3):292-9.
564. Kong, Von E., Zur Pertussisimpfung und ihren Gegenindikationen. *Helv Paediatr Acta.* 1953 Mar;8(1):90-8. The summary is given in German, French, Italian and English.
565. Kulenkampff, M., Schwartzman, J. S., Wilson, J., Neurological complications of pertussis inoculation. *Arch Dis Child.* 1974 Jan;49(1):46-9.
566. Centers for Disease Control, Recommendations of the Immunization Practices Advisory Committee (ACIP): Misconceptions Concerning Contraindications to Vaccination. *MMWR Morb Mortal Wkly Rep.* 1989 Apr 7;38(13):223-4.
567. Baraff, L.J., Cody, C.L., Cherry, J.D., DTP-Associated Reactions: An Analysis by Injection Site, Manufacturer, Prior Reactions, and Dose. *Pediatrics.* 1984 Jan;73(1):31-6.
568. Sen, S., Cloete, Y., et al., Adverse events following vaccination in premature infants. *Acta Paediatr.* 2001 Aug;90(8):916-20.
569. Lewis, K., Cherry, J. D., et al., The effect of Prophylactic Acetaminophen Administration on Reactions to DTP Vaccination. *Am J Dis Child.* January 1988 Jan;142(1):62-5.
570. Ipp, M.M., Gold, R., et al., Acetaminophen prophylaxis of adverse reactions following vaccination of infants with diphtheria-pertussis-tetanus toxoids-polio vaccine. *Pediatr Infect Dis J.* 1987 Aug;6(8):721-5.
571. Paracetamol Increases Immunisation Compliance. *Current Therapeutics.* 1988 Sep;29(9):12.
572. Strom J., Further Experience of Reactions, Especially of a Cerebral Nature, in Conjunction with Triple Vaccination: A Study Based on Vaccinations in Sweden 1959 - 65. *Brit Med J.* 1967 Nov 11;4(5575):320-3.
573. Van Der Horst, R.L., On teething in infancy. *Clin Pediatr (Phila).* 1973 Oct;12(10):607-10.
574. Cerri, P.S., Pereira-Júnior, J.A., et al., Mast cells and MMP-9 in the lamina propria during eruption of rat molars: quantitative and immunohistochemical evaluation. *J Anat.* 2010 Aug;217(2):116-25.
575. Schilling, L., Wahl, M., Opening of the blood-brain barrier during cortical superfusion with histamine. *Brain Res.* 1994 Aug 8;653(1-2):289-96.
576. Abbott, N.J., Inflammatory mediators and modulation of blood-brain barrier

permeability. *Cell Mol Neurobiol.* 2000 Apr;20(2):131-47.

577. Stamatovic, S.M., Keep, R.F., Andjelkovic, A.V., Brain Endothelial Cell-Cell Junctions: How to "Open" the Blood Brain Barrier. *Curr Neuropharmacol.* 2008 September;6(3): 179-92.
578. Berg, J.M., Neurological Complications of Pertussis Immunization. *Brit Med J.* 1958 Jul 5;2(5087)24-7.
579. Keith, L.S., Jones, D.E., Chou, C.H., Aluminum toxicokinetics regarding infant diet and vaccinations. *Vaccine.* 2002 May 31;20 Suppl 3:S13-7.
580. Finn, T.M., Egan, W., *Vaccine additives and manufacturing residuals in the United States*, in Plotkin, S.A., Orenstein, W., Offit, P.A., *Vaccines*, 6th Edition. Elsevier Saunders, 2013, printed in China.
581. Shivasharan, B.D., Nagakannan, P., et al., Protective Effect of Calendula officinalis L. Flowers Against Monosodium Glutamate Induced Oxidative Stress and Excitotoxic Brain Damage in Rats. *Indian J Clin Biochem.* 2013 Jul;28(3):292-8.
582. *Vaccines Not Mercury Free.* Health Advocacy in the Public Interest, Press Release, August 12, 2004.
583. Austin, D.W.,Shandley, K.A.,Palombo, E.A., Mercury in vaccines from the Australian childhood immunization program schedule. *J Toxicol Environ Health A.* 2010;73(10):637-40.
584. Shin, J., Wood, D., et al., WHO informal consultation on the application of molecular methods to assure the quality, safety and efficacy of vaccines, Geneva, Switzerland, 7–8 April 2005. *Biologicals.* 2007 Mar;35(1):63-71.
585. Plotkin, S.A., Orenstein, W., Offit, P.A., *Vaccines,* 6th Edition. Elsevier Saunders, 2013, printed in China.
586. Koyama, K., Deisher, T.A., *Spontaneous Integration of Human DNA Fragments into Host Genome.* Sound Choice Pharmaceutical Institute, Seattle, WA.
587. Murnane, J.P., Yezzi, M.J., Young, B.R., Recombination events during integration of transfected DNA into normal human cells. *Nucleic Acids Res.* 1990 May 11;18(9):2733-8.
588. Ma, B., He, L.F., et al., Characteristics and viral propagation properties of a new human diploid cell line, Walvax-2, and its suitability as a candidate cell substrate for vaccine production. *Hum Vaccin Immunother.* 2015;11(4):998-1009.
589. Limerick, S.R., Sudden infant death in historical perspective. *J Clin Pathol.* 1992 Nov;45(11 Suppl):3-6.
590. Stewart-Brown, S., Cot death and sleeping position. *BMJ.* 1992 Jun 6;304(6840):1508.
591. Hiley, C., Babies' sleeping position. *BMJ.* 1992 Jul 11;305(6845):115.
592. Statement to the National Vaccine Advisory Committee by Barbara Loe Fisher, Co-Founder & President National Vaccine Information Center September 26, 1994. *NVIC News.* November 1994;4(2).
593. Keens, T.G., Ward, S.L., et al., Ventilatory Pattern Following Diphtheria-Tetanus-Pertussis Immunization in Infants at Risk for Sudden Infant Death Syndrome. *Am J Dis Child.* 1985 Oct;139(10):991-4.

594. Hoffman, H.J., Hunter, J.C., et al., Diphtheria-Tetanus-Pertussis Immunization and Sudden Infant Death: Results of the National Institute of Child Health and Human Development Cooperative Epidemiological Study of Sudden Infant Death Syndrome Risk Factors. *Pediatrics*. 1987 Apr;79(4):598-611.
595. Brotherton, J.M., Hull, B.P., et al., Probability of coincident vaccination in the 24 or 48 hours preceding sudden infant death syndrome death in Australia. *Pediatrics*. 2005 Jun;115(6):643-6.
596. Griffin, M.R., Wayne, M.P.H., et al., Risk of Sudden Infant Death Syndrome after immunization with the diptheria-tetanus-pertussis vaccine. *New Engl J Med*. 1988 Sep 8;319(10):618-23.
597. Editor's note in reply to letter from Wendy Baldock, *Little Treasures*, Christmas '90;53.
598. Medical Research Council Committee on Inoculation Procedures and Neurological Lesions, Poliomyelitis and Prophylactic Inoculation Against Diphtheria, Whooping-cough and Smallpox. *Lancet*. 1956 Dec 15;268(6955):1223-31.
599. Offit, P. A., Bell, L.M., *Vaccines: What every parent should know*. IDG Books, New York, 1999, 41.
600. Vennemann, M.M., Butterfaß-Bahloul, T., et al., Sudden infant death syndrome: No increased risk after immunization. *Vaccine*. 2007 Jan 4;25(2):336-40.
601. Vennemann, M.M., Findeisen, M., et al., Infection, health problems, and health care utilisation, and the risk of sudden infant death syndrome. *Arch Dis Child*. 2005 May;90(5):520-2.
602. Horvarth, C.H.G., Sudden infant death syndrome. *NZ Med J*. 1990 Mar 14;107.
603. Hirvonen, J., Jantti, M., et al., Hyperplasia of Islets of Langerhans and Low Serum Insulin in Cot Deaths. *Forensic Sci Int*. 1980 Nov-Dec;16(3)::213-26.
604. Read, D.J.C., Williams, A.L., et al., Sudden Infant Deaths: Some Current Research Strategies. *Med J Aust*. 1979 Sep 8;2(5):236-8, 240-1, 244.
605. Aynsley-Green, A., Polak, J.M., et al., Averted Sudden Neonatal Death Due to Pancreatic Nesidioblastosis. *Lancet*. 1978 Mar 11;311(8063):550-1.
606. Cox, J.N., Guelpa, G., Terrapon, M., Islet-cell Hyperplasia and Sudden Infant Death. *Lancet*. 1976 Oct 2;2(7988):739-40.
607. Hannik, C.A., Cohen, H., Changes in plasma insulin concentration and temperature of infants after Pertussis vaccination. 4th International Symposium on Pertussis, Bethesda, Md. USA, IABS Special publication, 1979, 297-299, cited in Hennessen, W., Quast, U., Adverse Reactions After Pertussis Vaccination. *Dev Biol Stand*. 1979;43:95-100.
608. Dhar, H.L., West, G.B., Sensitization procedures and the blood sugar concentration. *J Pharm Pharmacol*. 1972 Mar;24(3):249-50.
609. Wilson, K., Potter, B., et al., Revisiting the possibility of serious adverse events from the whole cell pertussis vaccine: Were metabolically vulnerable

children at risk? *Med Hypotheses*. 2010 Jan;74(1):50-4.
610. Soldatenkova, V.A., Why case-control studies showed no association between Sudden Infant Death Syndrome and vaccinations. *Medical Veritas*. 2007;4:1411-3.
611. Findeisen,M., Vennemann, M.M., et al. German study on sudden infant death (GeSID): design, epidemiological and pathological profile. *Int J Legal Med.* 2004 Jun;118(3):163-9.
612. Palmiere, C., Mangin, P., Postmortem chemistry update part I. *Int J Legal Med.* 2012;126(2):187-98.
613. Bernier, R.H., Frank, J.A., et al., Diphtheria-tetanus toxiods-pertussis vaccination and sudden infant deaths in Tennessee. *J Pediatr*. 1982 Sep;101(3):419-21.
614. Apnoea and Unexpected Child Death. *Lancet*. 1979 Aug 18;2(8138):339-40.
615. National Institutes of Health Consensus Development Conference on Infantile Apnea and Home Monitoring, Sept 29 to Oct 1, 1986. *Pediatrics*. 1987;79:292-9.
616. www.freeyurko.bizland.com
617. Harasawa R., Tomiyama T., Evidence of Pestivirus RNA in Human Virus Vaccines. *J Clin Microbiol*. 1994 Jun;32(6);1604-5.
618. Potts, B. J., Sever, J.L., et al., Possible role of pestiviruses in microcephaly. *Lancet*. 1987 Apr 25;i(8539):972-973.
619. Yolken, R., Dubovi, E., Infantile gastroenteritis associated with excretion of pestivirus antigens. *Lancet*. 1989 Mar 11;i(8637):517-520.
620. Seeff, L.B., Beebe, G.W., et al., A serologic follow-up of the 1942 epidemic of post-vaccination hepatitis in the United States Army. *New Engl J Med.* 1987 Apr 16;316(16):965-70.
621. Time Magazine, Monday, 3 August, 57-8, 1942.
622. Theiler, M., Smith, H.H., Use of yellow fever virus modified by in vivo cultivation for human immunization. *J Exp Med.* 1937 May 31;65(6):787-800.
623. Fenner, F., Henderson, D.A., et al., *Smallpox and its Eradication*. World Health Organization, Geneva, 1988, 264-5.
624. Dey, S.K., Choudhury, T.K., A case of tuberculoid leprosy following small pox vaccination. *Indian J Dermatol.* 1985 Jul;30(3):39-41.
625. Sehgal, V.N., Rege, V.L., Vadiraj, S.N., Inoculation leprosy subsequent to small-pox vaccination. *Dermatologica*. 1970;141(6):393-6.
626. Wilson, Graham S., *The Hazards of Immunization.* The Athlone Press, London, 1967, 238.
627. Schippell, T.M., Let us Face the Facts. Herald of Health, August 1955. Reprinted in McBean, E., *The Poisoned Needle*, Health Research, 1974, 160.
628. Martin, W.J., Zeng, L.C., et al., Cytomegalovirus-related sequences in an atypical cytopathic virus repeatedly isolated from a patient with the chronic fatigue syndrome. *Am J Pathol.* 1994 Aug;45(2):440-51.

629. Martin, W.J., Ahmed, K.N., et al., African green monkey origin of the atypical cytopathic stealth virus isolated from a patient with chronic fatigue syndrome. *Clin Diagn Virol.* 1995 Jul;4(1):93-103.
630. Sweet, B.H., Hilleman, M.R., The vacuolating virus, S.V. 40. *Proc Soc Exp Biol Med.* 1960 Nov;105:420-7.
631. Eddy, B.E., Borman, G.S., et al., Identification of the oncogenic substance in rhesus monkey kidney cell cultures as simian virus 40. *Virology.* 1962 May;17:65-75.
632. Girardi, A.J., Sweet, B.H., et al., Development of tumors in hamsters inoculated in the neonatal period with vacuolating virus, SV40. *Proc Soc Exp Biol Med.* 1962 Mar;109:649-60.
633. Closing in on Polio, *Time*, 29 March 1954, 30.
634. Carbone, M., Pass, H.I., et al., New developments about the association of SV40 with human mesothelioma. *Oncogene.* 2003 Aug 11;22(33):5173-80.
635. Dang-Tan, T., Mahmud, S.M., et al., Polio vaccines, Simian Virus 40, and human cancer: the epidemiologic evidence for a causal association. *Oncogene.* 2004 Aug 23;23(38):6535-40.
636. Hooper, E., *The River: A Journey to the Source of HIV and AIDS.* Little, Brown and Company, Boston, New York, London, 1999. ISBN0-316-37261-7 (hc) In the same year it was published in Britain by Allen Lane, The Penguin Press, with the same page numbering. ISBN0-713-99335-9.
637. Courtois, G., Flack, A., et al., Preliminary Report on Mass Vaccination of man with live attenuated poliomyelitis virus in the Belgian Congo and Ruanda-Urundi. *Brit Med J.* 1958 July 26;2(5090):187-90.
638. Nahmias, A.J., Weiss, J., et al., Evidence for Human Infection with an HTLV III/LAV-Like Virus in Central Africa, 1959. *Lancet.* 1986 May 31;1(8492):1279-80.
639. *The Sunday Times Magazine,* June 21, 1987, 66.
640. Brown, P., Polio vaccine 'did not cause AIDS epidemic'. *New Sci.* 1992 Oct 31;136(1845):8.
641. Technology, Determination Win Against Implacable Enemy. *Dateline:CDC.* October 1979;11(10):2, 8.
642. Hooper, E., *The River: A Journey to the Source of HIV and AIDS.* Little, Brown and Company, Boston, New York, London, 1999, 307.
643. Fenner, F., Henderson, D.A., et al., *Smallpox and its Eradication.* World Health Organization, Geneva, 1988, 911.
644. Rappaport, J., News Blackout on pox vaccine link to AIDS protecting WHO (World Health Organization)? *Easy Reader*, 4 June 1987. Reprinted in *Report to the Consumer.* September 1987;396:1.
645. Hooper, E., *The River: A Journey to the Source of HIV and AIDS.* Little, Brown and Company, Boston, New York, London, 1999, 329.
646. Smits, Tinus, *Autism; Beyond Despair.* Emryss Publishers, Netherlands, 2012.
647. Compton Burnett, J., *Vaccinosis* (reprint), 1960, Health Science Press.
648. Zafrir, Y., Agmon-Levin, N., et al., Autoimmunity following hepatitis B

vaccine as part of the spectrum of 'Autoimmune (Auto-inflammatory) Syndrome induced by Adjuvants' (ASIA): analysis of 93 cases. *Lupus*. 2012 Feb;21(2):146-52.
649. Santoro, D., Stella, M., et al., Lupus nephritis after hepatitis B vaccination: an uncommon complication. *Clin Nephrol*. 2007 Jan;67(1):61-3.
650. Israeli, E., Agmon-Levin, N., et al., Adjuvants and autoimmunity. *Lupus*. 2009 Nov;18(13):1217-25.
651. Tomljenovic, L., Shaw, C.A., Mechanisms of aluminum adjuvant toxicity and autoimmunity in pediatric populations. *Lupus*. 2012 Feb;21(2):223-30.
652. Tomljenovic, L., Shaw, C.A., Do aluminum vaccine adjuvants contribute to the rising prevalence of autism? *J Inorg Biochem*. 2011 Nov;105(11):1489-99.
653. Shepherd, D., *Homoeopathy in Epidemic Diseases*. Health Science Press, Rustington, Sussex, 1967, 92-4.
654. Gilbert, D.A., *Temporal Organisation, Reorganisation, and Disorganisation in Cells*, in, Edmunds, L.N., (ed), *Cell Cycle Clocks*. Marcel Dekker, Inc., New York and Basel, 1984.
655. Personal communication, Don Gilbert, Department of Biochemistry, University of the Witwatersrand, 20th February 1990.
656. Doshi, P., The unofficial vaccine educators: are CDC funded non-profits sufficiently independent? *BMJ*. 2017 Nov 7;359.

Printed in Great Britain
by Amazon

62454563R00190